Dental Instruments

A POCKET GUIDE

THIRD EDITION

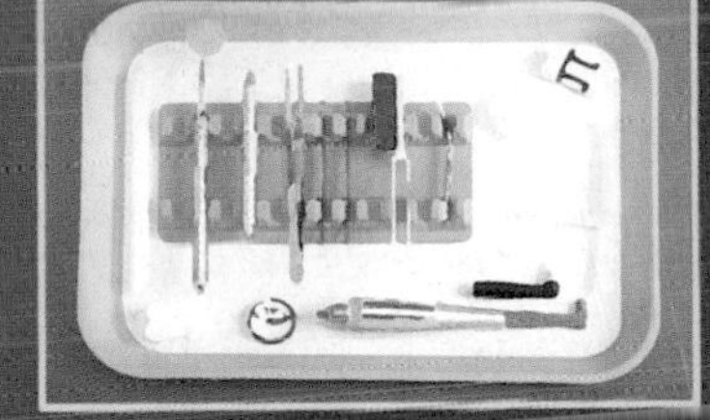

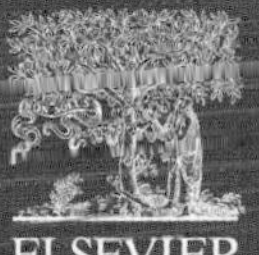

Linda R. Bartolomucci Boyd, CDA, RDA, BA

Dental Assisting Program
Diablo Valley College
Pleasant Hill, California

SAUNDERS
ELSEVIER

11830 Westline Industrial Drive
St. Louis, Missouri 63146

DENTAL INSTRUMENTS: A POCKET GUIDE ISBN: 978-1-4160-4619-6

978-1-4160-4619-6

Vice President and Publisher: Linda Duncan
Senior Editor: John Dolan
Developmental Editor: Courtney Sprehe
Publishing Services Manager: Patricia Tannian
Project Manager: John Casey
Designer: Julia Dummitt

Printed in China

Last digit is print number: 9 8 7 6 5 4 3 2

To my brother and sister-in-law, Ray and Meri,
for all of their love and support.

To all dental students,
your zest for learning has encouraged my ongoing passion for dentistry.

Preface

It is a great privilege to write the third edition of this dental instrument guide. As dentistry continues to evolve, so does the technology, and it is my goal to keep this book current by adding new instruments and equipment. Dental instruments and equipment remain an intricate part of the dental practice. Through the years, basic dental instruments have remained relatively unchanged, but design modifications have been made to accommodate new developments in the dental field. An example of this can be seen in the special coatings available on some instruments (i.e., the titanium coating found on composite instruments) that allow these instruments to be adapted to the different types of materials used in today's dental practice.

It is imperative that the clinician have a thorough knowledge and understanding of all instruments, since dental practices rely on them, equipment, and tray setups for efficient procedures. This text helps students, as well as employees in the dental office, master the identification and use of dental instruments. It includes both common and specialty instruments. Certain chapters focus on the instruments used in all dental practices, such as the components of the basic tray setup, the anesthetic syringe and its parts, evacuation devices, dental dams, handpieces, burs, and sterilization equipment. Other chapters are designed around various dental procedures, such as the instruments used in hygiene, amalgam, and composite procedures. The dental specialty chapters include instruments used in orthodontics, endodontics, and periodontics. Two chapters focus on oral surgery—one chapter addresses the general instruments used in oral and periodontal surgery, and the other focuses on extraction and implant instruments.

Most chapters feature one or more examples of a tray setup, which includes the instruments presented in that particular chapter. Tray setups are an important and intricate part of the dental office. Knowledge and understanding of the identification and functions of the instruments on the tray setups are imperative to the organization and efficiency of the dental office.

NEW TO THIS EDITION

As the world's technology has evolved, so has the technology for the instruments and equipment used in dentistry. To meet these ever-changing needs, the third edition of *Dental Instruments: A Pocket Guide* has incorporated three new chapters: Chapter 13, Preventive and Sealant Instruments and Bleaching Trays; Chapter 19, Dental Materials Equipment; and Chapter 20, Dental Radiography Equipment.

Along with the addition of these chapters, the number of instruments and equipment has been expanded, and new tray setups have been added to Chapter 12, Hygiene Instruments; Chapter 14, Orthodontic Instruments; and Chapter 17, Oral Surgery Extraction Instruments.

Many of the photos from the previous edition have been retaken to further enhance the usability of the text. Included in the new photos are all of the tray setups plus the photos in Chapter 2, Enamel Cutting Instruments (with close-ups of the working end), as well as several other new photos taken of the instruments featured in the previous editions.

The third edition features a *Sterilization Note* for each instrument, easily identified by the sterilization icon Ⓢ in front of the note. This note details the sterilization, infection control, and/or disposal protocol for each instrument and/or equipment presented in the chapter. These guidelines have been taken from the most current issue of Guidelines for Infection Control in Dental Health-Care Settings–2003 (Centers for Disease Control and Prevention. *MMWR* 2003;52[No. RR–17]:1 to 48, US Department of Health and Human Services, Atlanta, GA 30333.) However, it is important to review and follow the local and state regulations in which you practice because each city and state may have their own regulations that must be followed.

Also included is a *Practice Note* that gives examples of the tray setup(s) in which a particular instrument can be found, as well any other useful information. This informative feature cross references the instrument to tray setups in other chapters and dental procedures.

FORMAT

Simplification is the key to studying and understanding each instrument/piece of equipment and its functions and characteristics. The flip-book, flashcard style of this text is designed for easy identification and memorization. A picture or illustration of an instrument (or group of instruments) or dental equipment is pictured on the top page; the name, functions, characteristics, practice note(s), and guidelines for sterilization/infection control/disposal are listed on the bottom page. Some instruments on the top page have numbered parts. In these cases, the bottom page identifies the parts by matching the numbers on the photo to the numbers on the description page. As you master the name, functions, and characteristics of an instrument or piece of equipment, you can then test yourself. Fold the book in half, showing only the picture. Then, from memory, try to identify the instrument and describe its functions and characteristics. Verify your answer by checking the bottom page.

After mastering the individual instruments, you must be able to select and place instruments in order of use for specific dental procedures. At the end of most chapters there is an example of a tray setup(s) that illustrates the instruments covered in that chapter. The tray setups may include instruments from other chapters as well. For example, some of the instruments from Chapter 1, such as the basic setup (i.e., mouth mirror, explorer, and cotton forceps), are included on most of the tray setups. Also, the tray setups in this text include only instruments and usually not the auxiliary items that would be used for dental procedures. This element of the text will certainly enhance your ability to set trays up and use the instruments according to the correct sequence of the procedure.

TO THE STUDENT

The design elements of flash card–style learning, comprehensive chapters for specific dental procedures, and examples of tray setups can help you master an important and intricate part of the dental practice. This text can also be used as a quick reference guide when working in the clinic or dental practice.

I am confident that this text will help you to more easily learn the dental instruments, dental equipment, and tray setups that clinicians use in dental practices. It is imperative that all dental students begin their career in the dental profession with a thorough knowledge of dental instruments and equipment, and this text will help you achieve that goal.

I wish you all success in the field of dentistry. I know you will be a great asset to the dental profession.

Linda R. Bartolomucci Boyd

About EVOLVE

An Evolve website is an additional learning tool and can greatly enhance the text for both students and instructors.

FOR THE STUDENT

Evolve Student Resources offers the following features:

- **Chapter Assessment Quizzes.** The chapter assessment quizzes allow students to test their instrument knowledge by answering true/false, multiple choice, and matching questions. A quiz is included for each chapter, and each quiz features 10 questions. After taking the exam, students can review their results and see the right answers for the questions they missed.
- **Drag-and-Drop Exercises.** The drag-and-drop exercises test the student's skill at selecting the correct instrument in the right order for specific tray setups. A selection of instruments is shown. The students must select the correct instruments and put them in the correct order for use on the specified tray.
- **"In Use" image collection.** This image collection features 115 photos of instruments and equipment being used in a clinical setting, as well as detailed drawings showing specifically how the instrument functions. The instruments and equipment that are included in this image collection are indicated by a thumbnail of the photo or illustration or by the Evolve icon evolve appearing on the description page.
- **Appendices.** Five appendices provide information on instrument grasps, a sterilization management system, operating zones, the anesthetic color codes, and hand exercises.
- **Weblinks.** A variety of weblinks are provided for students to pursue further study.

FOR THE INSTRUCTOR

Evolve Instructor Resources offers the following features (instructors also have access to all of the student resources):

- **Image Collection.** This image collection includes every instrument/equipment image in the book, making it easy to include a photo or drawing in a lecture or quiz.
- **Teaching Tips.** The author has compiled a list of helpful tips for each chapter that are designed to help the instructor enhance and refine his or her own course.
- **Testbank in ExamView.** A 200-question testbank is included along with the correct answers. These questions can be sorted by chapter or randomly, making the creation of quizzes and exams much easier.
- **Tray Setup Quizzes.** These exams are designed to test students' knowledge of which instruments are used on specific tray setups. An answer key is provided.

Acknowledgments

I would like to express my deepest appreciation to all of my colleagues, dentist affiliations, professors, and my dearest family and friends for all of their insight, support, love, and prayers during the writing of this third edition. Of course, I appreciate and value each and every student, as their zest and enthusiasm for learning give me such encouragement to write a text that will enhance their learning.

I am extremely grateful to Courtney Sprehe for her perseverance in developing the third edition of this text, as her vision and mine were always the same. John Dolan, I thank you, for your expertise as editor in overseeing and publishing this third edition.

Two key people have played an important role in the photography in this edition. First and foremost I have the greatest respect and appreciation for the photographer, Jeff McMillan. His artistic ability and incredible photography skills have enhanced this text remarkably. Second, these photographs would not be possible without Andrew Hartzell, President of G. Hartzell & Son, Inc., who allowed us to borrow most of the instruments to photograph. Thank you, Andy!

Also, a special thank you goes to Professor Marylou Pineda, MS, CDA, RDA, from Diablo Valley College in Pleasant Hill, California, for allowing me to use the radiography devices for the photographs in Chapter 20. Don Colombana, Executive Director of Medical Imaging and Radiation Oncology Services at John Muir Health in Concord, California, was very gracious with his time to consult with me regarding digital radiography, I thank you! Thank you Sarah Brown for allowing me to borrow your high-tech camera for a few photographs.

An extended thank you to Phyllis Martina, RDH, BSDH, MBA, West Regional Representative of Schools & Institutions, from Hu-Friedy Instrument Manufacturing Company, who was always there to answer questions regarding equipment or instruments and connecting me with Hu-Friedy marketing for any photographs that I needed for this text.

I express boundless thanks to, **Joyce M. Litch, RDH, DDS, MSD, a consultant to the book**, who was willing at any time of the day to answer questions regarding the periodontal and hygiene chapters. I thank you for always being there for me! The bur chapter would not be as comprehensive without the consultation from Wayne Joseph, DDS. His insight into this chapter has been appreciated from the first edition to the third. Thank you to Ann Marie Gorczyca, DMD, MPH, MS, and her assistant, Jolene Genetti, RDA, who helped with the expansion of the Chapter 14, Orthodontic Instruments.

I would like to express my deepest and sincere appreciation to Cathy Clarke, RDA, my colleague, who spent numerous hours consulting with me regarding the new feature of this text, the Sterilization Note. Thank you Cathy for the many hours you devoted to this text! I cannot go without saying thank you to all of my colleagues for their support during the development of this text, especially Anna Nelson, MS, CDA, RDA, Yvonne Carter, BA, CDA, RDA, and Sharon Campton, MS, CDA, RDA, who reviewed the second edition to help bring the third edition to the next level.

I could not have written this third edition without the love, support, and prayers from my family: my sons, Michael and Matthew, who always gave me a nudge of encouragement; my daughter-in-law, Rebecca for her love and for being a model; my cousin Elaine Strizzi for her gentle and loving encouragement; my brother and sister-in-law, Ray and Meri, for the nourishment of my body and soul during this process; and Nick Reina, SDB, for your prayers of wisdom. Last, but certainly not least, are the wonderful, refreshing moments with my grandsons, Christian and Collin, and my new granddaughter, Alexis, that teach me the simplicity, enthusiasm, and zest for learning that encourages my writing.

Linda R. Bartolomucci Boyd

Consultant
Joyce Litch, RDH, DDS, MSD

For information about the author or to ask questions about the text, please visit www.lindaboyd.info/

Contents

Photo/Illustration Credits

Third edition photographer: Jeff McMillan, McMillan Studios, Livermore, California

First and Second editions photographer:
Kenneth B. Cook II, Pleasanton, California

3M ESPE Dental Products, Eagan, Minnesota
Automixer (3M ESPE Pentamix 2 Mixing Unit)

Alfa Medical, Hempstead, New York (www.sterlizers.com)
Sterilizer—Dry Heat (Static Air)
Sterilizer—Dry Heat (Rapid Heat Transfer)

Baum L, Phillips RW, Lund MR: *Textbook of Operative Dentistry*, ed 3, Philadelphia, 1995, Saunders.
Round Bur (inset photo)
Pear-Shaped Bur (inset photo)
Inverted Cone Bur (inset photo)

Bird DL, Robinson DS: *Torres and Ehrlich Modern Dental Assisting*, ed 9, St. Louis, 2009, Saunders.
Cotton Forceps (Pliers) (inset photo)
Recapping Device (inset photo)
High-Volume (Velocity) Evacuator (HVE) Tip (inset photo)
Low-Volume (Velocity) Saliva Ejector Tip (inset photo)
Disposable Prophy Angle Attachments for Slow-Speed Handpiece/Motor (inset photo)
Bur Shanks
Dental Dam Forceps (inset photo)
Amalgam Carrier (inset photo)
Discoid-Cleoid Carver (insert photo)
Wooden Wedge (inset photo)
Curing Light—Electronic (insert photo)
Gingival Retraction Cord Instrument (inset photo)
Implant Scaler (Disposable Tip)
Implant Scaler (Disposable Tip) (inset photo)
Three-Number Instrument (right photo)
Ultrasonic Scaling Unit (Power Scaler) (inset photo)
Disposables—Cotton Roll (inset photo)
Scissors—Short Blade (inset photo)
Vacuum Form
Band Pusher (inset photo)
Protective Mask (inset photo)
Protective Glasses/Eye Wear (inset photo)
Examination Gloves
Overgloves
Vibrator for Laboratory
Model Trimmer
Flexible Mixing Spatula (inset photo)

X-Ray Film—Various Sizes
Extraoral X-Ray Film—Cephalometric and Panoramic Radiographs
Film Holders—Periapical X-Ray
X-Ray Manual Developing Unit
X-Ray Rack (inset)

Carestream Health, Inc., Rochester, New York
Package of X-Ray Film
Extraoral X-Ray Film

Cohen S, Hargreaves KM: *Pathways of the Pulp*, ed 9, St. Louis, 2006, Mosby.
Endodontic Explorer (inset photo)
Endodontic Plugger (insert photo)

Colténe/Whaledent, Cuyahoga Falls, Ohio
Gutta-Percha

Cranin AN, Klein M, Simons AM: *Atlas of Oral Implantology*, ed 2, St. Louis, 1999, Mosby.
Tissue Forceps
Rongeurs
Bone File

Danville Materials, Inc., San Ramon, California
Air Abrasion Unit and Handpiece Attachment

DENTSPLY Caulk, Milford, Delaware
Matrix Band System

DENTSPLY Professional, York, Pennsylvania
Prophy Slow-Speed Handpiece/Motor with Disposable Prophy Angle Attachment
Prophy Angle Slow-Speed Handpiece/Motor and Attachments
Electric Handpiece Unit and Handpiece Attachments
Bur
Round Bur
Pear-Shaped Bur
Inverted Cone Bur
Straight Fissure Bur—Plain Cut
Tapered Fissure Bur—Plain Cut
Straight Fissure Bur—Crosscut
Tapered Fissure Bur—Crosscut
Finishing Bur
Diamond Bur—Flat-End Taper
Diamond Bur—Flat-End Cylinder
Diamond Bur—Flame
Diamond Bur—Wheel
Ultrasonic Scaling Unit (Power Scaler)

DENTSPLY Rinn, Elgin, Illinois
X-Ray Rack
X-Ray View Luminator
X-Ray Duplicator
Rinn XCP Holders for Digital Radiography

Dux Dental, Oxnard, California
Fluoride Tray—Disposable
Fluoride Tray—Disposable (inset photo)
Metal Perforated Full Arch Impression Trays
Alginator
Alginator (inset photo)
Reversible Hydrocolloid Unit

Irreversible Hydrocolloid Water-Cooled Impression Trays and Hoses
Paper Mixing Pads
Lead Aprons

DynaFlex, St. Louis, Missouri
Elastic Separators
Brass Wire Separators
Ligature Ties (stainless steel and silicone)

Garrison Dental Solutions, Spring Lake, Michigan
Sectional Matrix System

Gendex Dental Systems, Lake Zurich, Illinois
Dental X-Ray Unit

G. Hartzell & Son, Concord, California
Provided many of the instruments used in the professional photography

Global Dosimetry Solutions, Irvine, California
X-Ray Monitoring Device

Graber TM, Vanarsdall RL, Vig KWL: *Orthodontics: Current Principles and Techniques*, ed 4, St. Louis, 2005, Mosby.
Orthodontic Band with Bracket and Tubing (right photo)
Orthodontic Brackets
Orthodontic (Shure) Scaler (inset photo)

Gutmann JL, Dumsha TC, Lovdahl PE: *Problem Solving in Endodontics*, ed 4, St. Louis, 2006, Mosby.
Scalpel Handle with Blade (inset photo)

Hu-Friedy, Chicago, Illinois
Recapping Device (right photo)
Anterior Clamp
Premolar Clamp
Universal Clamp—Maxillary
Universal Clamp—Mandibular
Endodontic Stand
Ultrasonic Scaler Instrument Tip—Supragingival
Ultrasonic Scaler Instrument Tip—Subgingival
Ultrasonic Scaler Instrument Tip—Furcation
Ultrasonic Scaler Instrument Tip—Universal
Battery Operated Sharpening Device
Nitrile Utility Gloves
Cassette
Color Coding System for Instruments
Parts Box for Sterilization
Cassette Wrap
Sterilization Pouches
Process Indicator Tape and Dispensing Unit
Sterilization Spore Check—In Office
Flexible Mixing Spatula
Ultrasonic Scaling Unit (Power Scaler)

Iannucci J, Jansen Howerton L: *Dental Radiography: Principles and Techniques*, ed 3, St. Louis, 2006, Saunders.
X-Ray Safelight
Automatic Film Processor
Parts of Automatic Film Processor

Ivoclar Vivadent, Inc., Amherst, New York
Amalgamator

KaVo Dental Corporation, Lake Zurich, Illinois
Fiberoptic High-Speed Handpiece
Slow-Speed Motor with Straight Handpiece Attachment
Surgical Electric Handpiece Unit and Handpiece
Diagnodent

Kerr Corporation, Orange, California
Mixing Gun for Final Impression Material

Malamed SF: *Handbook of Local Anesthesia*, ed 5, St. Louis, 2004, Mosby.
Anesthetic Aspirating Syringe

Midmark Corp., Versailles, Ohio
Ultrasonic Cleaning Unit
Sterilizer—Autoclave (Saturated Steam)

Newman MG, Takei HH, Klokkevold PR, Carranza FA: *Carranza's Clinical Periodontology*, ed 10, St. Louis, 2006, Saunders.
Sharpening Stones
Back-Action Hoe (inset photo)

Nobel Biocare, Yorba Linda, California
Implant System

Obtura Spartan, Fenton, Missouri
Gutta-Percha Warming Unit

Patterson Dental Companies, Inc., St. Paul, Minnesota
Steel Spring Separators

Perry DA, Beemsterboer PL: *Periodontology for the Dental Hygienist*, ed 3, St. Louis, 2007, Saunders.
Furcation Probe (inset photo)
Implant

Practicon Dental, Greenville, North Carolina
Protective Mask
Protective Glasses/Eye Wear

Premier Dental, Plymouth Meeting, Pennsylvania
Reamer
Endodontic File—K Type
Endodontic File—Hedstrom

Proffit WR, Fields HW, Sarver DM: *Contemporary Orthodontics*, ed 4, St. Louis, 2007, Mosby.
Posterior Band Remover (inset photo)

Rosenstiel SF, Land MF, Fujimoto J: *Contemporary Fixed Prosthodontics*, ed 4, St. Louis, 2006, Mosby.
Dental Dam (inset photo)
Shade Guides
Gates Glidden Bur or Drill (inset photo)

SciCan, Toronto, Ontario
Sterilizer—Autoclave ("Flash")

Sirona Dental Systems LLC, Charlotte, North Carolina
Laser Handpiece Unit and Laser Handpiece Attachment
Cerec Machine
Cerec Machine (inset photo)

Digital Intraoral X-Ray Unit
Intraoral Sensors for Digital Radiography
Digital Panoramic Imaging Unit and Digital Cephalometric Imaging Unit

SybronEndo, Orange, California
Electronic Apex Locator
Vitalometer/Pulp Tester

Thermo Fisher Scientific, Dubuque, Iowa
Sterilizer—Chemiclave (Unsaturated Chemical Vapor)

Vident, Brea, California
Digital Shade Guide
Digital Shade Guide (inset photo)

Young AP, Kennedy DB: *Kinn's The Medical Assistant: An Applied Learning Approach,* ed 9, St. Louis, 2003, Saunders.
Needle Holder (inset photo)

CHAPTER 1

Basic Dental Instruments

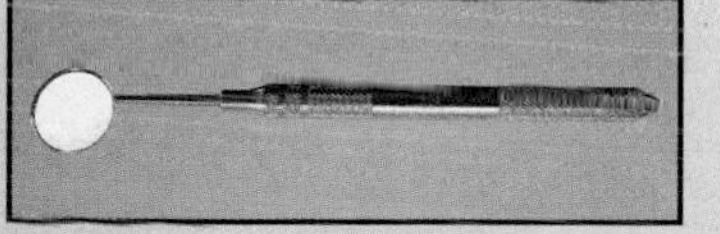

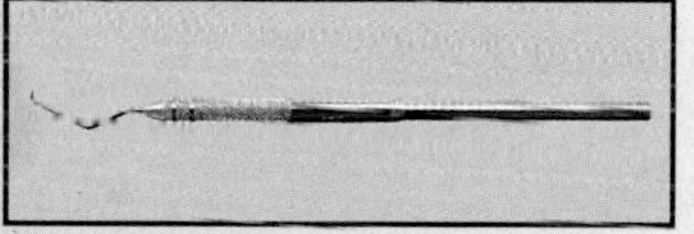

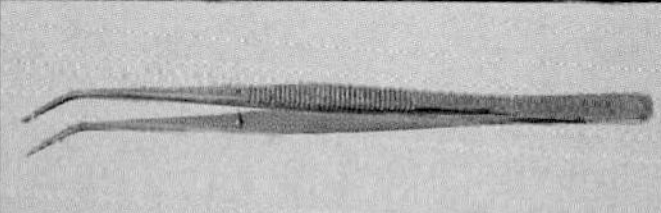

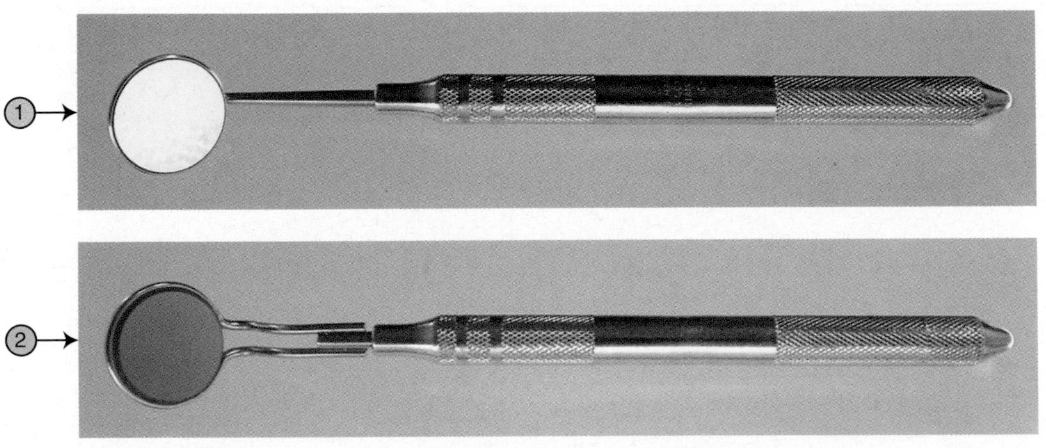
1
2

INSTRUMENT

Mouth Mirror evolve

FUNCTIONS

To provide indirect vision
To retract lips, cheeks, and tongue
To reflect light into the mouth

CHARACTERISTICS

(1) Front surface mirrors—Accurate, distortion-free image
(2) Double-sided mirrors—Used to retract tongue or cheek and view intraoral cavity simultaneously
Flat surface mirrors—Used in disposable models
Concave mirrors—Magnify image
Range of sizes
Commonly used sizes: no. 4 and no. 5
Single ended
Different mirror handles available

PRACTICE NOTE

Mouth Mirror is used on most tray setups.

(S) Mouth Mirror must be cleaned, bagged individually or bagged/wrapped in a tray setup, and then sterilized. A chemical/steam indicator device should be included in the wrapping.

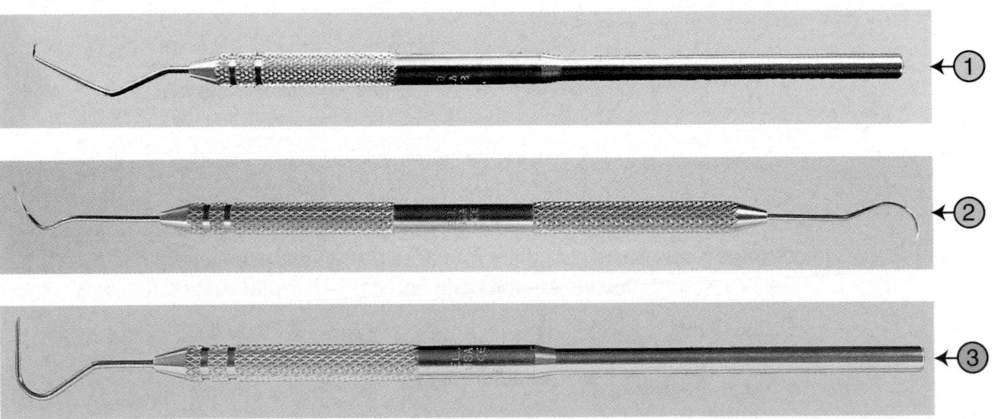
1
2
3

INSTRUMENT

Explorers

evolve

FUNCTION To examine teeth for decay (caries), calculus, furcations, or other abnormalities

CHARACTERISTICS Pointed tips; sharp, thin, flexible

Single or double ended

- Double-ended models—May have different styles of working ends; may also have explorer on one end and periodontal probe on the other

Variety of sizes and types:

1. Orban
2. Pigtail
3. Shepherd's hook

PRACTICE NOTE Explorer is used on most tray setups.

S Explorer must be cleaned, bagged individually or bagged/wrapped in a tray setup, and then sterilized. A chemical/steam indicator device should be included in the wrapping.

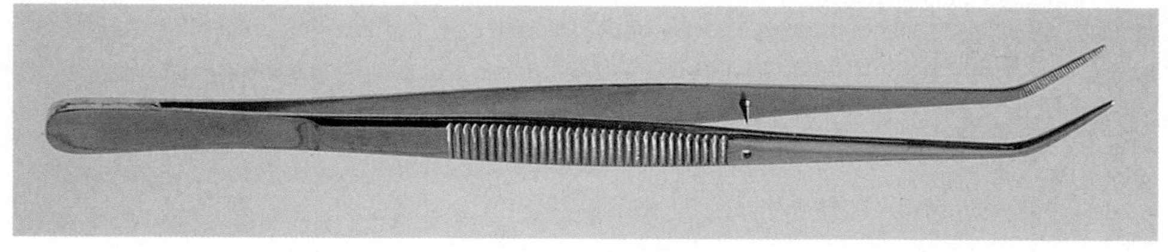

INSTRUMENT

Cotton Forceps (Pliers)

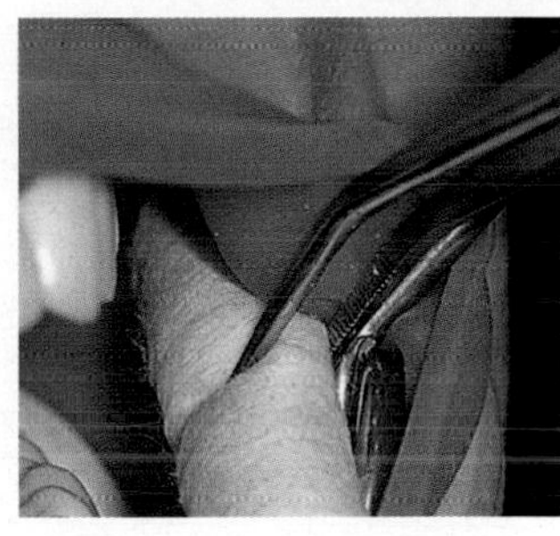

FUNCTION To grasp or transfer items and/or material into and out of the oral cavity

CHARACTERISTICS Plain or serrated tips
Pointed or rounded tips
Locking forceps (see Chapter 11: Endodontic Instruments)
Range of sizes available

PRACTICE NOTE Cotton Forceps is used on most tray setups.

Ⓢ Cotton Forceps must be cleaned, bagged individually or bagged/wrapped in a tray setup, and then sterilized. A chemical/steam indicator device should be included in the wrapping.

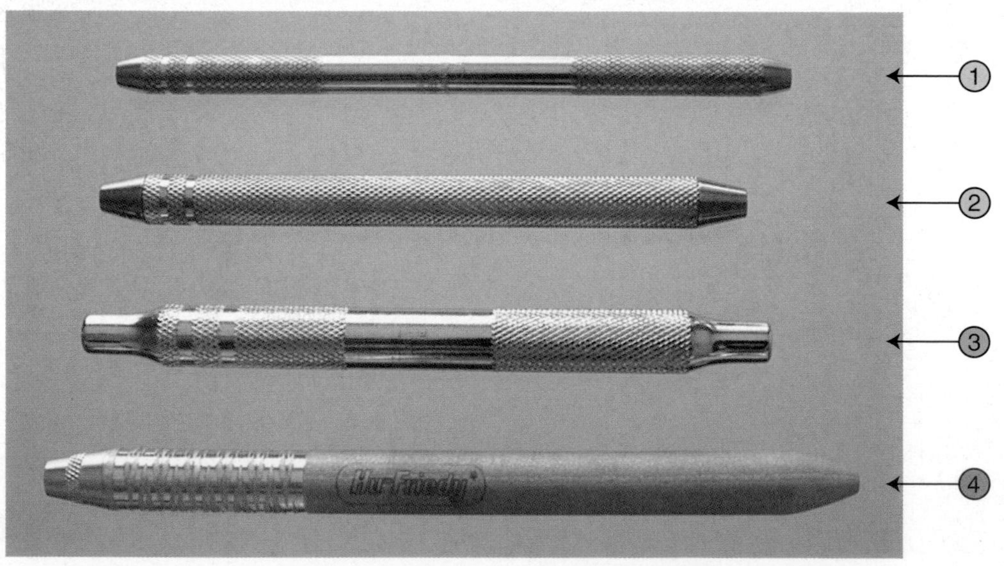
1
2
3
4
Hu-Friedy

INSTRUMENT

Instrument Handles

FUNCTION To hold (grasp) instrument

CHARACTERISTICS Single or double ended

Removable working ends (replaceable and interchangeable)

Examples: Mouth mirror, scaler

Nonremovable working ends also available

Larger diameter models—Help lighten grasp and maximize control

Alternating diameter models—Lessen stress associated with carpal tunnel syndrome

Lighter weight models—Minimize fatigue

Variety of sizes, styles, and textures:

1. Small, round 1/4-inch stainless steel
2. Standard, hollow 5/16-inch stainless steel
3. Lightweight, 3/8-inch slip-resistant pattern
4. Satin Steel model—Lightweight, ergonomically designed

S When working end is attached to the handle, the instrument must be cleaned, bagged individually or bagged/wrapped in a tray setup, and then sterilized. A chemical/steam indicator device should be included in the wrapping.

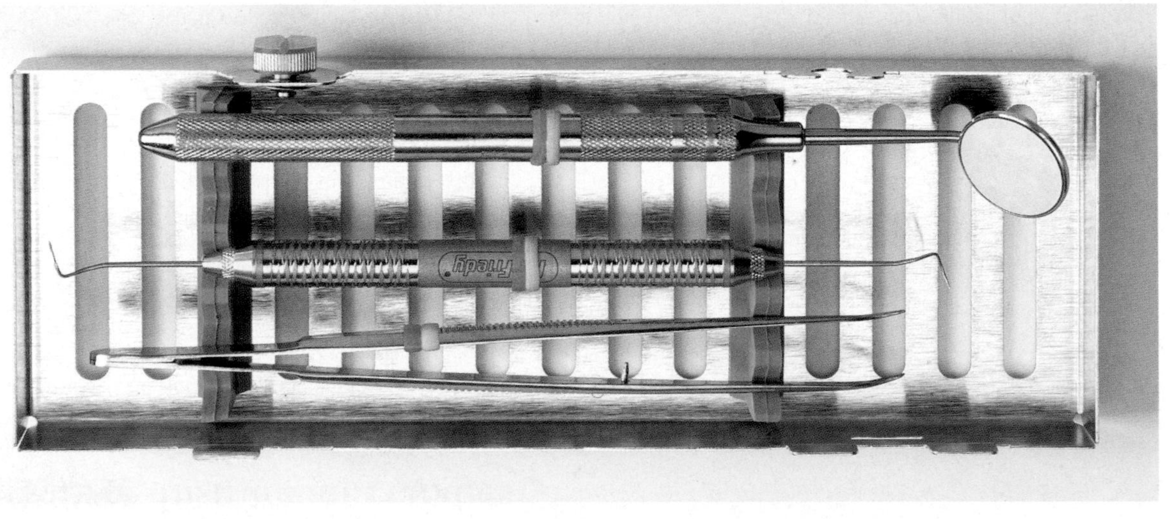
Friedy

TRAY SETUP

Basic

FROM TOP TO BOTTOM

Mouth Mirror, Pigtail Explorer, Cotton Forceps (example of color-coded instruments in a cassette)

PRACTICE NOTE Basic setup is found on most all dental tray setups.

Basic Setup Instruments must be cleaned, bagged as a tray setup or in a cassette (as shown in picture) and then sterilized. A chemical/steam indicator device should be included in the wrapping.

CHAPTER 2

Enamel Cutting Instruments

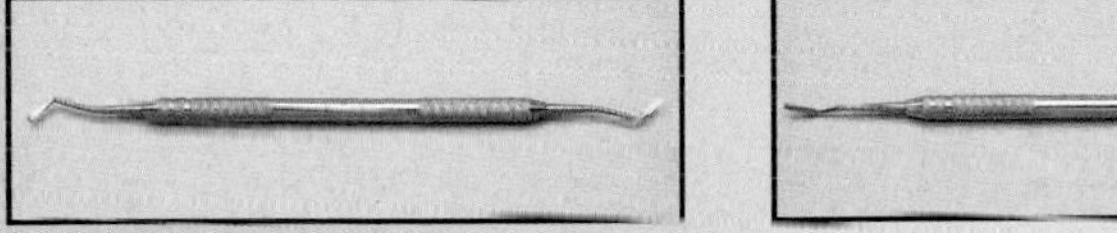

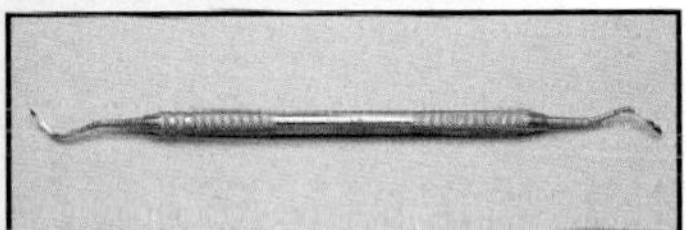

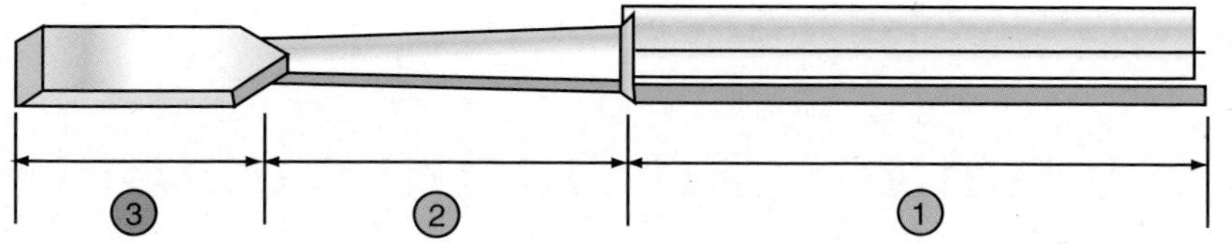
3
2
1

Parts of an Instrument

① **HANDLE**	Grasping end of instrument Variety of sizes and styles Handle styles (refer to page 9)
② **SHANK**	Connects handle to working end of instrument May be straight or may have one or more angles to accommodate specific areas of the mouth
③ **WORKING END**	May have cutting edge, blade, bevel, point, nib, or beaks

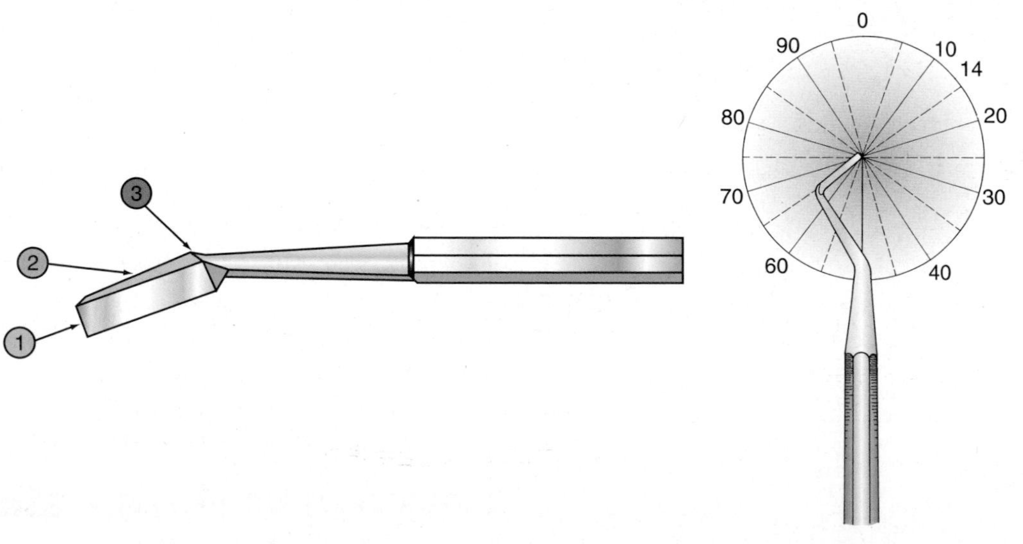

3
2
1
0
90
10
14
80
20
70
30
60
40

INSTRUMENT

Three-Number Instrument*

FUNCTION Numbers on handle indicate width, length, and angle of blade

① Indicates width of blade in tenths of millimeters

Example: 20 indicates a width of 2 mm

② Indicates length of blade in millimeters

Example: 8 indicates a length of 8 mm

③ Indicates angle of blade from long axis of shaft

Example: 12 indicates an angle of 12 degrees

The designation for the instrument described above is 20-8-12.

Examples of three-numbered instruments: Enamel Hatchet, Enamel Hoe, Wedelstaedt

* The instrument number formula was designed by Dr. G.V. Black, Northwestern University.

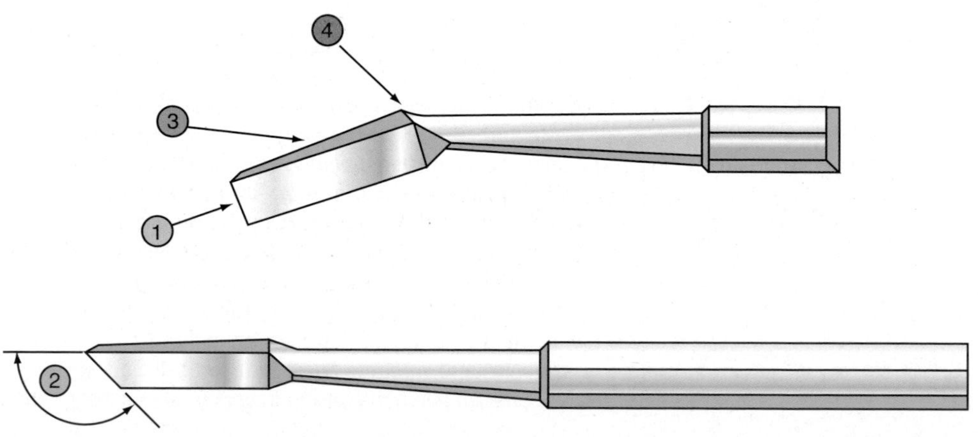
4
3
1
2

INSTRUMENT

Four-Number Instrument*

FUNCTION Numbers on handle indicate width of blade, angle of cutting edge, length of blade, and angle of blade

① Indicates width of blade in tenths of millimeters

Example: 20 indicates a width of 2 mm

② Indicates angle of cutting edge of blade in relation to handle

Example: 95 indicates a cutting edge angle of 95 degrees

③ Indicates length of blade in millimeters

Example: 8 indicates a length of 8 mm

④ Indicates angle of blade from long axis of shaft

Example: 12 indicates a blade angle of 12 degrees

The designation for the instrument described above is 20-95-8-12.

Examples of four-numbered instruments: Angle Former, Gingival Margin Trimmers—Mesial and Distal

* The instrument number formula was designed by Dr. G.V. Black, Northwestern University.

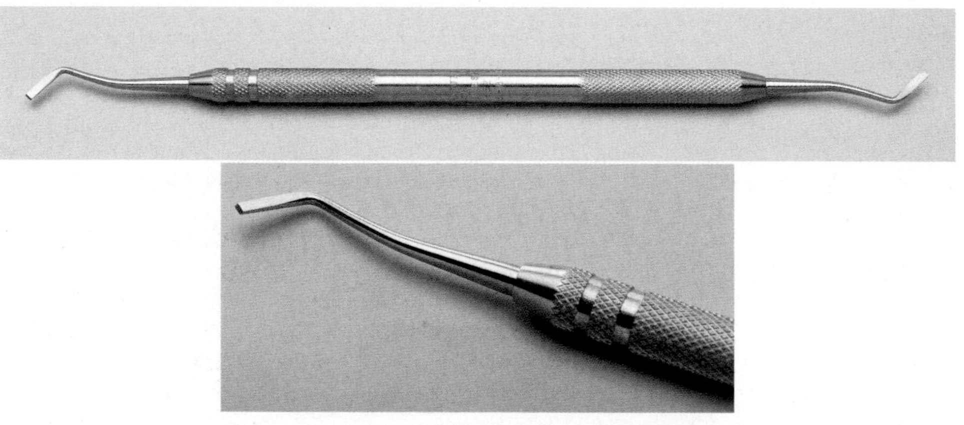

INSTRUMENT

Enamel Hatchet

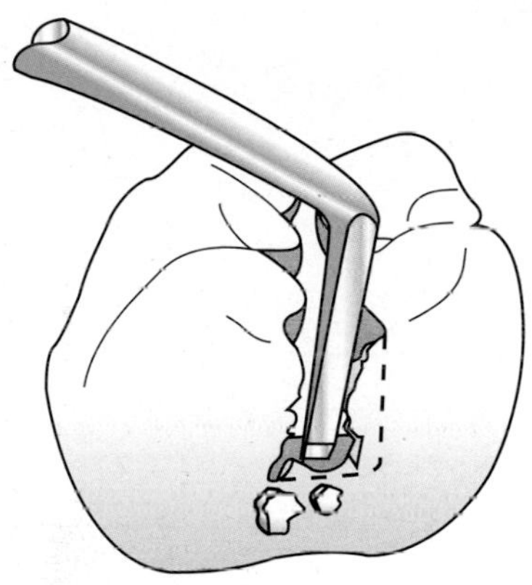

FUNCTIONS

To clean and smooth walls in cavity preparation
To remove enamel not supported by dentin

CHARACTERISTICS

Used with push motion
Cutting edge on same plane as handle
Single or double ended
Is a three-numbered instrument

Examples of instrument numbers:

20-9-14
15-8-14
15-8-12

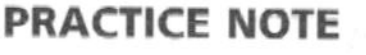

PRACTICE NOTE

Enamel Hatchet is used on restorative tray setups.

Ⓢ Enamel Hatchet must be cleaned, bagged individually or bagged/wrapped in a tray setup, and then sterilized. A chemical/steam indicator device should be included in the wrapping.

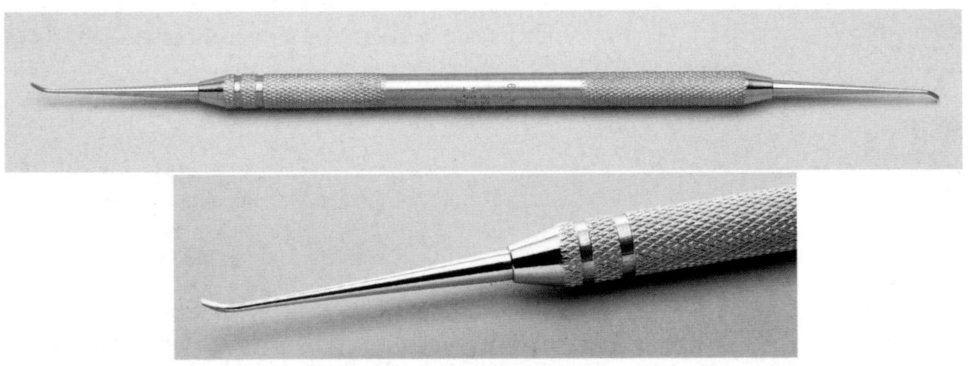

INSTRUMENT

Enamel Hoe

evolve

FUNCTIONS

To clean and smooth floor and walls in cavity preparation
To form or accentuate line angles in cavity preparation

CHARACTERISTICS

Used with pulling motion
Cutting edge or blade almost perpendicular to handle
Is a three-numbered instrument

Examples of instrument numbers:

10-4-8
10-4-14

PRACTICE NOTES

Enamel Hoe is used on restorative tray setups.

Ⓢ Enamel Hoe must be cleaned, bagged individually or bagged/wrapped in a tray setup, and then sterilized. A chemical/steam indicator device should be included in the wrapping.

24

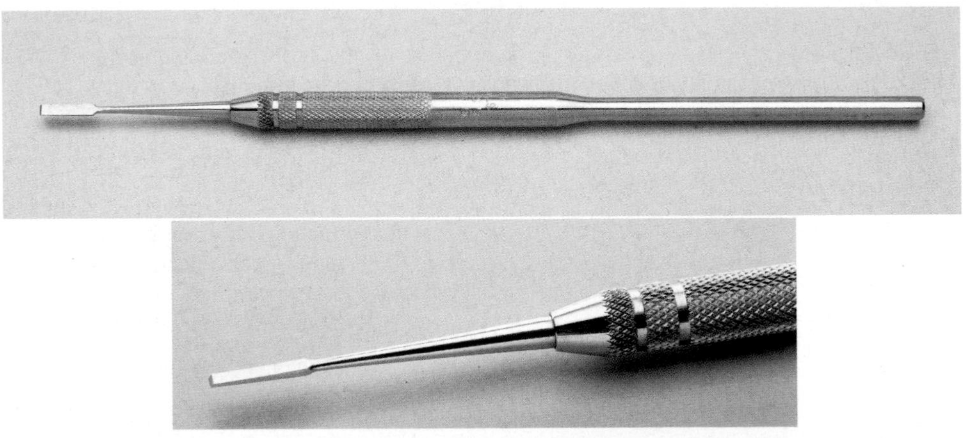

INSTRUMENT

Straight Chisel

FUNCTION To plane and cleave enamel in cavity preparation

CHARACTERISTICS Used with push motion
Single-bevel cutting edge
Single or double ended

Examples of instrument numbers:
15
20

PRACTICE NOTE Straight Chisel is used on restorative tray setups.

S Straight Chisel must be cleaned, bagged individually or bagged/wrapped in a tray setup, and then sterilized. A chemical/steam indicator device should be included in the wrapping.

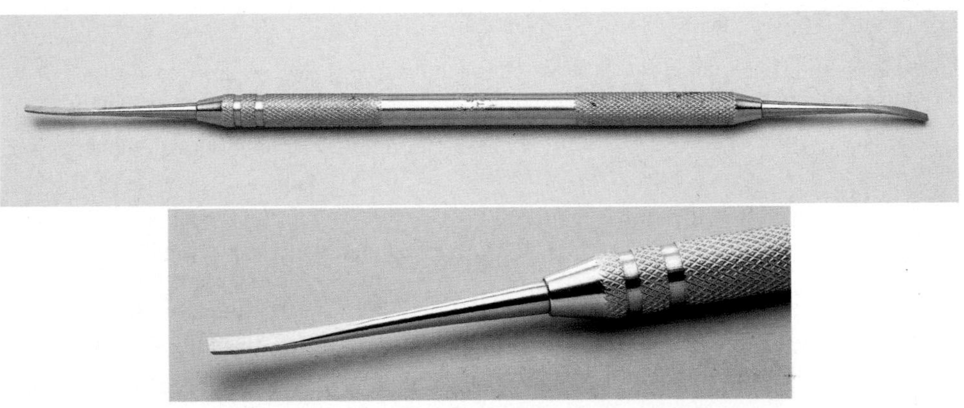

INSTRUMENT

Wedelstaedt Chisel

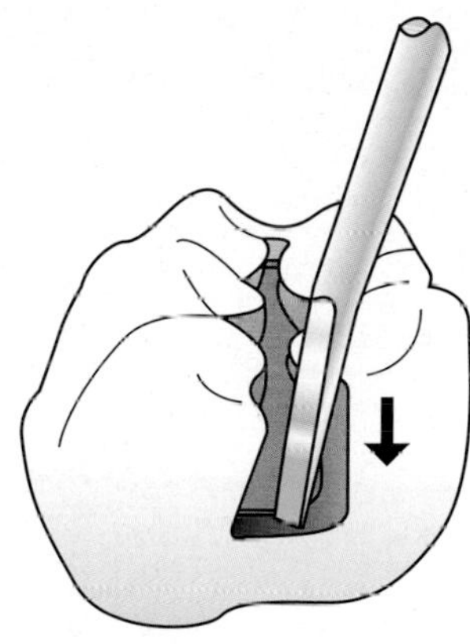

FUNCTION To plane and cleave enamel in cavity preparation

CHARACTERISTICS Used with push motion
Curved blade
Single-bevel cutting edge
Single or double ended
Is a three-numbered instrument

Examples of instrument numbers:
15-15-3
11.5-15-3

PRACTICE NOTE Wedelstaedt Chisel is used on restorative tray setups.

S Wedelstaedt Chisel must be cleaned, bagged individually or bagged/wrapped in a tray setup, and then sterilized. A chemical/steam indicator device should be included in the wrapping

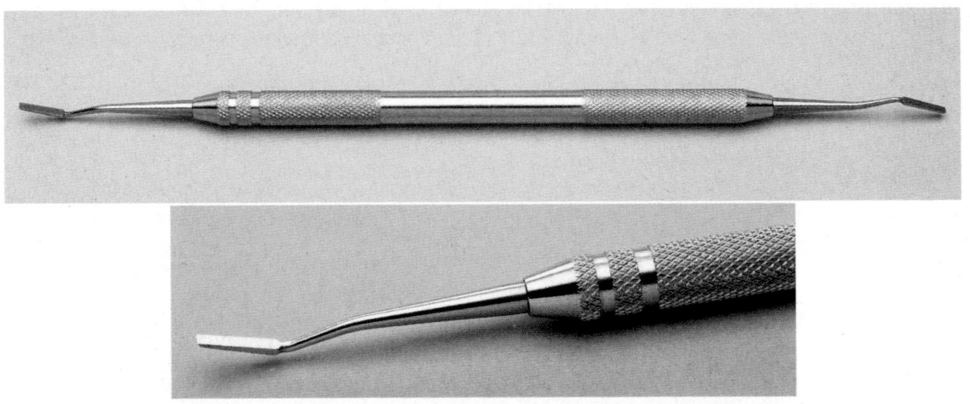

INSTRUMENT

Binangle Chisel

FUNCTION To plane and cleave enamel in cavity preparation

CHARACTERISTICS Used with push motion
Two angles in the shank
Single or double ended
Is an example of three-numbered instrument

Examples of instrument numbers:

20-9-8
15-8-8

PRACTICE NOTE Binangle Chisel is used on restorative tray setups.

Ⓢ Binangle Chisel must be cleaned, bagged individually or bagged/wrapped in a tray setup, and then sterilized. A chemical/steam indicator device should be included in the wrapping.

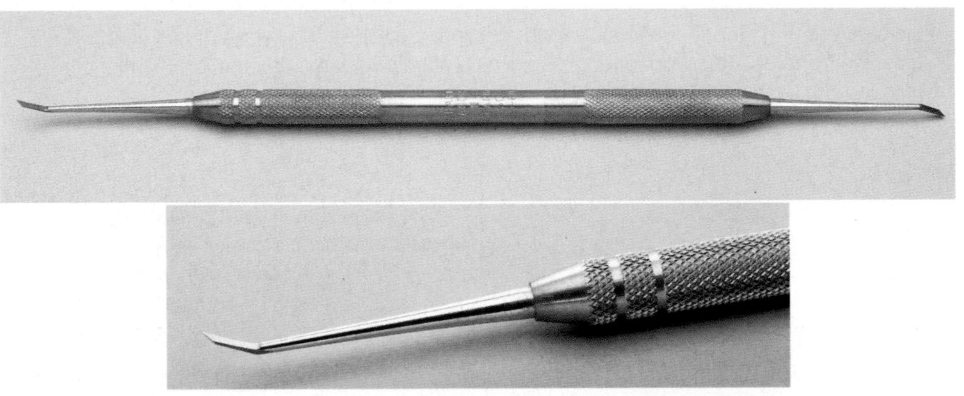

INSTRUMENT

Angle Former

evolve

FUNCTION To accentuate line and point angles in internal outline and retention in cavity preparation

CHARACTERISTICS Cutting edge at an angle
Single or double ended
Is a four-numbered instrument

Examples of instrument numbers:

12-80-5-8
9-80-4-8

PRACTICE NOTE Angle Former is used on restorative tray setups.

Ⓢ Angle Former must be cleaned, bagged individually or bagged/wrapped in a tray setup, and then sterilized. A chemical/steam indicator device should be included in the wrapping.

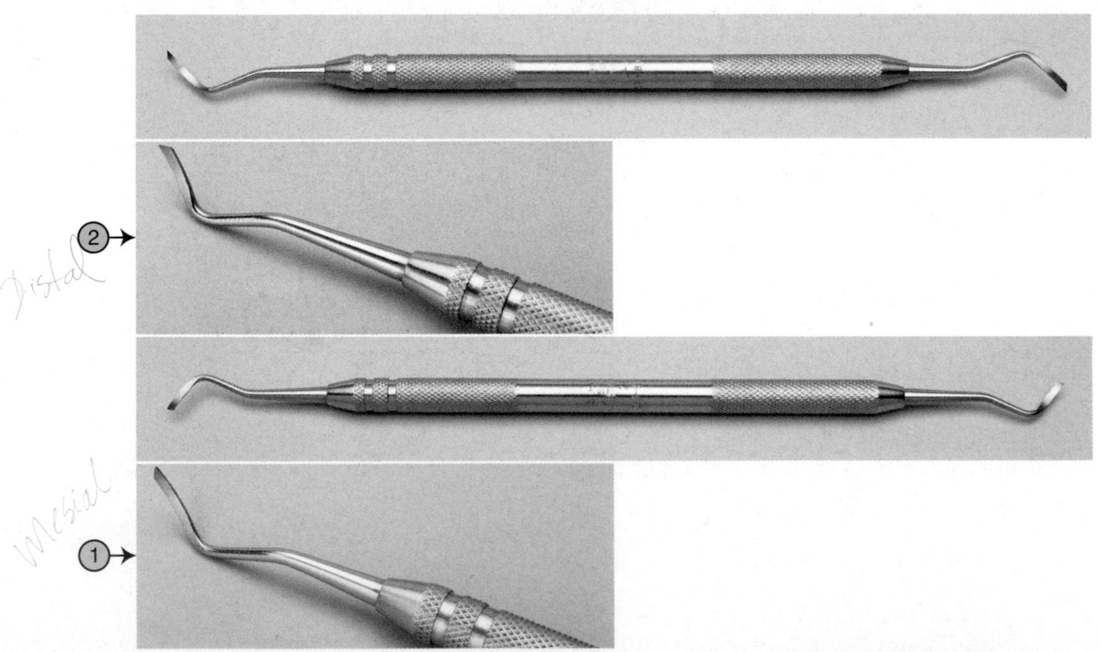
2
1

INSTRUMENT

Gingival Margin Trimmer—Mesial and Distal

evolve

FUNCTION To bevel cervical walls of mesial and distal retention areas

CHARACTERISTICS

① Mesial: To place bevels on the mesial cervical margin of the preparation
② Distal: To place bevels on the distal cervical margin of the preparation
Curved blade
Cutting edge at angle to blade
Double ended (one end curves to the right, the other to the left)
Is a four-numbered instrument

Examples of instrument numbers:
Mesial: 13-80-8-14 or 15-80-8-12
Distal: 13-95-8-14 or 15-95-8-12

PRACTICE NOTES

Gingival Margin Trimmer is used on restorative tray setups.
Gingival Margin Trimmer is placed on tray setups in pairs; mesial and distal.
Refer to the Amalgam tray setup in Chapter 8.

Ⓢ Gingival Margin Trimmer must be cleaned, bagged individually or bagged/wrapped in a tray setup, and then sterilized. A chemical/steam indicator device should be included in the wrapping.

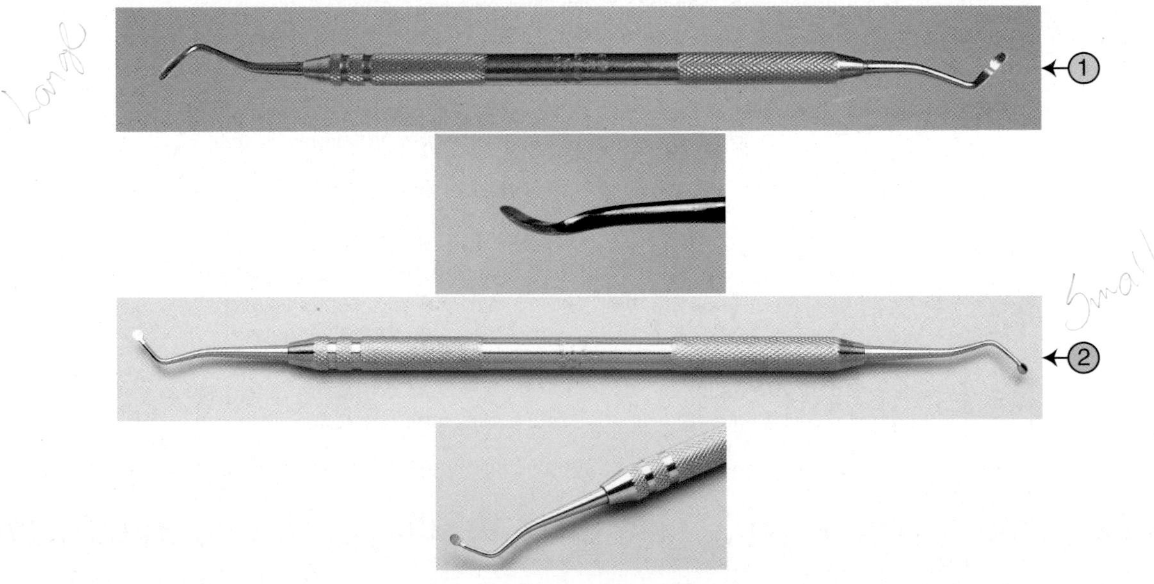
1
2

INSTRUMENT

Spoon Excavators evolve

FUNCTION To remove carious dentin

Secondary functions:

- To remove temporary crowns
- To remove temporary cement in temporary restoration
- To remove permanent crown during try in

CHARACTERISTICS Concave design, spoon-shaped with cutting edge

Range of sizes:

- ① Large—Curved blade
- ② Small—Round blade

Single or double ended

PRACTICE NOTE Spoon Excavator is used on restorative tray setups.

Refer to the Amalgam tray setup (see Chapter 8), Composite tray setups (see Chapter 9), and Crown and Bridge Restorative tray setups (see Chapter 10)

Ⓢ Spoon Excavators must be cleaned, bagged individually or bagged/wrapped in a tray setup, and then sterilized. A chemical/steam indicator device should be included in the wrapping.

CHAPTER 3

Local Anesthetic Syringe and Components

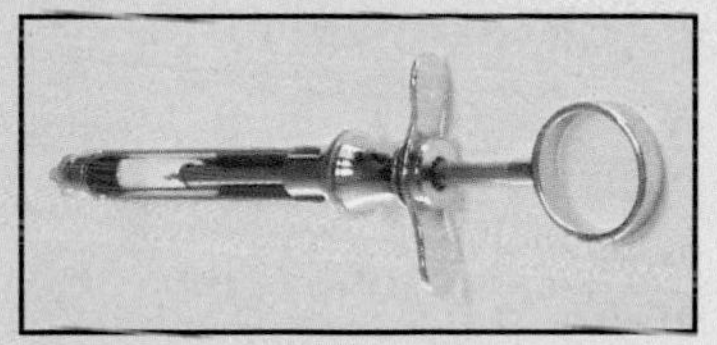

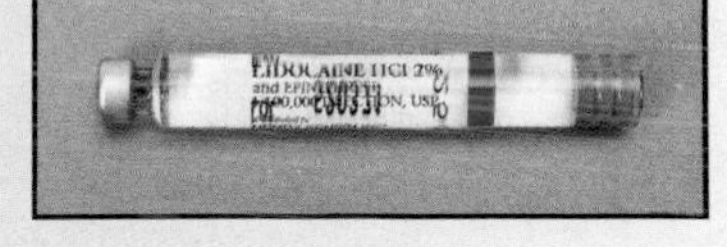

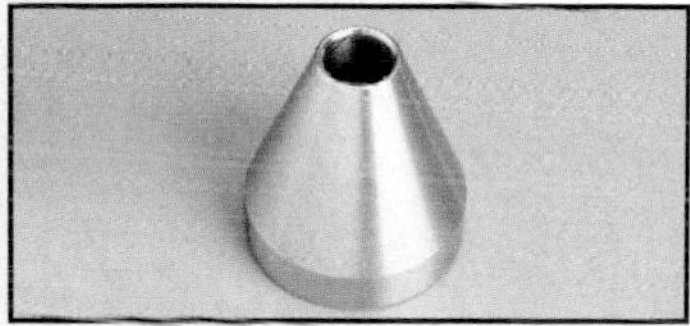

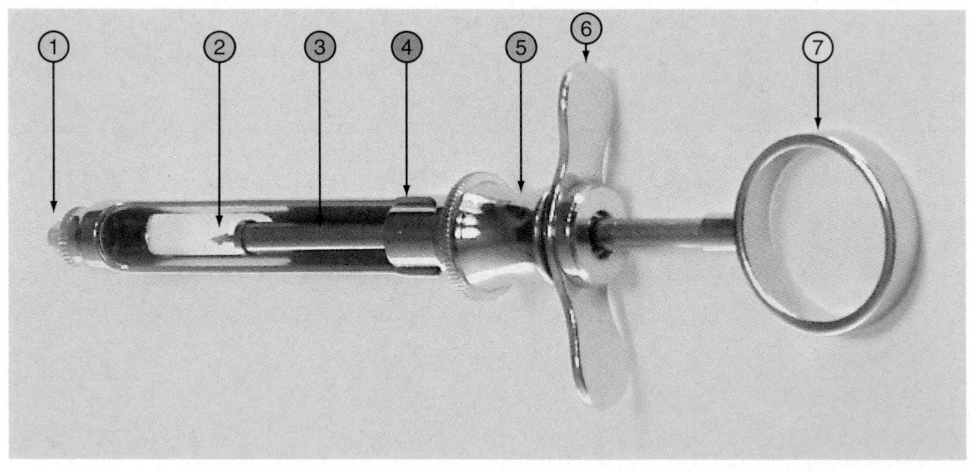
1
2
3
4
5
6
7

INSTRUMENT

Anesthetic Aspirating Syringe

FUNCTION
To administer a local anesthetic

CHARACTERISTICS
Parts:
- ① Threaded tip
- ② Harpoon
- ③ Piston rod
- ④ Barrel of syringe
- ⑤ Finger grip
- ⑥ Finger bar
- ⑦ Thumb ring

PRACTICE NOTES
Syringes with harpoons are considered aspirating syringes.
Disposable syringes equipped with needles and preloaded with anesthetic are available.
Anesthetic Aspirating Syringe is used on most tray setups.

S Anesthetic Aspirating Syringe must be cleaned, bagged individually or bagged/wrapped in a tray setup, and then sterilized. A chemical/steam indicator device should be included in the wrapping. Disposable preloaded syringes with needle must be disposed of in a Sharps container.

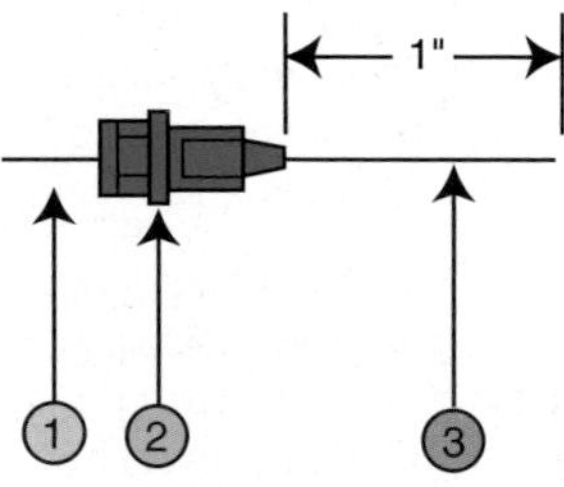
1"
1
2
3

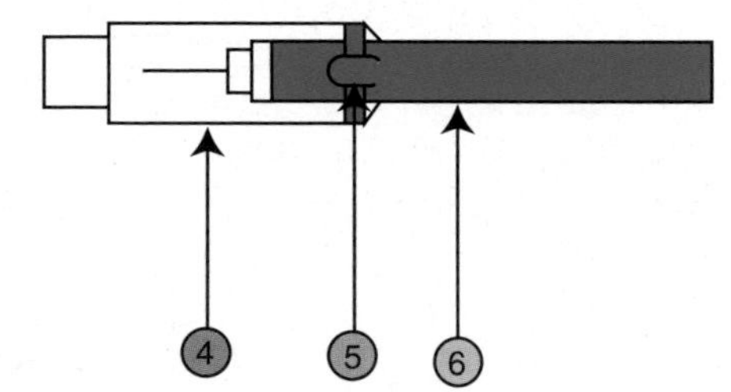
4
5
6

INSTRUMENT

Short Needle

FUNCTION To administer anesthetic by infiltration injection on maxillary arch

CHARACTERISTICS Parts:

① Cartridge end of needle
② Needle hub
③ Injection end of needle
④ Protective cap
⑤ Seal on cap
⑥ Needle guard

1 inch long

Variety of gauges:

- Gauge number—Identifies diameter (thickness) of needle
- Larger gauge number—Indicates thinner needle (e.g., 30 gauge is thinner than 25 gauge)

PRACTICE NOTE Local anesthetic syringe setup is used on most tray setups (see page 50).

Ⓢ Short Needle must be disposed of in a Sharps container. Single use only.

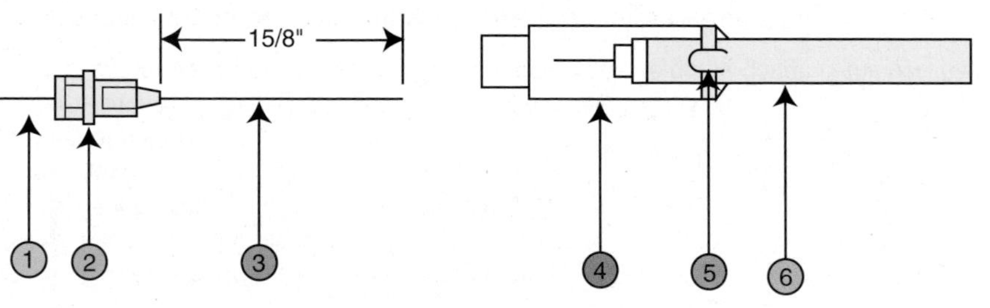
15/8"
1
2
3
4
5
6

INSTRUMENT

Long Needle

FUNCTION To administer anesthetic by block injection on mandibular arch

CHARACTERISTICS Parts:

① Cartridge end of needle ② Needle hub
③ Injection end of needle ④ Protective cap
⑤ Seal on cap ⑥ Needle guard

1⅝ inches long

Variety of gauges:

- Gauge number—Identifies diameter (thickness) of needle
- Larger gauge number—Indicates thinner needle (e.g., 30 gauge is thinner than 25 gauge)

PRACTICE NOTE Local anesthetic syringe setup is used on most tray setups (see page 50).

Ⓢ Long Needle must be disposed of in a Sharps container. Single use only.

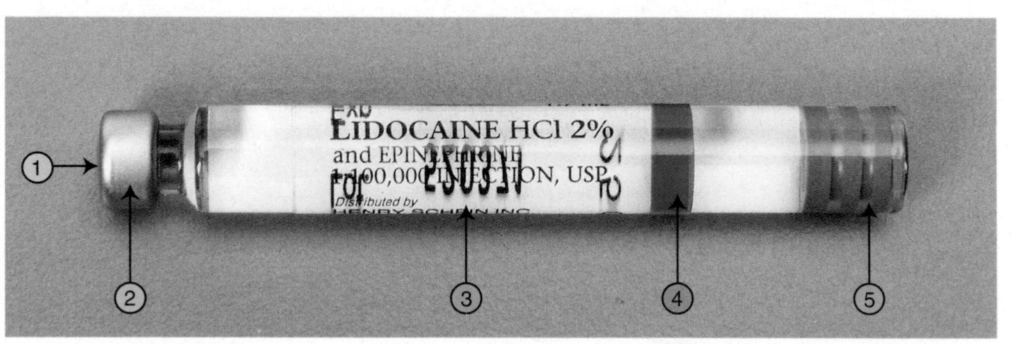
1
2
3
4
5
LIDOCAINE HCl 2%
and EPINEPHRINE
1:100,000 INJECTION, USP
Distributed by

INSTRUMENT

Anesthetic Cartridge evolve

FUNCTION To hold liquid anesthetic for local injection in the oral cavity

CHARACTERISTICS Parts:

① Rubber diaphragm—Syringe needle is inserted into the diaphragm to penetrate into the cartridge
② Aluminum cap holds the rubber diaphragm in place
③ Glass cartridge (also referred to as a carpule)
④ Color-coded band indicating type of anesthetic (required by the American Dental Association [ADA], June 2003)
⑤ Silicon rubber plunger—Harpoon of syringe inserts into silicon rubber plunger

Composition of solution in cartridge—Contains 1.7 to 1.8 ml of anesthetic solution
Plunger slightly indented from rim of glass

PRACTICE NOTES Type of anesthetic used depends on patient's health history and dental procedure performed.
Local anesthetic syringe setup is used on most tray setups (see page 50).

Ⓢ Anesthetic cartridge must be disposed of in a Sharps container. Refer to local and state recommendations for disposal of cartridge. Single use only.

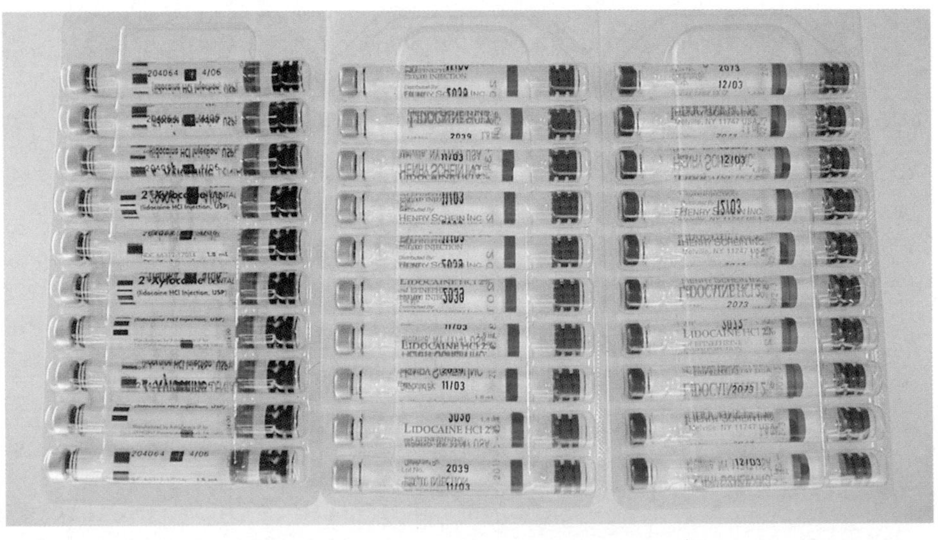
204064 4/06
(lidocaine HCl Injection, USP)
LIDOCAINE HCl 2%
HENRY SCHEIN INC.
2039
11/03
12/03
2073

INSTRUMENT

Anesthetic Cartridges/Blister Packs

FUNCTION To hold liquid anesthetic for injection

CHARACTERISTICS Several types of anesthetic solution available
Each cartridge is labeled
Color code system on cartridge—Identifies type of anesthetic (required by the American Dental Association [ADA], June 2003)
Type of anesthetic used depends on patient's health history and dental procedure performed:

- Ratio of epinephrine: the lower the second number, the higher the percentage of vasoconstrictor. Information printed on cartridge. Example of common anesthetic for routine dental procedures 1:100,000.
- Longer-lasting anesthetic has a higher percentage of vasoconstrictor. Example: 1:50,000.
- Anesthetic is available without a vasoconstrictor.

PRACTICE NOTES Remove each cartridge from blister pack as needed for each procedure and place cartridge on tray setup. Local anesthetic syringe setup is used on most tray setups (see page 50).

Ⓢ Anesthetic Cartridge must be disposed of in a Sharps container. Refer to local and state recommendations for disposal of cartridge. Each Anesthetic Cartridge single use only.

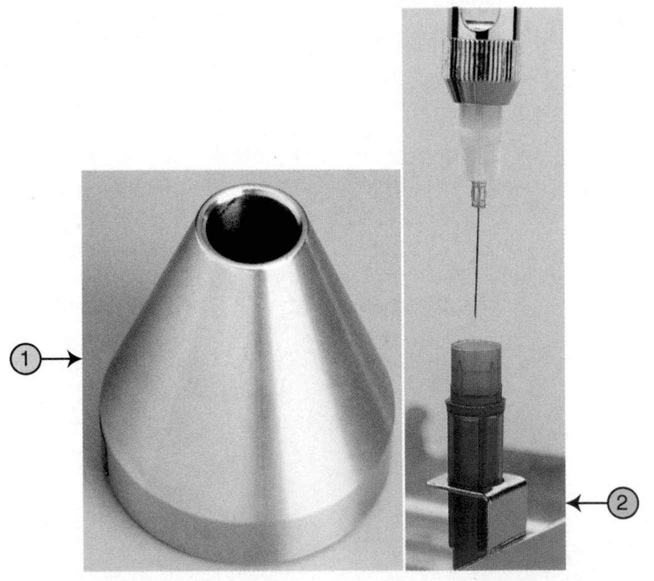
1
2

INSTRUMENT

Recapping Device

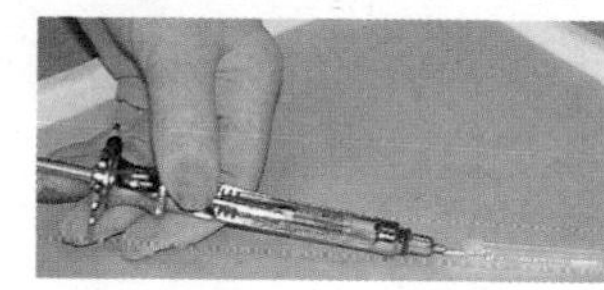

FUNCTION To hold needle sheath for one-hand recapping after injection

CHARACTERISTICS ① Low center of gravity for stability in recapping—Jenker
② Needle Cap Holder attached to cassette
Helps prevent needle stick accidents
Different styles of needle stick protectors available

PRACTICE NOTE Needle stick protector is used on most tray setups.

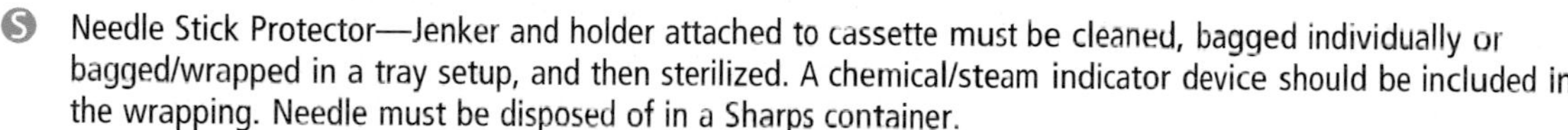

Ⓢ Needle Stick Protector—Jenker and holder attached to cassette must be cleaned, bagged individually or bagged/wrapped in a tray setup, and then sterilized. A chemical/steam indicator device should be included in the wrapping. Needle must be disposed of in a Sharps container.

The scoop technique is shown in photo at top right.

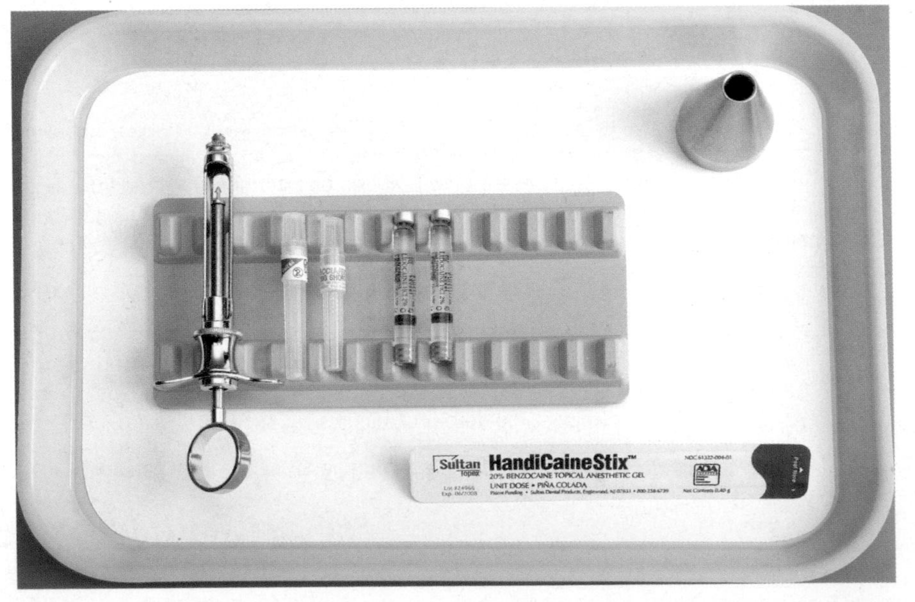
Sultan
HandiCaineStix™
20% BENZOCAINE TOPICAL ANESTHETIC GEL
UNIT DOSE • PIÑA COLADA

TRAY SETUP

Local Anesthetic Syringe

FROM LEFT TO RIGHT

Anesthetic aspirating syringe, long needle, short needle, anesthetic cartridges, needle stick protector (top right), topical anesthetic (bottom right)

PRACTICE NOTE Local anesthetic syringe setup is found on most tray setups.

Ⓢ Anesthetic Syringe and Needle Stick Protector must be cleaned, bagged individually or bagged/wrapped in a tray setup, and then sterilized. A chemical/steam indicator device should be included in the wrapping. Anesthetic cartridge must be disposed of in a Sharps container. Refer to local and state recommendations for disposal of cartridge. Needles must be disposed of in a Sharps container. Single use only. Topical anesthetic should be disposed of in the garbage. Single use only.

CHAPTER 4

Evacuation Devices and Air/Water Syringe Tip

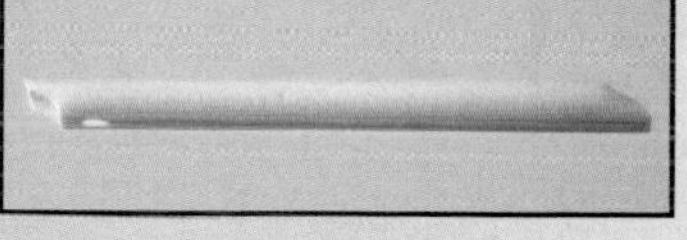

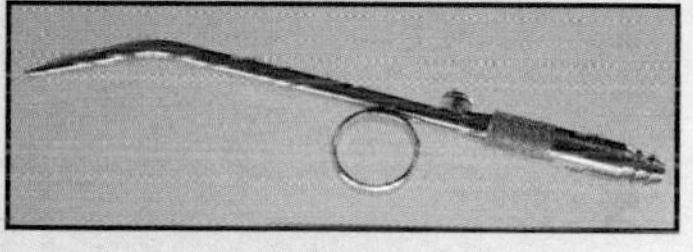

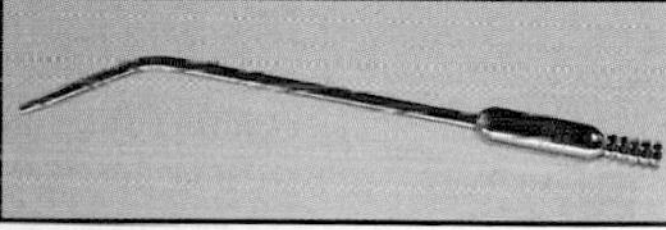

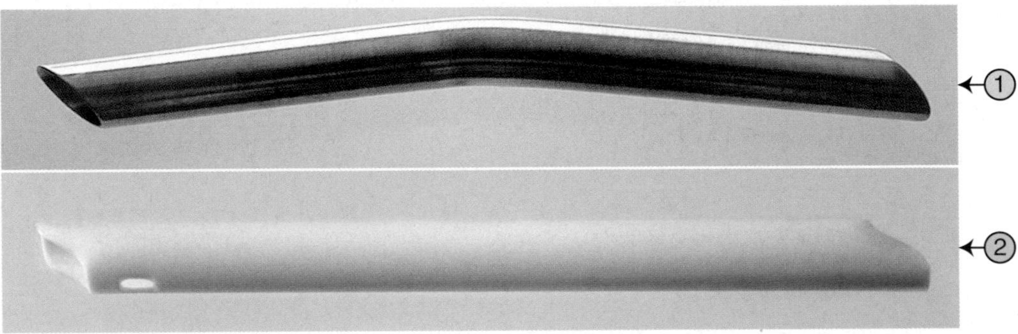
1
2

INSTRUMENT

High-Volume (Velocity) Evacuator (HVE) Tip

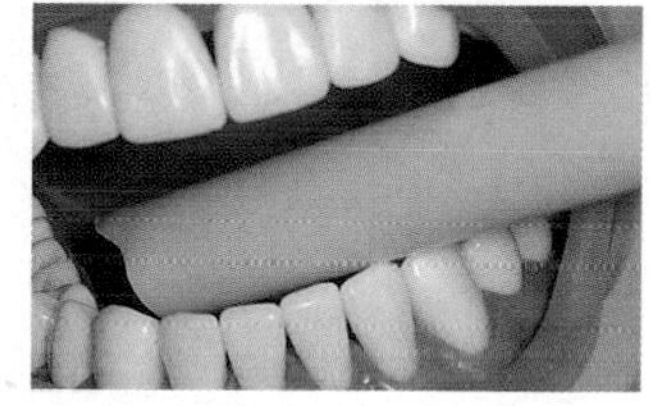

FUNCTION To evacuate large volumes of fluid and debris from the oral cavity

CHARACTERISTICS
① Stainless steel evacuator tip
② Plastic evacuator tip—Disposable plastic
Straight or slightly angled at one or both ends
Also available in plastic that may be sterilized

PRACTICE NOTES Evacuator tip attaches to high-velocity tubing on dental unit.
HVE tip is used on most tray setups.

Ⓢ HVE Tip must be cleaned, bagged individually or bagged/wrapped in a tray setup, and then sterilized. A chemical/steam indicator device should be included in the wrapping. Disposable plastic HVE Tip should be disposed of in the garbage. Single use only.

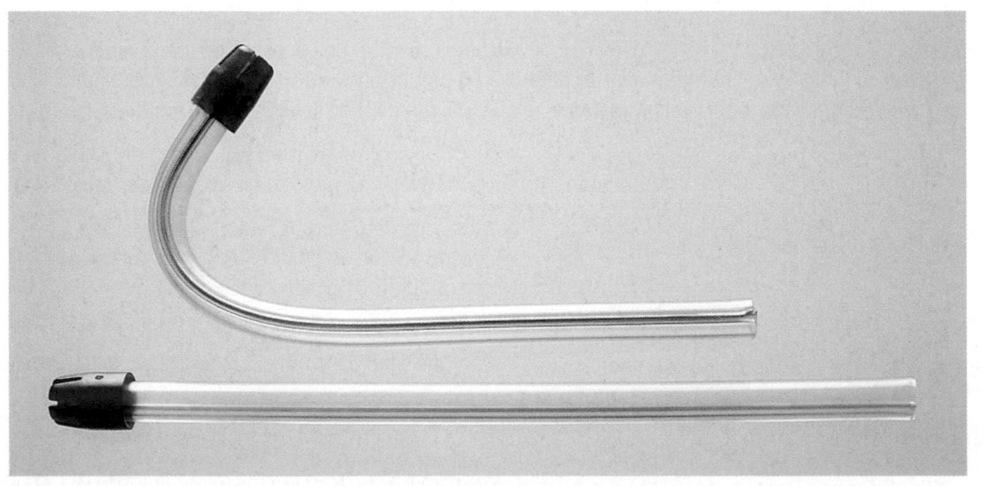

INSTRUMENT

Low-Volume (Velocity) Saliva Ejector Tip

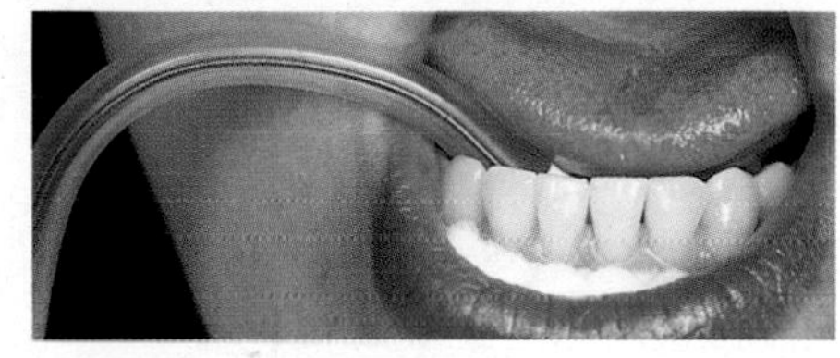

FUNCTION To evacuate smaller volumes of fluid from the oral cavity

CHARACTERISTICS Disposable plastic for single use only
Can be bent for placement under tongue and in other areas of mouth or can be used straight
Variety of styles

PRACTICE NOTES Attaches to low-velocity tubing on dental unit
Saliva Ejector Tip is used on most tray setups.

S Disposable Saliva Ejector Tip should be disposed of in the garbage. Single use only.

58

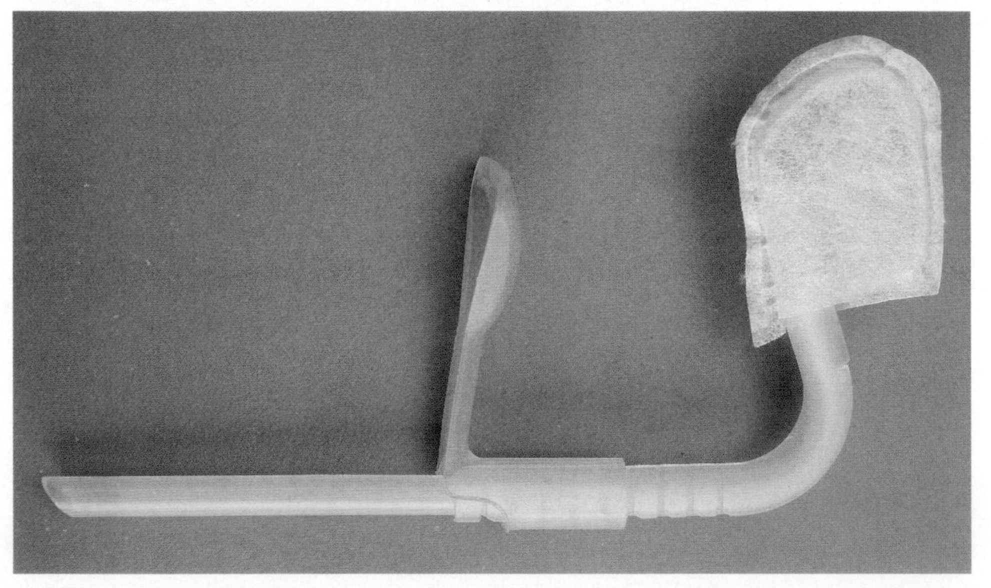

INSTRUMENT

Low-Volume (Velocity) Mandibular Evacuator

FUNCTIONS

To evacuate smaller volumes of fluid from the oral cavity
To use on mandibular arch
To retract tongue during evacuation

CHARACTERISTICS

Blade for retraction of tongue is covered for patient comfort
Device to place under patient's chin to hold evacuator in place
Disposable plastic for single use only
Also available in metal referred to as a Sveptoper

PRACTICE NOTES

Attaches to low-velocity tubing on dental unit
Disposable Low-Volume Mandibular Evacuator is used on Sealant tray setups (see page 361) and on procedures for mandibular arch when operator is working without an assistant.

Ⓢ Disposable Low-Volume Mandibular Evacuator (pictured) should be disposed of in the garbage. Low-Volume Mandibular Evacuator (Svedopter) must be cleaned, bagged individually or bagged/wrapped in a tray setup, and then sterilized. A chemical/steam indicator device should be included in the wrapping.

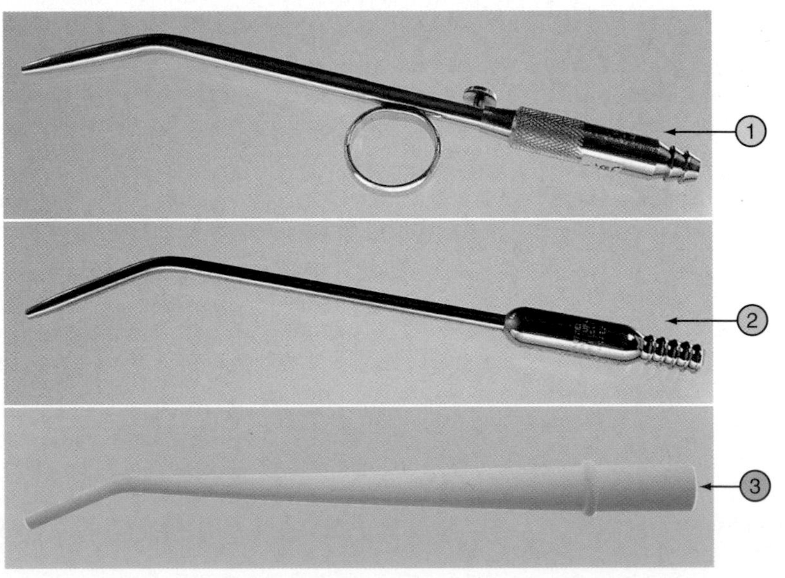
1
2
3

INSTRUMENT

High-Volume (Velocity) Surgical Evacuation Tip evolve

FUNCTION To evacuate fluid from oral cavity and surgical site

CHARACTERISTICS Stainless steel, autoclavable plastic, disposable plastic:

1. Stainless steel self-cleaning evacuation tip
2. Stainless steel evacuation tip
3. Plastic disposable tip

Narrowed tip accommodates surgical site

PRACTICE NOTES Surgical Evacuation Tip attaches to high-velocity tubing on dental unit
May require connecting tube for adaptation to surgical evacuation tip
Some stainless steel surgical tips narrow at insertion of tubing; additional tubing is necessary to connect to high velocity tubing on dental unit.
Surgical Evacuation Tip is used on most surgical tray setups.

S Surgical Evacuation Tips must be cleaned, bagged individually or bagged/wrapped in a tray setup, and then sterilized. A chemical/steam indicator device should be included in the wrapping. Disposable Surgical Evacuation Tip should be disposed of in the garbage. Single use only.

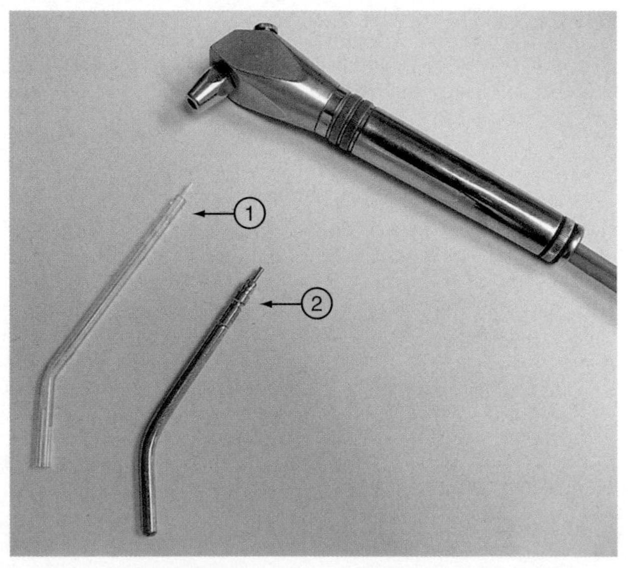
1
2

INSTRUMENT

Air/Water Syringe with Removable Tip

FUNCTION To rinse and dry specific teeth or entire oral cavity

CHARACTERISTICS Air/Water Syringe is also referred to as Three-Way syringe

Characteristics of buttons on Air/Water Syringe:

Push left button on Air/Water Syringe and it expels water only

Push right button on Air/Water Syringe and it expels air only

Push both buttons on Air/Water Syringe and it expels spray

Types of tips:

① Disposable plastic syringe tip for single use

② Metal syringe tip

PRACTICE NOTES Syringe Tip—Attaches to air/water syringe

Air/Water Syringe attaches to the tubing on the dental unit

Ⓢ Air/Water Syringe Tip must be cleaned, bagged individually or bagged/wrapped in a tray setup, and then sterilized. A chemical/steam indicator device should be included in the wrapping. Disposable Air/Water Syringe Tip should be disposed of in the garbage. Single use only. Air/Water Syringe that the tip is attached to must be disinfected according to the manufacturer's recommendation.

CHAPTER 5

Dental Handpieces

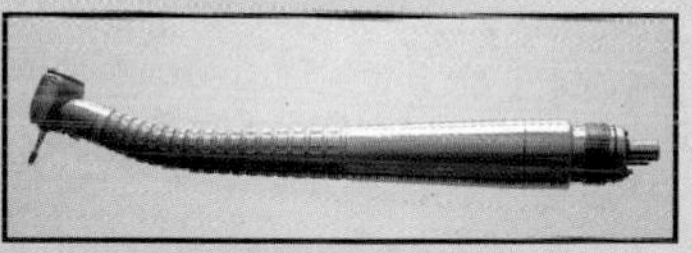

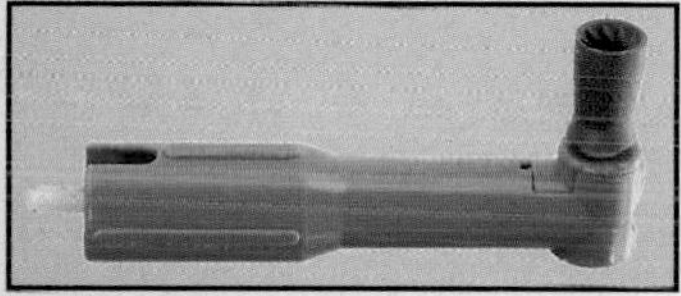

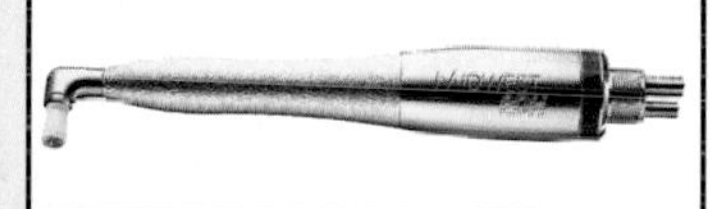

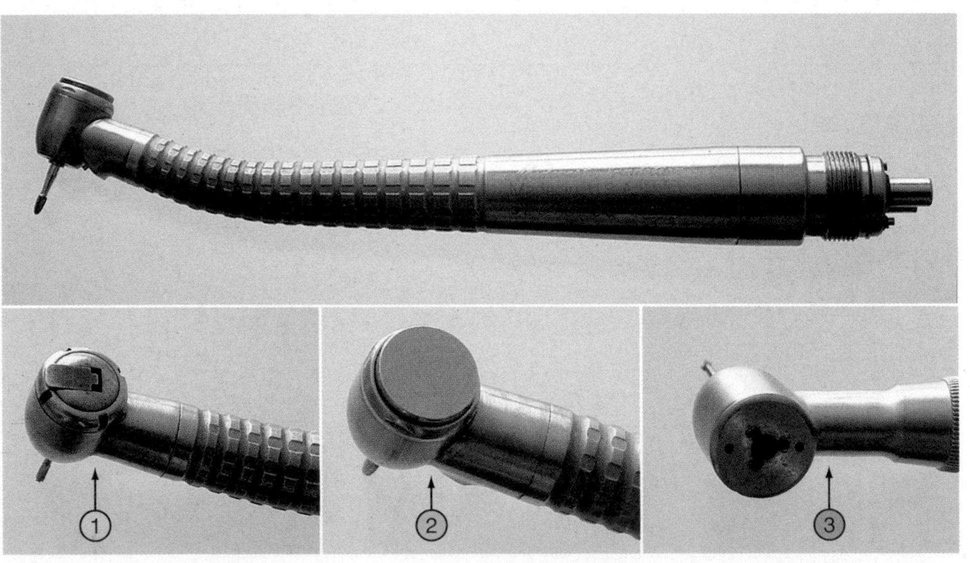
1
2
3

INSTRUMENT

High-Speed Handpiece evolve

FUNCTIONS

To use with bur to cut tooth with decay or other dental anomalies

Example: Cavity preparation for restoration or crown

To use with bur for adjusting crowns and bridges for final fit

CHARACTERISTICS

Handpiece is run by air pressure at a maximum speed of 450,000 rotations per minute.

On high-speed handpiece, bur generates extreme amount of heat.

Instrument sprays water/air or air on bur for cooling purposes to prevent damage to pulp.

Different styles of securing bur are available:

① Power level chuck
② Push-button chuck
③ Conventional chuck

PRACTICE NOTE

Handpiece attaches to tubing on dental unit

Ⓢ High-Speed Handpiece must be lubricated according to the manufacturer's recommendation, cleaned, bagged individually, and then sterilized. A chemical/steam indicator device should be included in the wrapping.

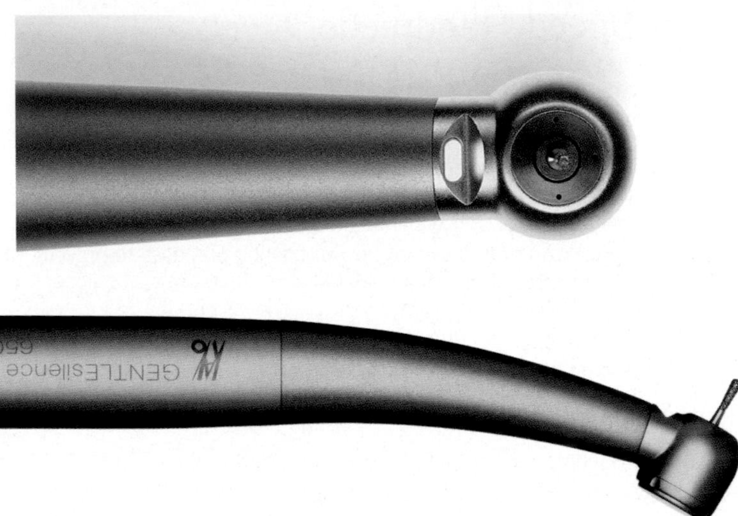
GENTLEsilence LUX
6500 B

INSTRUMENT

Fiberoptic High-Speed Handpiece

FUNCTIONS

To illuminate tooth during preparation for restoration
To provide light intraorally during use of handpiece

CHARACTERISTICS

Light(s) at head of handpiece
Lights up working area while handpiece rotates
Same characteristics as high-speed handpiece

PRACTICE NOTE

Handpiece attaches to tubing on dental unit

S Fiberoptic High-Speed Handpiece must be lubricated according to the manufacturer's recommendation, cleaned, bagged individually, and then sterilized. A chemical/steam indicator device should be included in the wrapping.

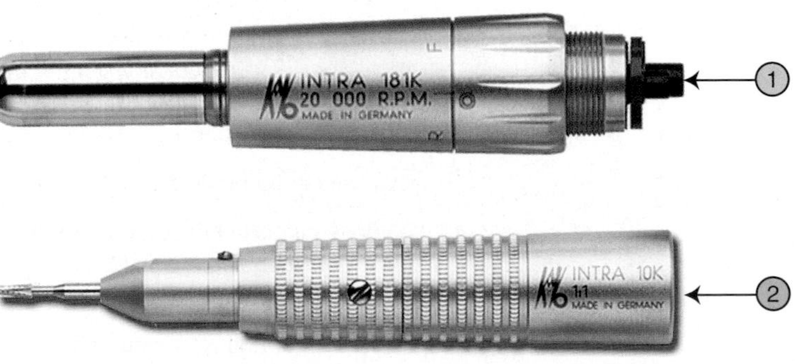
INTRA 181K
20 000 R.P.M.
MADE IN GERMANY
F
R
1
INTRA 10K
1:1
MADE IN GERMANY
2

INSTRUMENT

Slow-Speed Motor with Straight Handpiece Attachment

FUNCTIONS

To use with slow-speed attachments
To use straight attachment with long-shank straight bur

① Slow-Speed Motor
② Straight Handpiece Attachment (with bur)

CHARACTERISTICS

Maximum speed of 30,000 rotations per minute; used as adjunct to high-speed handpiece
Contra-angle or prophy angle attachments—Designed for intraoral use
Straight attachment—Usually used outside oral cavity

PRACTICE NOTE

Slow-Speed Motor attaches to tubing on dental unit

Ⓢ Slow-Speed Motor with Straight Handpiece Attachment must be lubricated according to the manufacturer's recommendation, cleaned, bagged individually, and then sterilized. A chemical/steam indicator device should be included in the wrapping.

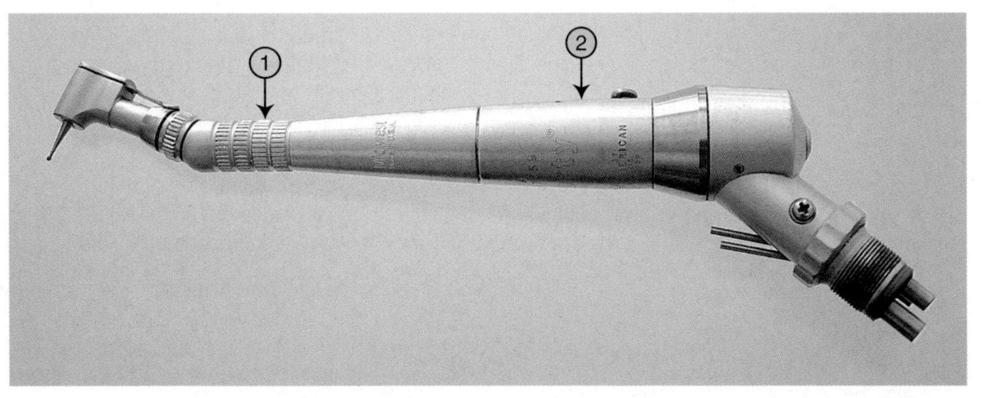
1
2

INSTRUMENT

Slow-Speed Motor with Contra-Angle Handpiece Attachment

FUNCTIONS To use with burs for intraoral and extraoral procedures:

- To remove decay
- To refine cavity preparation
- To adjust occlusal restorations
- To polish amalgam restorations
- To adjust provisional and permanent crowns and bridges
- To adjust partials and dentures

CHARACTERISTICS

① Contra-Angle Handpiece Attachment
② Slow-Speed Motor

Contra-Angle attaches to straight handpiece or to Slow-Speed Motor

Types of Contra-Angle Attachments:

- Latch type (pictured)—Latch-type bur or latch-type prophylaxis polishing cup or brush
- Friction grip—Friction-grip bur

PRACTICE NOTE Slow-Speed Motor attaches to tubing on unit

Ⓢ Slow-Speed Motor and Contra-Angle Handpiece Attachment must be lubricated according to the manufacturer's recommendation, cleaned, bagged individually, and then sterilized. A chemical/steam indicator device should be included in the wrapping.

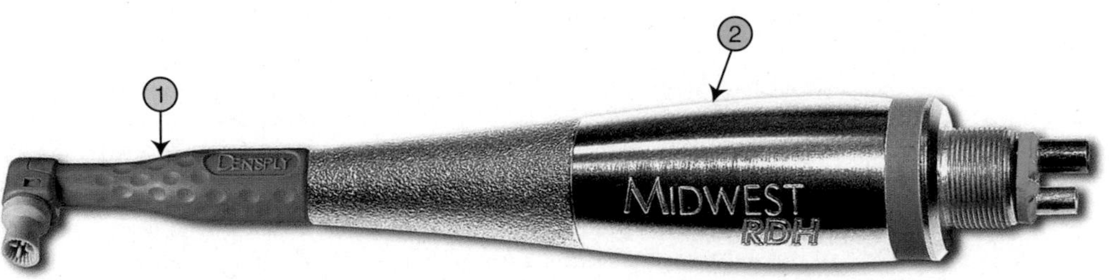
1
2
DENSPLY
MIDWEST
RDH

INSTRUMENT

Prophy Slow-Speed Handpiece/Motor* with Disposable Prophy Angle Attachment

FUNCTION To polish teeth with prophylaxis/prophy cup or brush attachment

CHARACTERISTICS
① Disposable Prophy Angle Attachment (with rubber polishing cup)
② Prophy Slow-Speed Handpiece/Motor
Prophy angle attaches to handpiece/motor
Lightweight design to reduce hand and wrist fatigue
Ergonomic shape for natural hand positioning

PRACTICE NOTE Prophy Handpiece/Motor attaches to tubing on dental unit

S Prophy Slow Speed Handpiece/Motor must be lubricated according to the manufacturer's recommendation, cleaned, bagged individually, and then sterilized. A chemical/steam indicator device should be included in the wrapping. Disposable Prophy Angle Attachment (with rubber polishing cup) must be disposed of in garbage. Single use only.

---

* Referred to as RDH (registered dental hygienist) *prophy handpiece.*
Pictured: MIDWEST RDH Hygiene Handpiece for Disposable Prophy Angles.

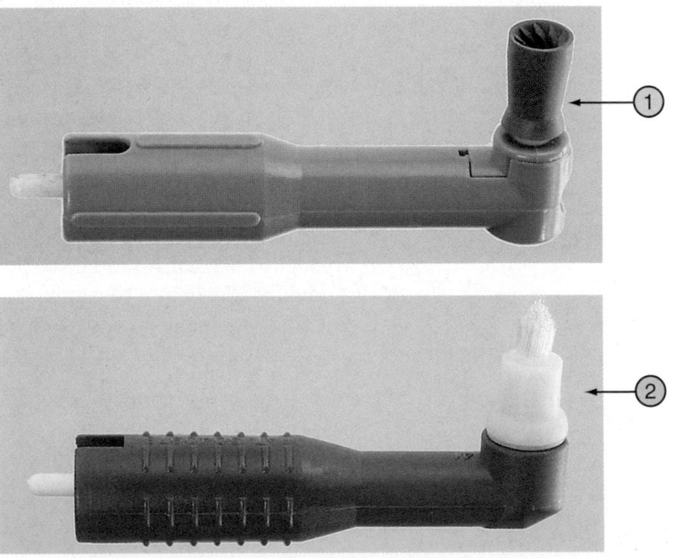
1
2

INSTRUMENT

Disposable Prophy Angle Attachments for Slow-Speed Handpiece/Motor

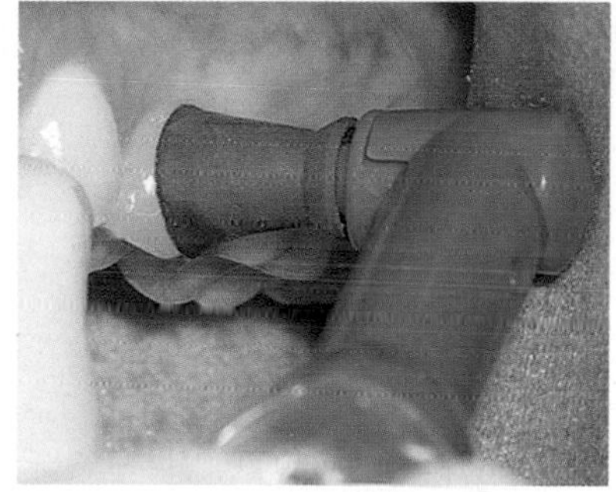

FUNCTION To polish teeth with prophylaxis/prophy cup or brush

CHARACTERISTICS Attaches to straight or Prophy Slow-Speed Handpiece/Motor

Types:

① Disposable prophy cup—For polishing all surfaces of teeth

② Disposable prophy brush—For polishing occlusal surfaces and deep grooves on lingual surfaces of anterior teeth

PRACTICE NOTE Disposable Prophy Angle Attachments are used mostly on prophylaxis and sealant tray setups.

Ⓢ Disposable Prophy Angle Attachments (rubber polishing cup or brush) must be disposed of in garbage. Single use only.

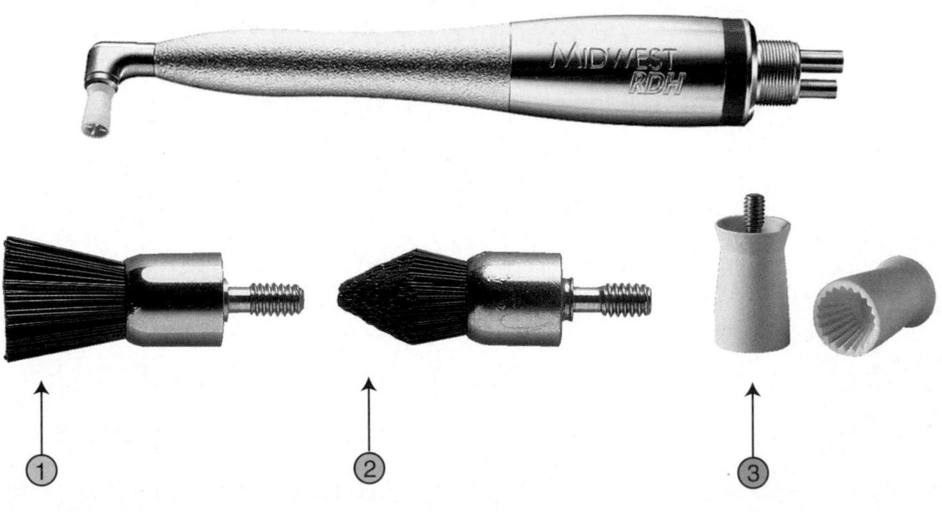
MIDWEST
RDH
1
2
3

INSTRUMENT

Prophy Angle Slow-Speed Handpiece/Motor* 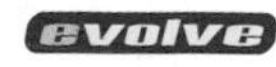

FUNCTION To polish teeth with prophylaxis/prophy cup or brush

CHARACTERISTICS Prophy Angle Slow-Speed Handpiece/Motor is one piece.
Disposable screw-type prophy cup or brush attaches to Prophy Angle Slow-Speed Handpiece/Motor.
Lightweight design to reduce hand and wrist fatigue.
Ergonomic shape for natural hand positioning.
Attachments:

① Flat-end brush
② Tapered-end brush
③ Prophy cup

PRACTICE NOTE Prophy Angle Slow-Speed Handpiece/Motor attaches to tubing on dental unit

Ⓢ Prophy Angle Slow-Speed Handpiece/Motor must be lubricated according to the manufacturer's recommendation, cleaned, bagged individually, and then sterilized. A chemical/steam indicator device should be included in the wrapping. Disposable prophy polishing cup or brush must be disposed of in garbage. Single use only.

---

*Referred to as RDH (registered dental hygienist) prophy handpiece.
Pictured: MIDWEST® RDH® Hygiene Handpiece with Prophy Right Angle.

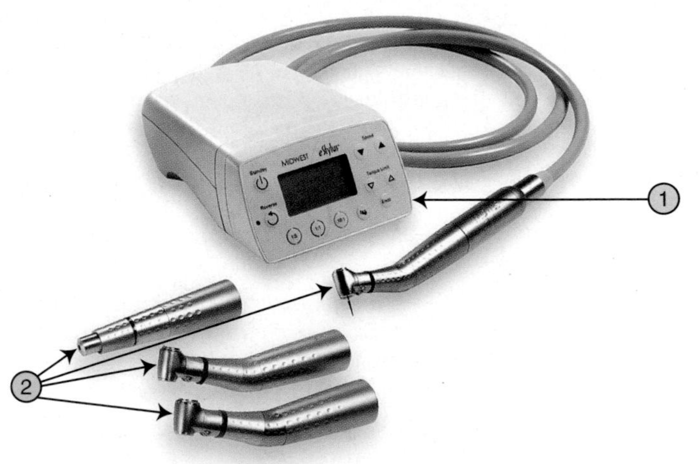
MIDWEST
eStylus
Speed
Torque Limit
Reverse
1
2

INSTRUMENT

Electric Handpiece Unit and Handpiece Attachments

FUNCTIONS

To use with bur for intraoral cavity preparation
To use with endodontic nickel-titanium rotary instruments
To use with bur for trimming of provisional crowns
To use with bur for adjusting permanent restorations, crowns, and bridges

CHARACTERISTICS

① Electric Handpiece Unit
② Electric Handpiece Attachments
Speed (i.e., rotations per minute [rpm]) can be set before procedure.

PRACTICE NOTES

Handpiece attaches to tubing on Electric Handpiece Unit
Electric Handpiece is used with restorative and endodontic tray setups.

Ⓢ Electric Handpiece Attachments must be lubricated according to the manufacturer's recommendation, cleaned, bagged individually, and then sterilized. A chemical/steam indicator device should be included in the wrapping. Barriers should be used on the unit and/or the manufacturer's recommendation should be followed for disinfecting the unit.

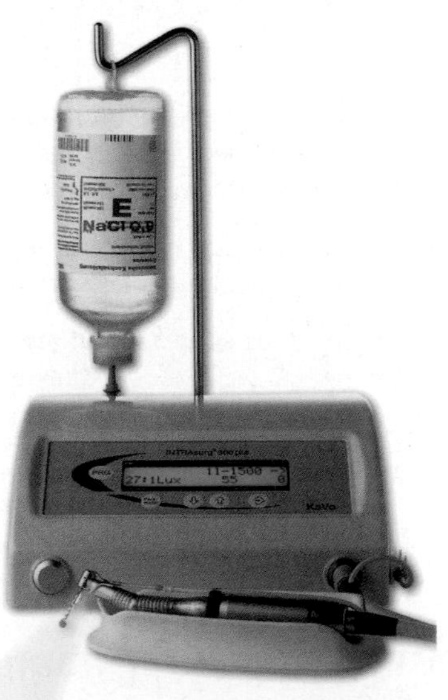
E
11-1500
27:1Lux 55 0
KaVo

INSTRUMENT

Surgical Electrical Handpiece Unit and Handpiece Attachments

FUNCTIONS
To use with depth drills for implants
To use with sterile water for cooling drilling system

CHARACTERISTICS
Straight and contra-angled (pictured) handpiece attachments available
Maximum speed of 40,000 rotations per minute (rpm)
Lower speed (e.g., 10–50 rpm) used for implant
Handpiece pictured includes a light

PRACTICE NOTE
Surgical Electric Handpiece Unit and Handpiece Attachments is used with surgical tray setups.

Ⓢ Surgical Electrical Handpiece Attachments must be lubricated according to the manufacturer's recommendation, cleaned, bagged individually, and then sterilized. A chemical/steam indicator device should be included in the wrapping. Barriers should be used on the unit and/or the manufacturer's recommendation should be followed for disinfecting the unit.

Pictured: KaVo INTRAsurg 300 plus. Information provided is specific to this unit.

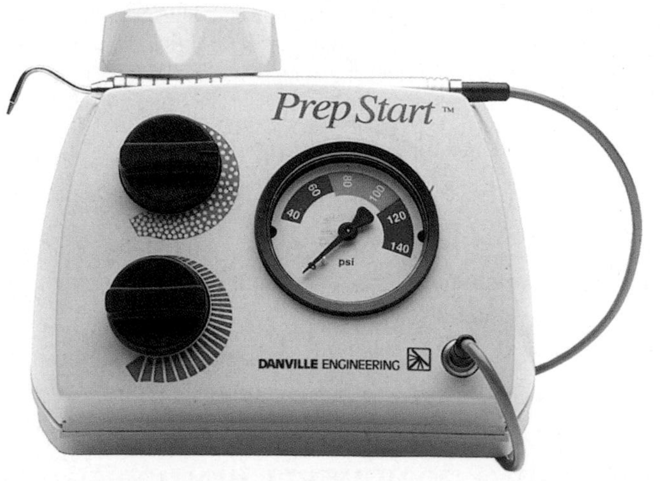

Prep Start ™
40
60
80
100
120
140
psi
DANVILLE ENGINEERING

INSTRUMENT

Air Abrasion Unit and Handpiece Attachment

FUNCTIONS

To use for class I or class VI cavity preparation
To use for preparation of occlusal surface for sealants

CHARACTERISTICS

Handpiece Attachment uses high pressure of alpha-alumina particles through small device that removes decay and/or prepares pit and fissures for sealants or restoration.
Minimal use of anesthesia is required.

PRACTICE NOTE

Air Abrasion Unit and Handpiece Attachment is used with class IV restorative tray setups and with sealant tray setups.

(S) Air Abrasion Handpiece Attachments must be lubricated according to the manufacturer's recommendation, cleaned, bagged individually, and then sterilized. A chemical/steam indicator device should be included in the wrapping. Barriers should be used on the unit and/or the manufacturer's recommendation should be followed for disinfecting the unit.

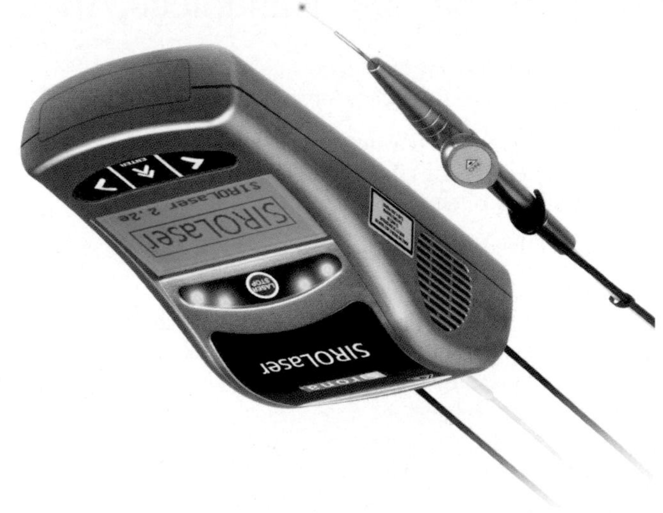
SIROLaser
SIROLaser 2.2e
SIROLaser

INSTRUMENT

Laser Handpiece Unit and Laser Handpiece Attachment

FUNCTION To cut, vaporize, or cauterize soft tissue

Examples:

To remove lesions or tumors
To reduce excess tissue
To control bleeding

CHARACTERISTICS New technological device
Works by means of a highly concentrated light source
SIROLaser (pictured) operates at a wavelength of 980 nanometers and has a power output varying from 0.5 to 7 watts.

PRACTICE NOTE Laser used with endodontics, periodontics, and/or oral surgery tray setups

Ⓢ Laser Handpiece Attachment must be cleaned, bagged individually, and then sterilized. A chemical/steam indicator device should be included in the wrapping. Barriers should be used on the unit and/or the manufacturer's recommendation should be followed for disinfecting the unit.

CHAPTER 6

Burs and Rotary Attachments for Handpieces

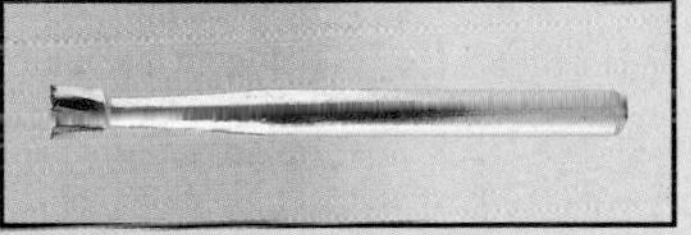

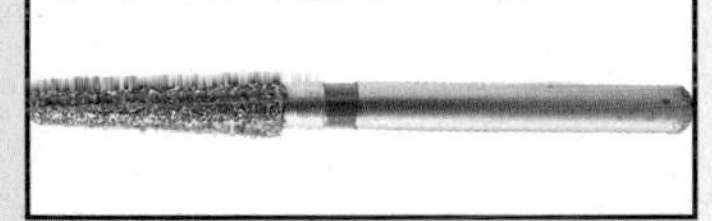

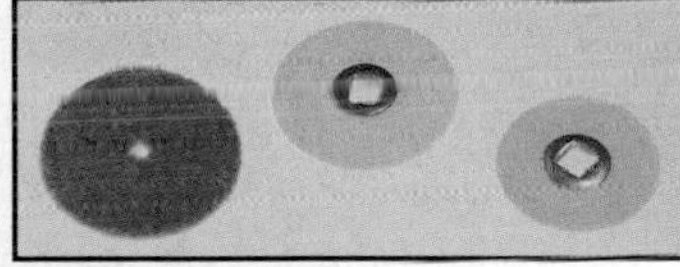

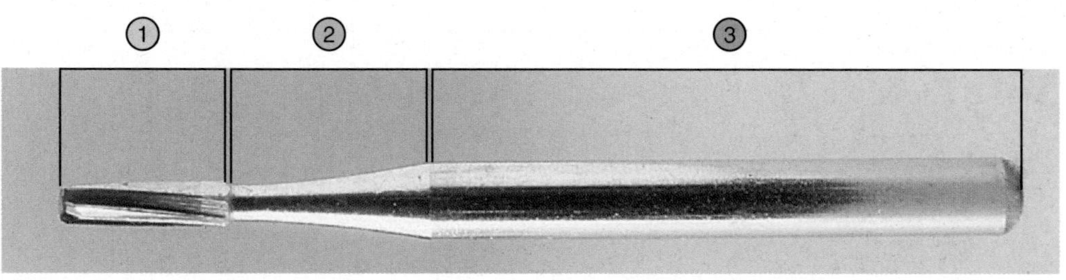
1
2
3

INSTRUMENT

Bur

FUNCTION To be used in high-speed or low-speed handpiece

CHARACTERISTICS Parts:

① Head: Part of bur that cuts, polishes, or finishes
Available in a variety of shapes and sizes

② Neck: Part of bur that tapers to connect shank to head

③ Shank: Part of bur that is inserted into the handpiece

- Length and style vary depending on handpiece used.
- Bur with straight, long shank fits into straight slow-speed handpiece.
- Bur with latch-type shank fits into contra-angle slow-speed handpiece.
- Friction grip bur fits into high-speed handpiece; chuck or lever tightens bur into the handpiece.

Pictured: MIDWEST Bur.

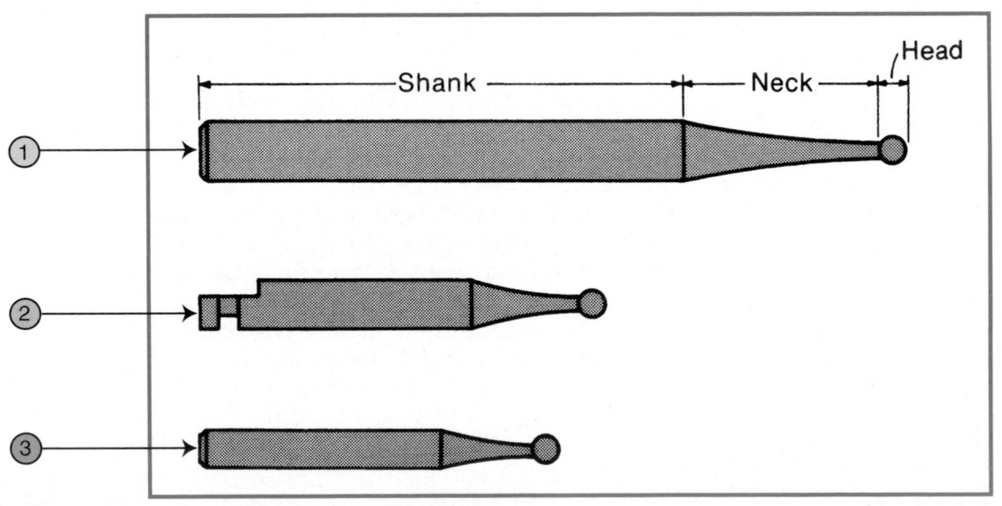
Shank
Neck
Head
1
2
3

INSTRUMENT

Bur Shanks

FUNCTION To insert shank part of bur into handpiece

CHARACTERISTICS Fit a variety of shanks into different styles of handpiece

Working or cutting end of the bur could be the same style and/or size, but shank could be different according to handpiece used.

Examples:

① No. 2 round bur in straight shank
② No. 2 round bur in latch-type shank
③ No. 2 round bur in friction grip shank

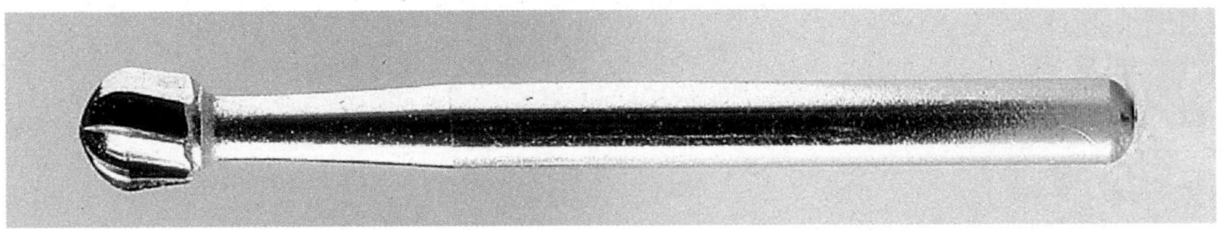

INSTRUMENT

Round Bur

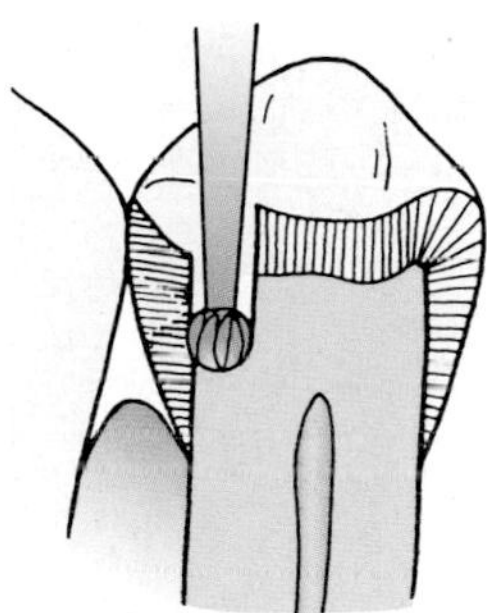

FUNCTIONS
To remove caries from tooth structure
To open tooth for endodontic treatment
To place retention in cavity preparation

CHARACTERISTICS
Range of sizes
Commonly used sizes: No. ¼ to no. 10

PRACTICE NOTES
Bur is inserted and secured in a handpiece.
Type of handpiece determines type of shank used.

Ⓢ Round Bur must be cleaned, bagged individually or bagged/wrapped in a tray setup, and then sterilized. A chemical/steam indicator device should be included in the wrapping, or the used Bur must be disposed of in a Sharps container.

Pictured: MIDWEST Round Bur.

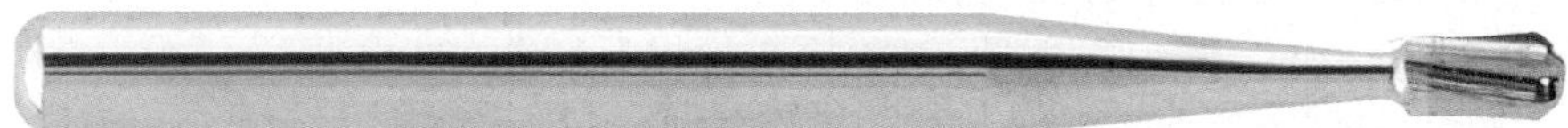

INSTRUMENT

Pear-Shaped Bur

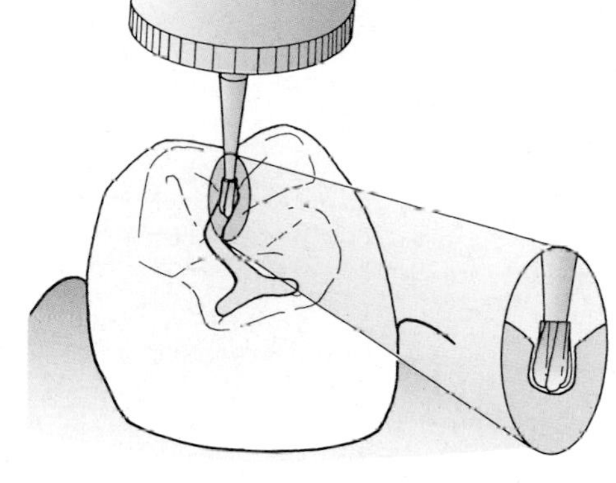

FUNCTIONS

To open tooth for a restoration
To remove caries

CHARACTERISTICS

Frequently used in preparation of composite restorations
Range of sizes
Commonly used sizes: No. 330 to no. 333
Bur head available in long
Example: No. 333L

PRACTICE NOTES

Bur is inserted and secured in a handpiece.
Type of handpiece determines type of shank used.

Ⓢ Pear-Shaped Bur must be cleaned, bagged individually or bagged/wrapped in a tray setup, and then sterilized. A chemical/steam indicator device should be included in the wrapping, or the used Bur must be disposed of in a Sharps container.

Pictured: MIDWEST Pear-Shaped Bur.

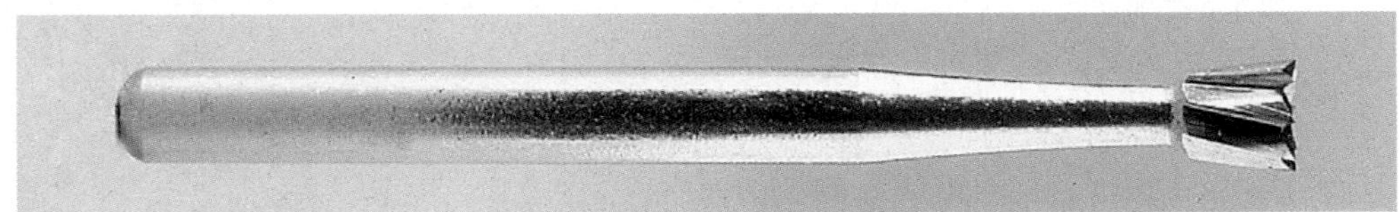

INSTRUMENT

Inverted Cone Bur

FUNCTIONS

To remove caries
To establish retention in tooth for cavity preparation

CHARACTERISTICS

Range of sizes
Commonly used sizes: No. 33½, no. 34, no. 37, no. 39

PRACTICE NOTES

Bur is inserted and secured in a handpiece.
Type of handpiece determines type of shank used.

Ⓢ Inverted Cone Bur must be cleaned, bagged individually or bagged/wrapped in a tray setup, and then sterilized. A chemical/steam indicator device should be included in the wrapping, or the used Bur must be disposed of in a Sharps container.

Pictured: MIDWEST Inverted Cone Bur.

100

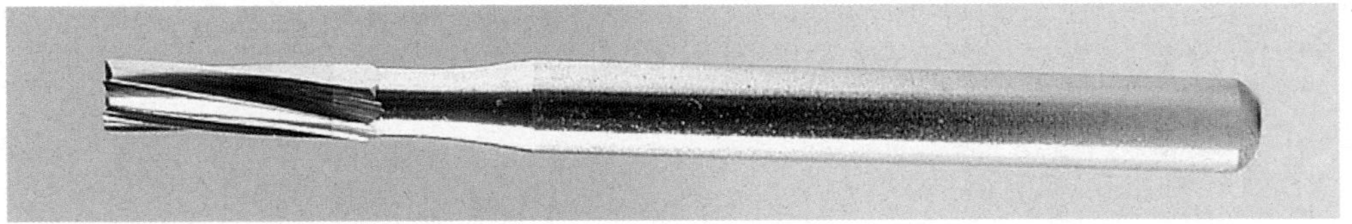

INSTRUMENT

Straight Fissure Bur—Plain Cut evolve

FUNCTIONS

To cut cavity preparation
To form inner walls of cavity preparation
To place retention grooves in walls of cavity preparation

CHARACTERISTICS

Cutting part of bur—Has parallel sides
Range of sizes
Commonly used sizes: No. 56, no. 57, no. 58
May have short or long shank for adaptation to a variety of cavity preparations; "S" at end of number indicates short shank, "L" indicates long shank
Examples of short and long shank friction grip burs: No. 56S, no. 56L

PRACTICE NOTES

Bur is inserted and secured in a handpiece.
Type of handpiece determines type of shank used.

S Straight Fissure Bur—Plain Cut must be cleaned, bagged individually or bagged/wrapped in a tray setup, and then sterilized. A chemical/steam indicator device should be included in the wrapping, or the used Bur must be disposed of in a Sharps container.

Pictured: MIDWEST Straight Fissure Bur—Plain Cut.

102

INSTRUMENT

Tapered Fissure Bur—Plain Cut evolve

FUNCTIONS

To cut cavity preparation
To form angles in walls of cavity preparation
To place retention grooves in walls of cavity preparation

CHARACTERISTICS

Cutting part of bur—Has tapered sides
Range of sizes
Commonly used sizes: No. 168, no. 169, no. 170, no. 171
May have short or long shank for adaptation to a variety of cavity preparations; "S" at end of number indicates short shank, "L" indicates long shank
Examples of short and long shank friction grip burs: No. 168S, no. 171L

PRACTICE NOTES

Bur is inserted and secured in a handpiece.
Type of handpiece determines type of shank used.

S Tapered Fissure Bur—Plain Cut must be cleaned, bagged individually or bagged/wrapped in a tray setup, and then sterilized. A chemical/steam indicator device should be included in the wrapping, or the used Bur must be disposed of in a Sharps container.

Pictured: MIDWEST Tapered Fissure Bur—Plain Cut.

104

INSTRUMENT

Straight Fissure Bur—Crosscut

FUNCTIONS

To cut cavity preparation
To form walls of cavity preparation
To place retention grooves in walls of cavity preparation

CHARACTERISTICS

Cutting part of bur—Has parallel sides with horizontal cutting edges
Range of sizes
Commonly used sizes: No. 556, no. 557, no. 558
May have long shank for adaptation to a variety of cavity preparations; "L" at end of number indicates long shank
Example of long shank friction grip bur: No. 556L

PRACTICE NOTES

Bur is inserted and secured in a handpiece.
Type of handpiece determines type of shank used.

Ⓢ Straight Fissure Bur—Crosscut must be cleaned, bagged individually or bagged/wrapped in a tray setup, and then sterilized. A chemical/steam indicator device should be included in the wrapping, or the used Bur must be disposed of in a Sharps container.

Pictured: MIDWEST Straight Fissure Bur—Crosscut

106

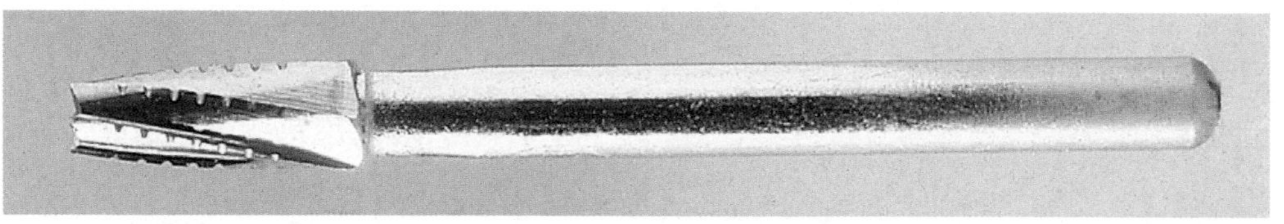

INSTRUMENT

Tapered Fissure Bur—Crosscut

FUNCTIONS

To cut cavity preparation
To form angles in walls of cavity preparation
To place retention grooves in walls of cavity preparation

CHARACTERISTICS

Cutting part of bur—Has tapered sides with horizontal cutting edges
Range of sizes
Commonly used sizes: No. 699, no. 700, no. 701, no. 702, no. 703
May have long shank for adaptation to a variety of cavity preparations; "L" at end of number indicates long shank
Example of long shank friction grip bur: No. 701L

PRACTICE NOTES

Bur is inserted and secured in a handpiece
Type of handpiece determines type of shank used.

S Tapered Fissure Bur—Crosscut must be cleaned, bagged individually or bagged/wrapped in a tray setup, and then sterilized. A chemical/steam indicator device should be included in the wrapping, or the used Bur must be disposed of in a Sharps container.

Pictured: MIDWEST Tapered Fissure Bur—Crosscut.

108

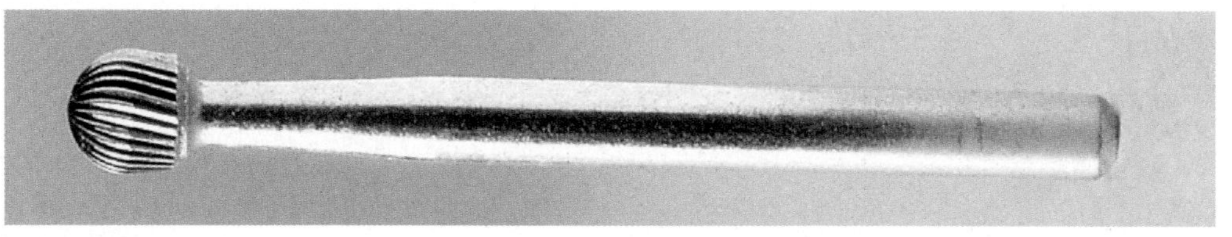

INSTRUMENT

Finishing Bur

FUNCTIONS

To finish composite restoration
To finish restoration by restoring anatomy in tooth
To equilibrate or adjust occlusion

CHARACTERISTICS

Variety of shapes and sizes

PRACTICE NOTES

Bur is inserted and secured in a handpiece.
Type of handpiece determines type of shank used.

Ⓢ Finishing Bur must be cleaned, bagged individually or bagged/wrapped in a tray setup, and then sterilized. A chemical/steam indicator device should be included in the wrapping, or the used Bur must be disposed of in a Sharps container.

Pictured: MIDWEST Finishing Bur.

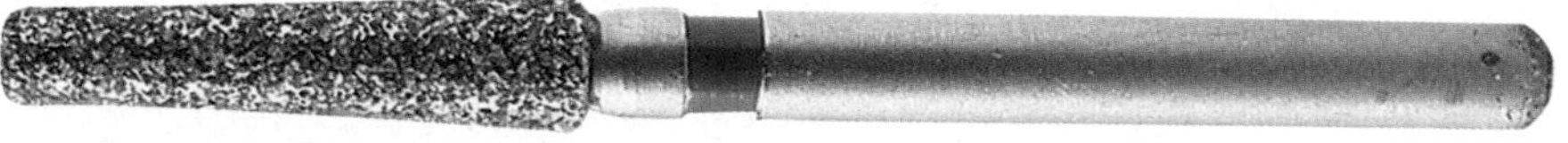

INSTRUMENT

Diamond Bur—Flat-End Taper

evolve

FUNCTION To reduce a tooth for crown preparation when a square shoulder is needed

CHARACTERISTICS Range of grits—Superfine to course; grit designated by color band on shank of diamond bur or by letter after name of diamond bur

Superfine diamond burs—Used for finishing restorations

Variety of shapes and sizes

PRACTICE NOTES Bur is inserted and secured in a handpiece.

Type of handpiece determines type of shank used.

S Diamond Bur—Flat-End Taper must be cleaned, bagged individually or bagged/wrapped in a tray setup, and then sterilized. A chemical/steam indicator device should be included in the wrapping, or the used Diamond Bur must be disposed of in a Sharps container.

Pictured: MIDWEST Diamond Bur—Flat-End Taper

112

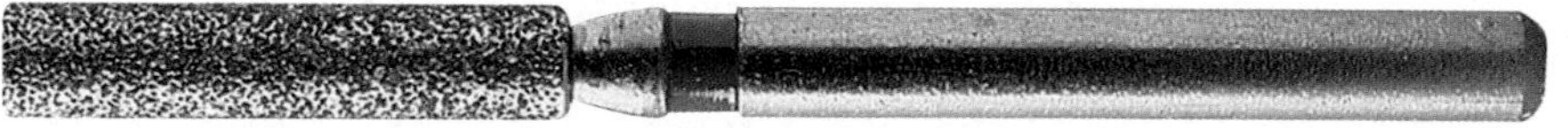

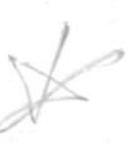

INSTRUMENT

Diamond Bur—Flat-End Cylinder

FUNCTION To reduce a tooth for crown preparation when parallel walls and flat floors are needed

CHARACTERISTICS Range of grits—Superfine to coarse; grit designated by color band on shank of diamond bur or by letter after name of diamond bur

Superfine diamond burs—Used for finishing restorations

Variety of shapes and sizes

PRACTICE NOTES Bur is inserted and secured in a handpiece.

Type of handpiece determines type of shank used.

S Diamond Bur—Flat-End Cylinder must be cleaned, bagged individually or bagged/wrapped in a tray setup, and then sterilized. A chemical/steam indicator device should be included in the wrapping, or the used Diamond Bur must be disposed of in a Sharps container.

Pictured: MIDWEST Diamond Bur—Flat-End Cylinder.

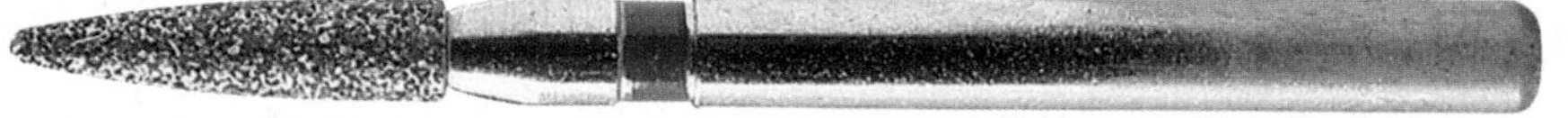

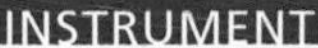

Diamond Bur—Flame

FUNCTION To reduce a tooth for crown preparation for subgingival margins

CHARACTERISTICS Range of grits—Superfine to coarse; grit designated by color band on shank of diamond bur or by letter after name of diamond bur
Superfine diamond burs—Used for finishing restorations
Variety of shapes and sizes

PRACTICE NOTES Bur is inserted and secured in a handpiece.
Type of handpiece determines type of shank used.

Diamond Bur—Flame must be cleaned, bagged individually or bagged/wrapped in a tray setup, and then sterilized. A chemical/steam indicator device should be included in the wrapping, or the used Diamond Bur must be disposed of in a Sharps container.

Pictured: MIDWEST Diamond Bur—Flame.

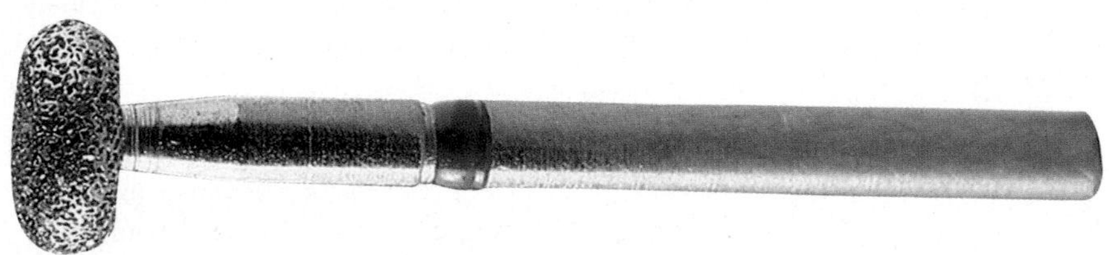

INSTRUMENT

Diamond Bur—Wheel evolve

FUNCTION To reduce a tooth for crown preparation on lingual aspect of anterior teeth and to reduce bulk of incisal edges

CHARACTERISTICS Range of grits—Superfine to coarse; grit designated by color band on shank of diamond bur or by letter after name of diamond bur

Superfine diamond burs—Used for finishing restorations

Variety of shapes and sizes

PRACTICE NOTES Bur is inserted and secured in a handpiece.

Type of handpiece determines type of shank used.

Ⓢ Diamond Bur—Wheel must be cleaned, bagged individually or bagged/wrapped in a tray setup, and then sterilized. A chemical/steam indicator device should be included in the wrapping, or the used Diamond Bur must be disposed of in a Sharps container.

Pictured: MIDWEST Diamond Bur—Wheel.

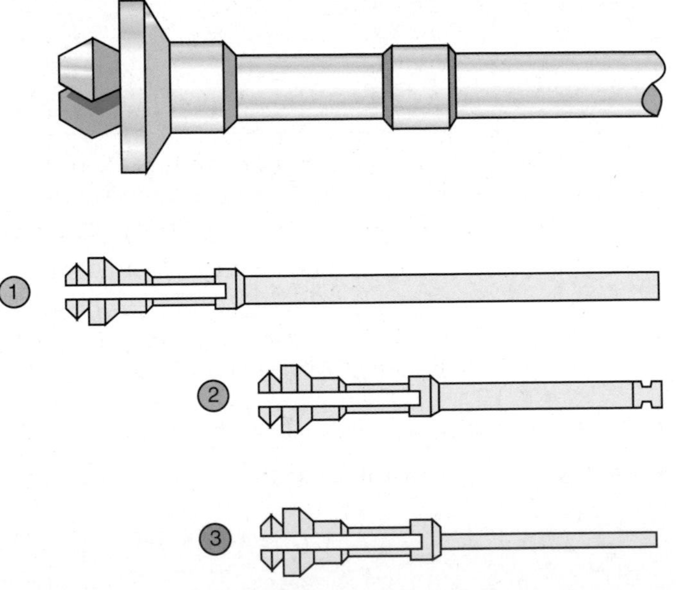
1
2
3

INSTRUMENT

Mandrel—Snap On

FUNCTION

To attach discs to Mandrel for finishing and polishing inside or outside oral cavity (Mandrel is inserted into handpiece)

CHARACTERISTICS

Shank types:

1. Long shank—For straight slow-speed handpiece
2. Short latch-type shank— For contra-angle slow-speed handpiece
3. Friction grip shank—For high-speed handpiece

Plastic disposable Snap-On Mandrels available

PRACTICE NOTES

Mandrel is inserted and secured in a handpiece.
Type of handpiece determines type of shank used.

Ⓢ Mandrel—Snap On must be cleaned, bagged individually or bagged/wrapped in a tray setup, and then sterilized. A chemical/steam indicator device should be included in the wrapping. Disposable Snap-On Mandrels should be disposed of in the garbage. Single use only.

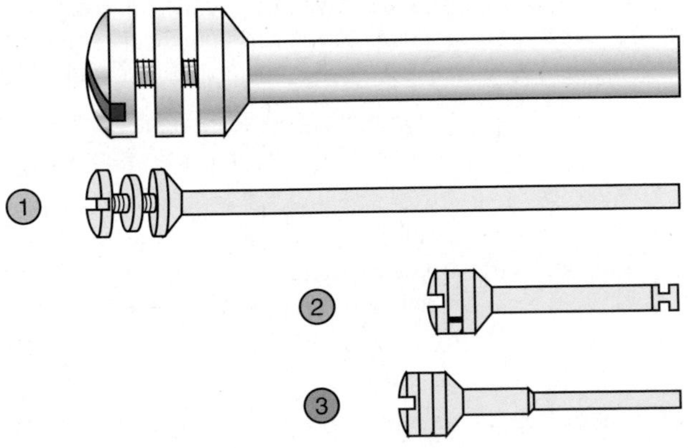
1
2
3

INSTRUMENT

Mandrel—Screw On

FUNCTION To attach discs to Mandrel for finishing and polishing inside or outside oral cavity (Mandrel is inserted into handpiece)

CHARACTERISTICS Shank types:

1. Long shank—For straight slow-speed handpiece
2. Short latch-type shank—For contra-angle or right-angle slow-speed handpiece
3. Friction grip shank—For high-speed handpiece

PRACTICE NOTES Mandrel is inserted and secured in a handpiece.
Type of handpiece determines type of shank used.

S Mandrel—Screw On must be cleaned, bagged individually or bagged/wrapped in a tray setup, and then sterilized. A chemical/steam indicator device should be included in the wrapping.

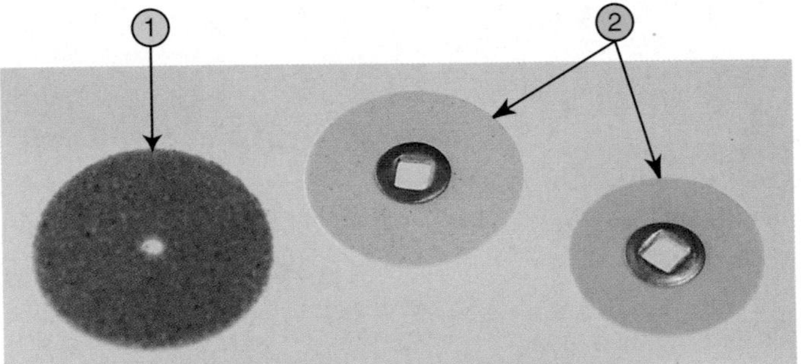
1
2

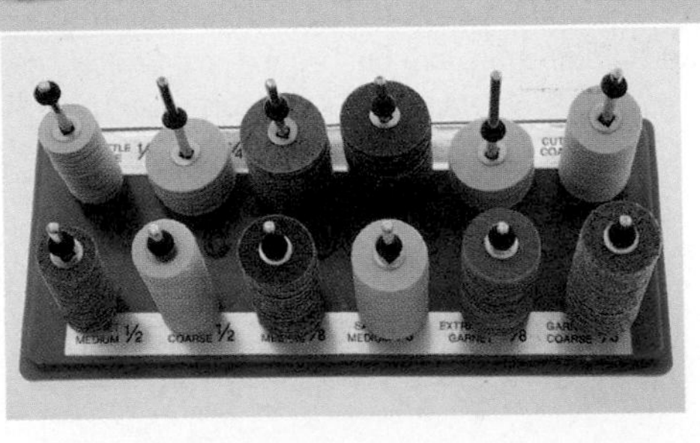
MEDIUM ½
COARSE ½

INSTRUMENT

Sandpaper Disc evolve

FUNCTIONS

To contour restorative material
To polish restorative material (extra fine grit)

CHARACTERISTICS

Range of grits (coarse to extra fine)
Two types:

① Screw on
② Snap on (metal center)

Sandpaper Disc organizer has a range of sizes and grits

PRACTICE NOTE

Sandpaper Disc is attached to either a snap-on mandrel or a screw-on mandrel depending on the type of Sandpaper Disc being used.

Disposable Sandpaper Discs should be disposed of in the garbage. Single use only

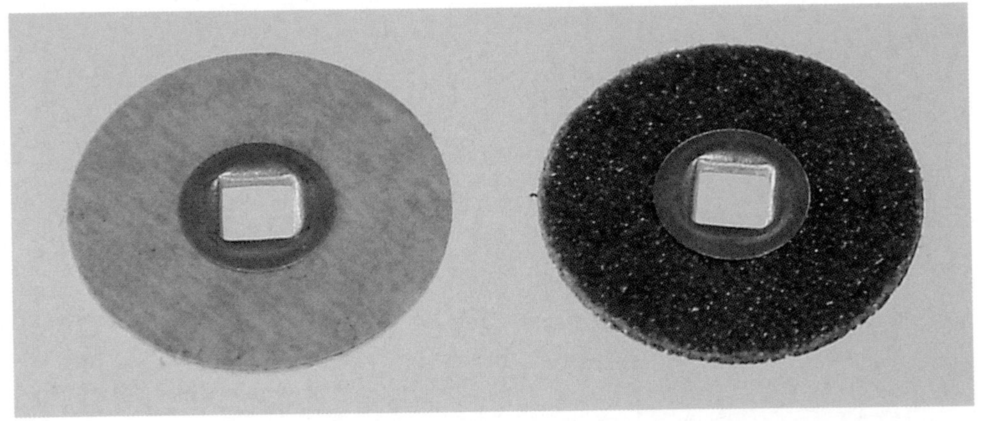

INSTRUMENT

Composite Disc

FUNCTIONS

To contour restorative material
To polish or smooth restorative material (extra fine grit)

CHARACTERISTICS

Made from synthetic material to accommodate composite restorations
Range of grits (coarse to extra fine)
Variety of sizes
Two types available:
- Snap on (pictured)
- Screw on

PRACTICE NOTE

Composite Disc is attached to either a snap-on mandrel or a screw-on mandrel depending on the type of Composite Disc being used.

S Disposable Composite Discs should be disposed of in the garbage. Single use only.

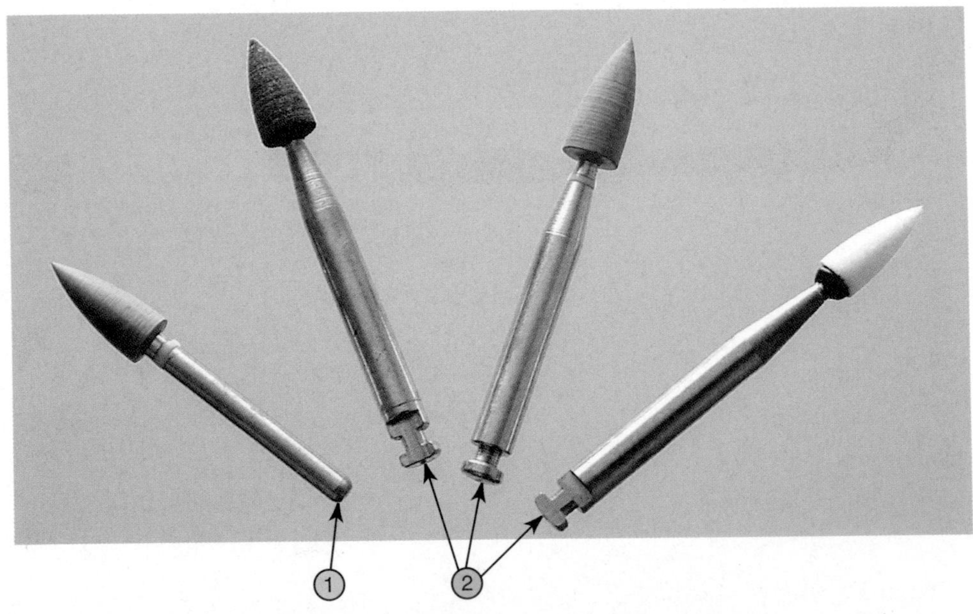
1
2

INSTRUMENT

Rubber Points evolve

FUNCTION To polish restorations, amalgam, composite, and gold

CHARACTERISTICS Types of polishing grits:

- Brown points (brownies)—Abrasive
- Green points (greenies)—Less abrasive than brownies
- White points—Polishing point

Variety of shanks available for all types of rubber points:

1. Friction grip
2. Latch type

PRACTICE NOTES Rubber Point is inserted and secured in a handpiece.
Type of handpiece determines type of shank used.

S Rubber Point must be cleaned, bagged individually or bagged/wrapped in a tray setup, and then sterilized. A chemical/steam indicator device should be included in the wrapping.

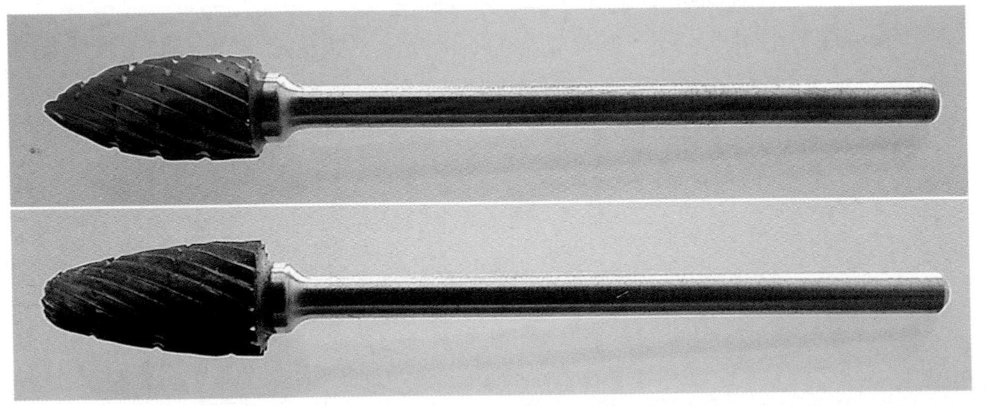

INSTRUMENT

Laboratory Bur—Acrylic Bur evolve

FUNCTION To cut models or trim acrylic in laboratory

CHARACTERISTICS Long shank—For attachment to straight handpiece
Variety of sizes and shapes

PRACTICE NOTE Laboratory Bur is inserted and secured in a slow-speed handpiece with a straight attachment.

Ⓢ Laboratory Bur—Acrylic Bur must be cleaned, bagged individually, and sterilized with a chemical indicator device included in the wrapping when used on any patient's appliances.

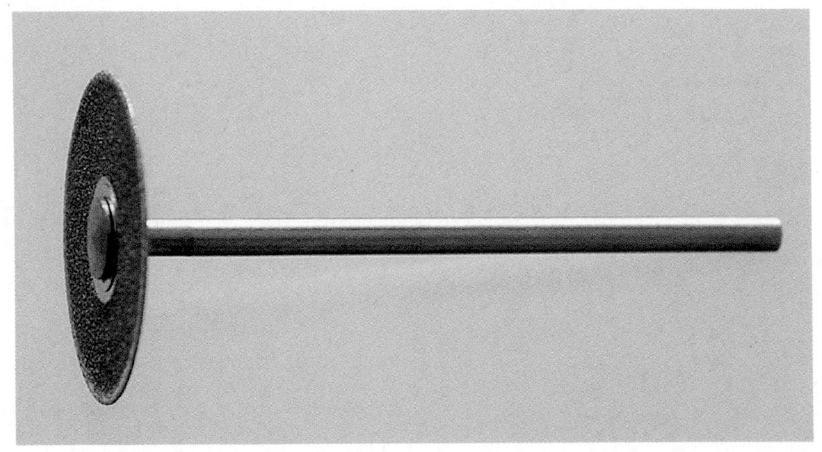

INSTRUMENT

Laboratory Bur—Diamond Disc

FUNCTION To contour or cut models in the laboratory

CHARACTERISTIC Single- or double-sided cutting edge

PRACTICE NOTE Laboratory Bur—Diamond Disc is inserted and secured in a slow-speed handpiece with a straight attachment.

S Laboratory Bur—Diamond Disc must be cleaned, bagged individually, and sterilized with a chemical indicator device included in the wrapping when used on any patient's appliances.

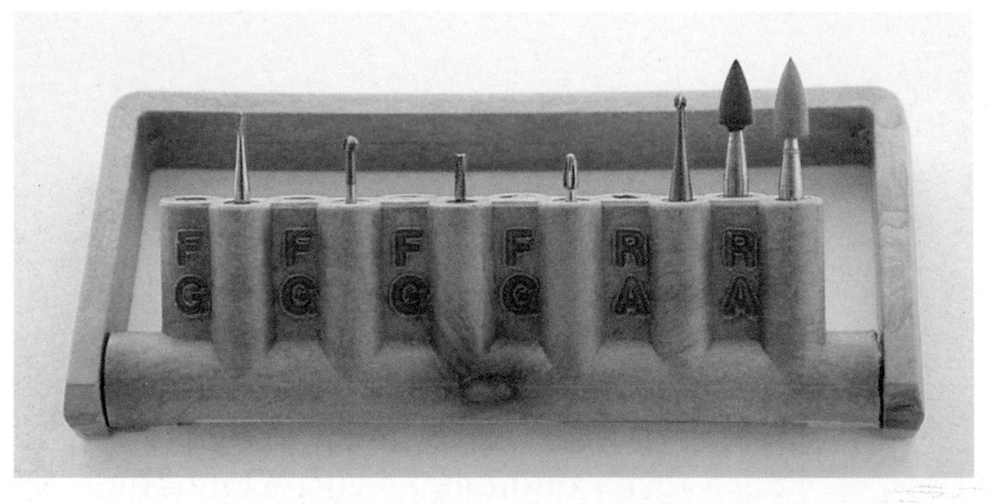
FG
FG
FG
FG
RA
RA

INSTRUMENT

Magnetic Bur Block with Burs

FUNCTION To be used on dental tray setups

CHARACTERISTICS Magnetic to hold burs in place
Holds friction grip and latch-type burs
Variety of shapes and sizes available
Various colors available to coordinate with color of tray

PRACTICE NOTE Magnetic Bur Blocks with Burs are used on most restorative tray setups.

S Magnetic Bur Block with Burs must be cleaned, bagged individually or bagged/wrapped in a tray setup, and then sterilized with a chemical indicator device included in the wrapping.

CHAPTER 7

Dental Dam Instruments

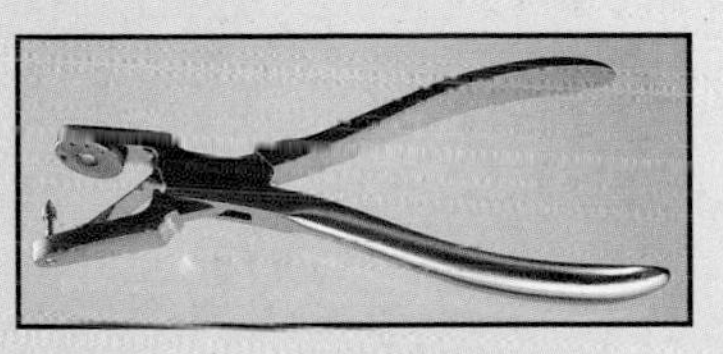

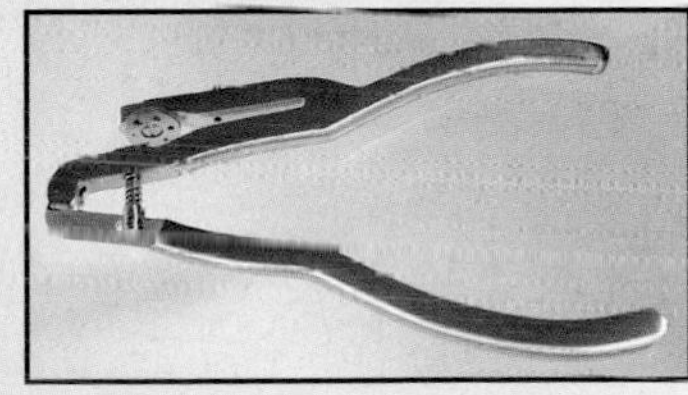

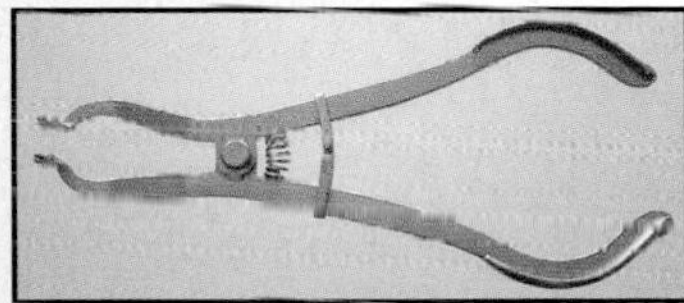

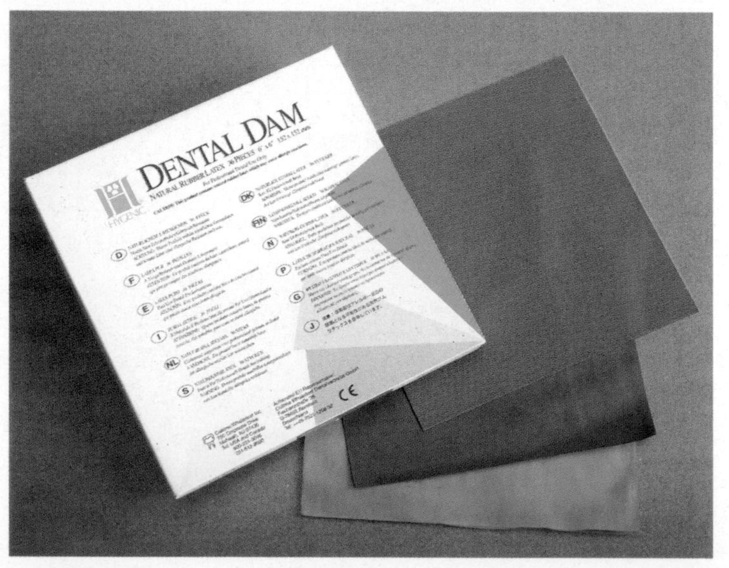
DENTAL DAM
HYGENIC

INSTRUMENT

Dental Dam

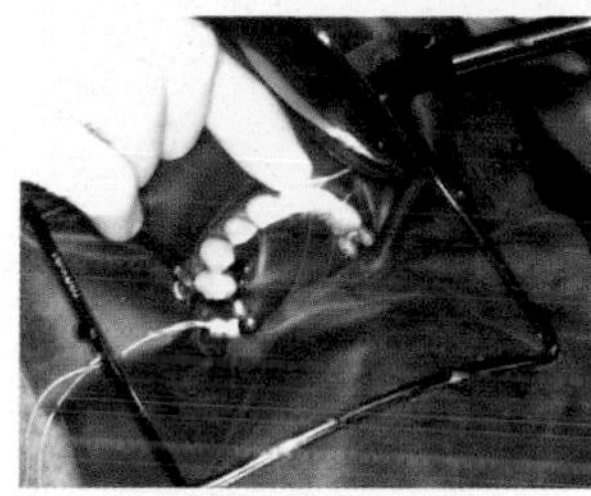

FUNCTION To isolate teeth for dental procedures

CHARACTERISTICS Sizes—4 × 4, 5 × 5, 6 × 6, or continuous roll
Gauge or thickness—Thin, medium, heavy
Colors—Gray, green, blue, pastels
Latex free—Purple

PRACTICE NOTE Latex-free dental dam (purple) is used for patients who have latex allergy.

S Dental Dam should be disposed of in garbage. Single use only.

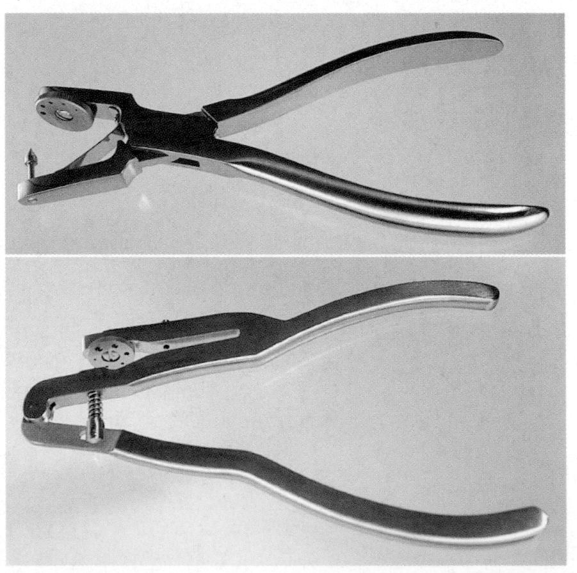

INSTRUMENT

Dental Dam Punch evolve

FUNCTION To punch holes in dental dam for each individual tooth

CHARACTERISTICS Designated hole size for each tooth for permanent dentition:

- No. 5—Anchor tooth (largest)
- No. 4—Molars
- No. 3—Premolars
- No. 2—Maxillary central and laterals. Maxillary and mandibular cuspids
- No. 1—Mandibular central and laterals (smallest)

PRACTICE NOTES The oral cavity is examined before holes are punched to accommodate the patient's specific dentition. A space of 3 to 3.5 mm is maintained between holes.

Ⓢ Dental Dam Punch must be cleaned, bagged individually or bagged/wrapped in a tray setup, and then sterilized. A chemical/steam indicator device should be included in the wrapping. Hinged instruments should be processed open and unlocked.

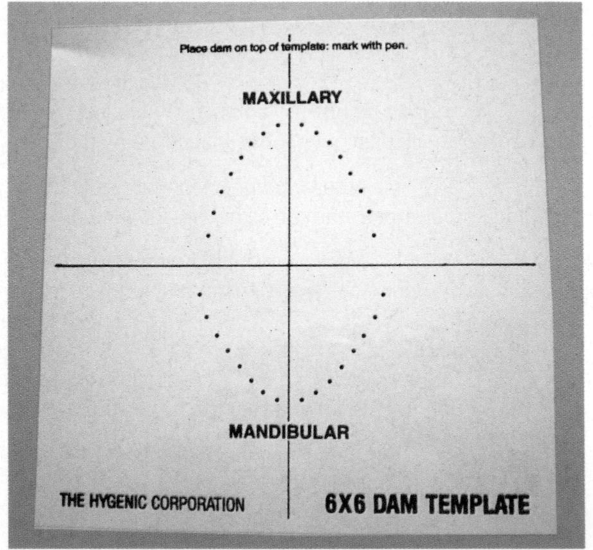
Place dam on top of template: mark with pen.
MAXILLARY
MANDIBULAR
THE HYGENIC CORPORATION
6X6 DAM TEMPLATE

INSTRUMENT

Dental Dam Template

FUNCTION To use as a guide for marking and punching holes in correct position on dental dam

CHARACTERISTICS Made of durable plastic

Has 32 dots that represent the adult dentition

PRACTICE NOTES The oral cavity is examined before holes are marked and punched to adjust positioning to the patient's specific dentition.

The dental dam is placed on the template, and the points where holes should be punched are marked with a pen.

S Dental Dam Template should be disinfected according to the manufacturer's recommendation.

142

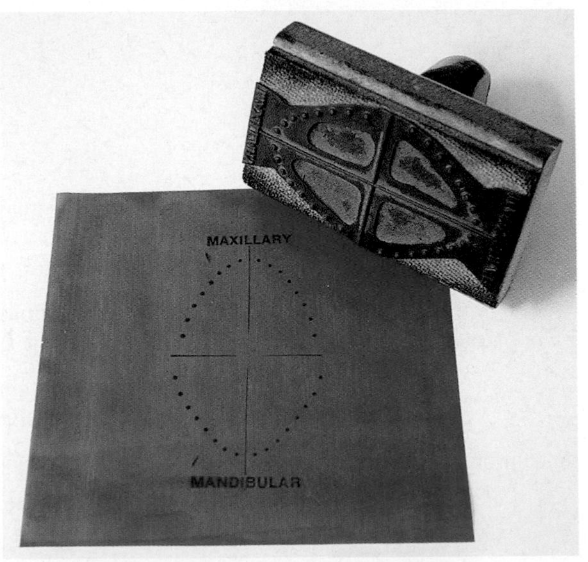

INSTRUMENT

Dental Dam Stamp

FUNCTION To mark holes on dental dam

CHARACTERISTICS Has 32 dots that represent the adult dentition
Used as guide for punching holes in correct position

PRACTICE NOTE The oral cavity is examined before holes are marked and punched to adjust positioning to the patient's specific dentition.

Ⓢ Dental Dam Stamp should be disinfected according to the manufacturer's recommendation.

144

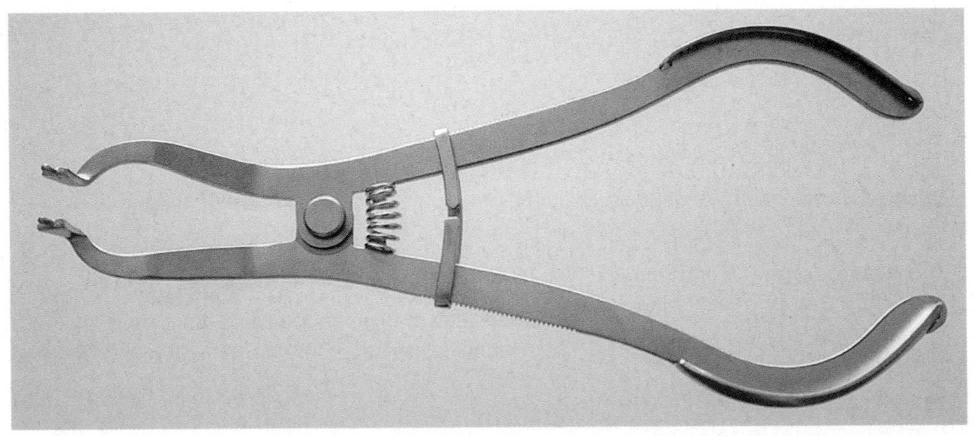

INSTRUMENT

Dental Dam Forceps

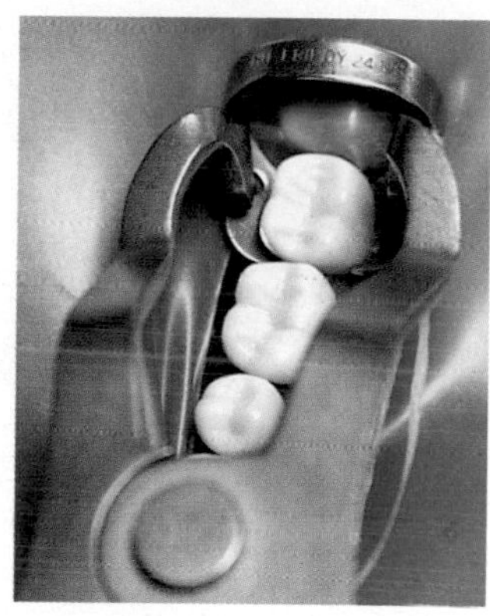

FUNCTION To place dental dam clamp on tooth and to remove clamp after procedure

CHARACTERISTICS Beaks on forceps fit into dental dam clamp
Forceps open with spring motion
Bar between handle holds forceps in place while clamp is seated

PRACTICE NOTE Squeeze handles on Dental Dam Forceps to open working end

S Dental Dam Forceps must be cleaned, bagged individually or bagged/wrapped in a tray setup, and then sterilized. A chemical/steam indicator device should be included in the wrapping. Hinged instruments should be processed open and unlocked.

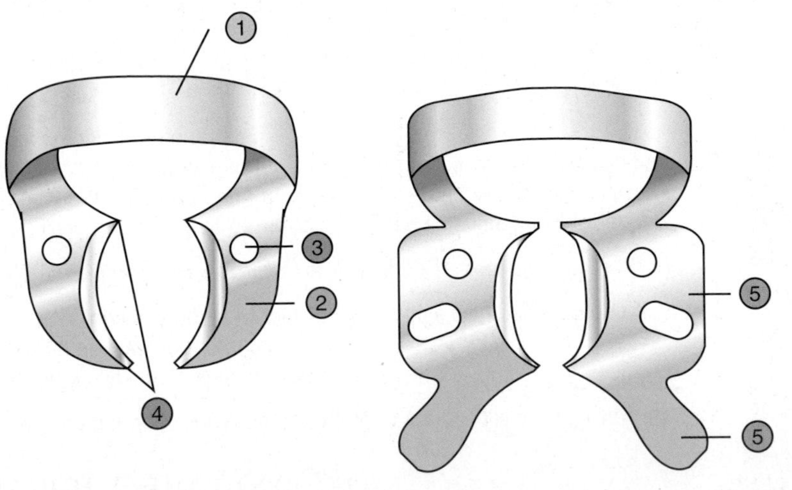
1
3
2
4
5
5

INSTRUMENT

Dental Dam Clamp

FUNCTION To anchor and stabilize dental dam

CHARACTERISTICS Parts:

1. Bow: Placed toward distal part of tooth
2. Jaws: Have four prongs that secure clamp on tooth
3. Holes: On jaws; designated for beaks on forceps to place clamp on tooth
4. Prongs: Designed to secure clamp on cervical part of tooth, beyond the height of contour
5. Winged clamps: Have extension of metal on jaws to hold dental dam away for better visibility (wingless clamps do not have extra extension of metal)

Ⓢ Dental Dam Clamp must be cleaned, bagged individually or bagged/wrapped in a tray setup, and then sterilized. A chemical/steam indicator device should be included in the wrapping.

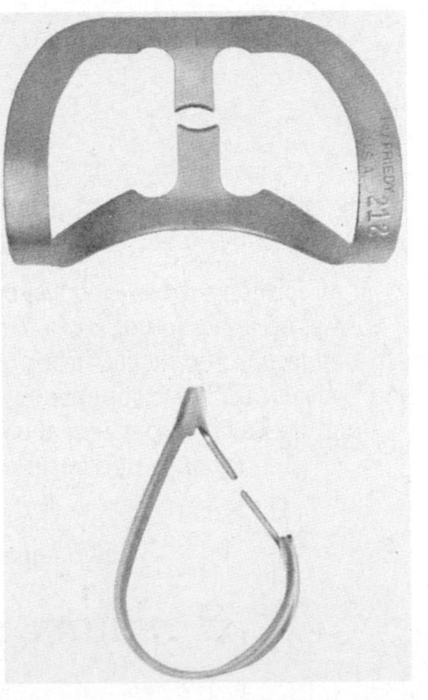

INSTRUMENT

Anterior Clamp evolve

FUNCTION To anchor and stabilize dental dam

CHARACTERISTICS Used only on anterior teeth

Example: Wingless clamp

Range of sizes available

PRACTICE NOTES Anterior Clamp is used on a dental dam setup for restorative and endodontic procedures.

Dental floss (ligature tie) must be attached to each dental clamp before each use for safety to allow for retrieval of clamp if dislodged and patient inhales or swallows.

S Anterior Clamp must be cleaned, bagged individually or bagged/wrapped in a tray setup, and then sterilized.

A chemical/steam indicator device should be included in the wrapping.

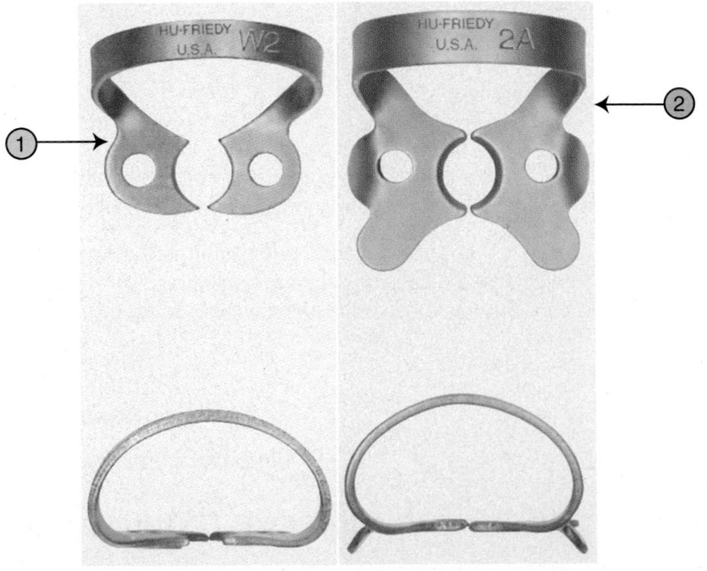
HU-FRIEDY
U.S.A.
W2
HU-FRIEDY
U.S.A.
2A
1
2

INSTRUMENT

Premolar Clamp

FUNCTION To anchor and stabilize dental dam

CHARACTERISTICS Clamp used is determined by tooth size
Range of sizes available
Variety of styles

Examples:
① Wingless clamp
② Winged clamp

PRACTICE NOTES Premolar Clamp is used on a dental dam setup for restorative and endodontic procedures.
Dental floss (ligature tie) must be attached to each dental clamp before each use to allow for retrieval of clamp if dislodged and patient inhales or swallows.

Ⓢ Premolar Clamp must be cleaned, bagged individually or bagged/wrapped in a tray setup, and then sterilized. A chemical/steam indicator device should be included in the wrapping.

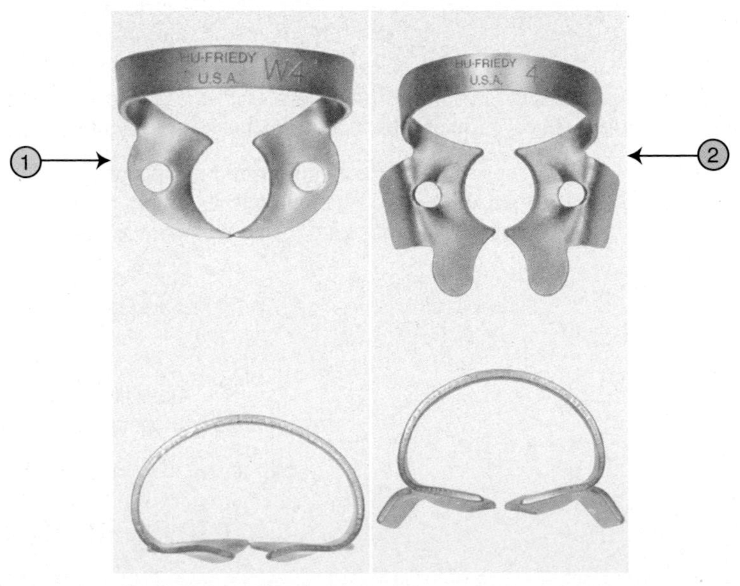
1
2
HU-FRIEDY
U.S.A.
W4
HU-FRIEDY
U.S.A.
4

INSTRUMENT

Universal Clamp—Maxillary

FUNCTION To anchor and stabilize dental dam

CHARACTERISTICS Used on right or left posterior molars
Range of sizes available
Variety of styles
Examples:
① Wingless clamp
② Winged clamp

PRACTICE NOTES Maxillary Clamp is used on a dental dam setup for restorative and endodontic procedures.
Dental floss (ligature tie) must be attached to each dental clamp before each use to allow for retrieval of clamp if dislodged and patient inhales or swallows.

Ⓢ Universal Maxillary Clamp must be cleaned, bagged individually or bagged/wrapped in a tray setup, and then sterilized. A chemical/steam indicator device should be included in the wrapping.

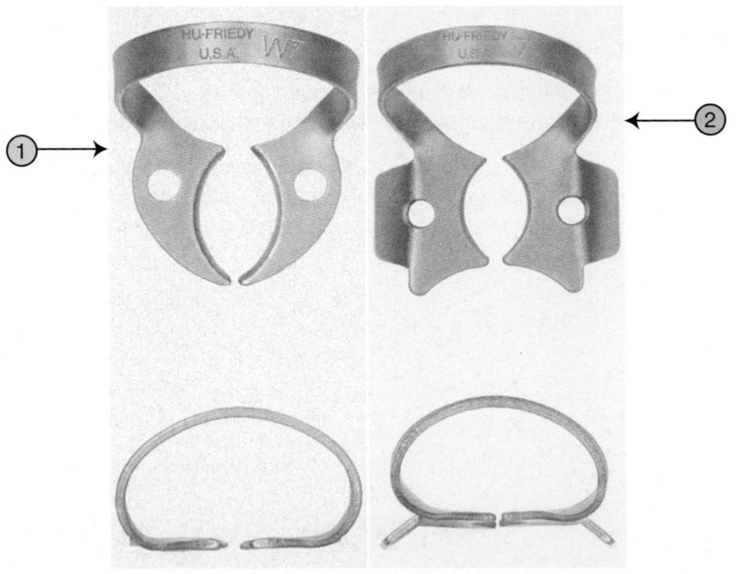
1
2
HU-FRIEDY
U.S.A.
W7
HU-FRIEDY
U.S.A.

INSTRUMENT

Universal Clamp—Mandibular

FUNCTION To anchor and stabilize dental dam

CHARACTERISTICS Used on right or left posterior molars
Range of sizes available
Variety of styles

Examples:

① Wingless clamp
② Winged clamp

PRACTICE NOTES Mandibular Clamp is used on a dental dam setup for restorative and endodontic procedures.
Dental floss (ligature tie) must be attached to each dental clamp before each use to allow for retrieval of clamp if dislodged and patient inhales or swallows.

Ⓢ Universal Mandibular Clamp must be cleaned, bagged individually or bagged/wrapped in a tray setup, and then sterilized. A chemical/steam indicator device should be included in the wrapping.

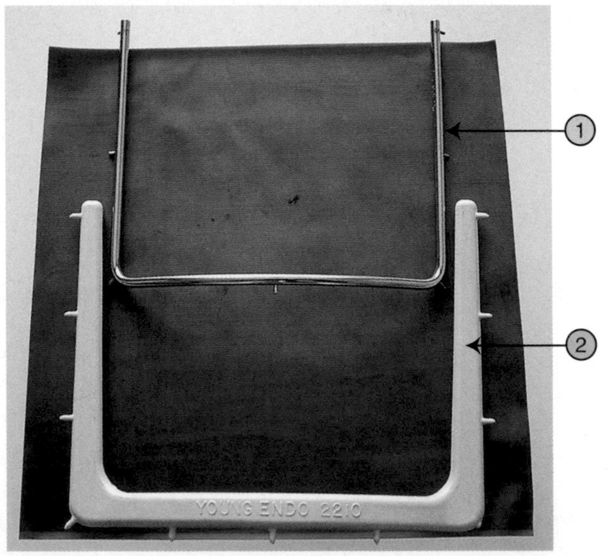
1
2
YOUNG ENDO 2210

INSTRUMENT

Dental Dam Frame

FUNCTION To hold dental dam away from teeth

CHARACTERISTICS ① Metal Frame
② Plastic Frame
Plastic frame—May be left on during radiographic exposures
Various styles of frames available

PRACTICE NOTE Dental Dam Frame is used on a dental dam setup for restorative and endodontic procedures.

Ⓢ Dental Dam Frame must be cleaned, bagged individually or bagged/wrapped in a tray setup, and then sterilized. A chemical/steam indicator device should be included in the wrapping.

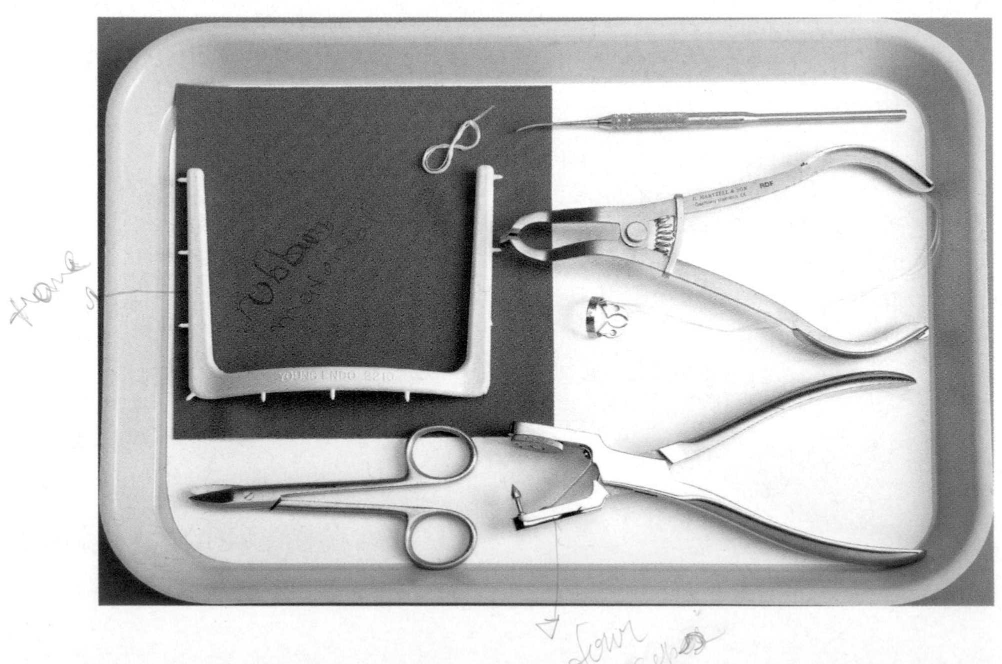
YOUNG ENDO 2210
RDF

TRAY SETUP

Dental Dam

LEFT (TOP TO BOTTOM)
Dental dam (latex free), dental floss, plastic dental dam frame, crown and bridge scissors (see Chapter 10)

RIGHT (TOP TO BOTTOM)
Beavertail burnisher used to invert dental dam (see Chapter 8), dental dam forceps, dental dam clamp with stabilizing ligature tie (dental floss), dental dam punch

S Refer to each picture for correct procedure for instrument sterilization or disposal of instrument or material.

CHAPTER 8

Amalgam Restorative Instruments

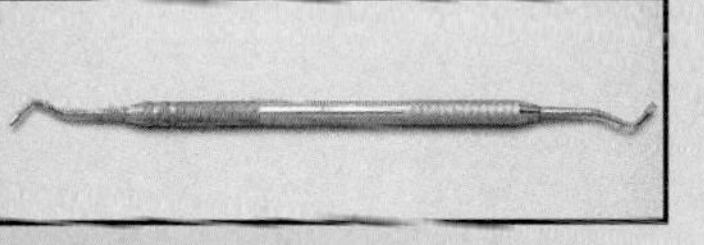

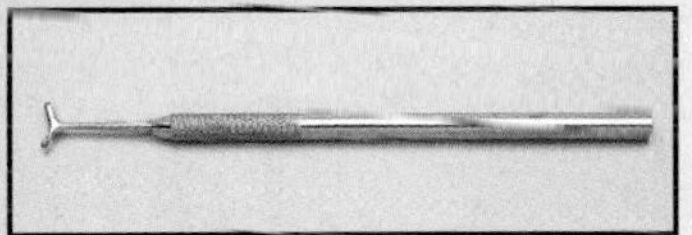

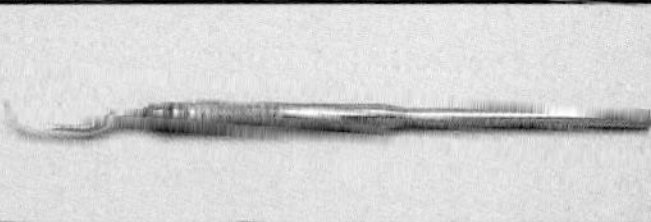

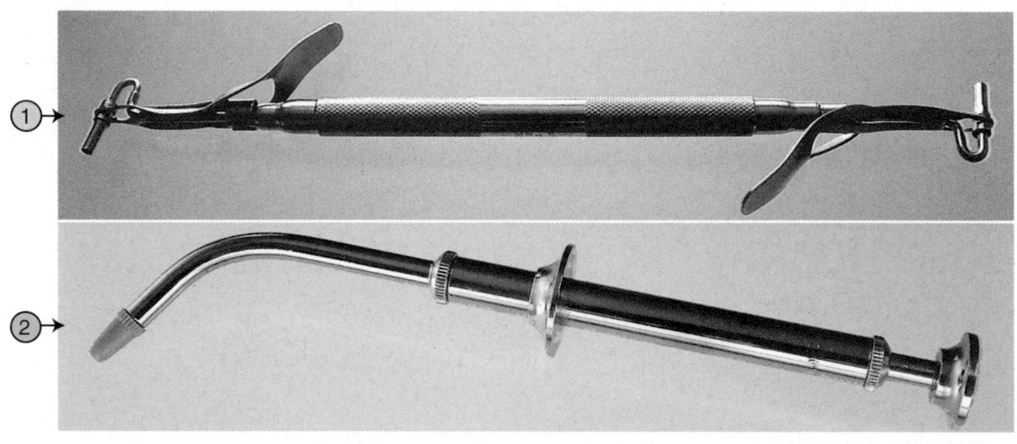
1
2

INSTRUMENT

Amalgam Carrier

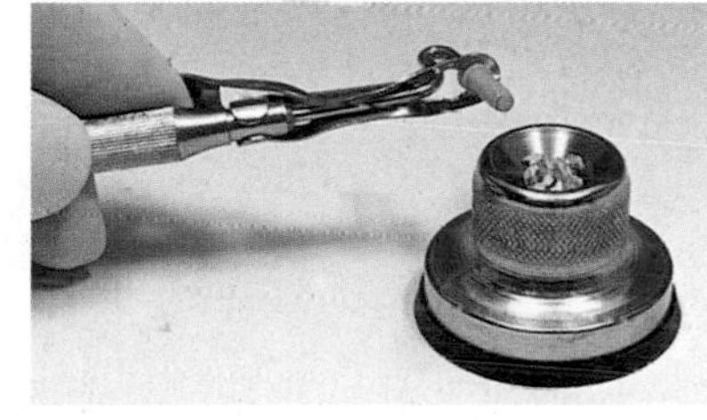

FUNCTION To carry and dispense amalgam for cavity preparation

CHARACTERISTICS Single or double ended:

① Double ended—One small end, one large end

② Single ended—Plunger style

The inside of the hollow tubes is coated with metal or Teflon.

PRACTICE NOTES Amalgam is placed in hollow tubes and then transferred to the cavity preparation.

Amalgam sticks in the carrier if it is not released immediately after the tubes are filled.

Amalgam Carrier is used exclusively on amalgam tray setups.

Ⓢ Amalgam Carrier must be cleaned, bagged individually or bagged/wrapped in a tray setup, and then sterilized. A chemical/steam indicator device should be included in the wrapping.

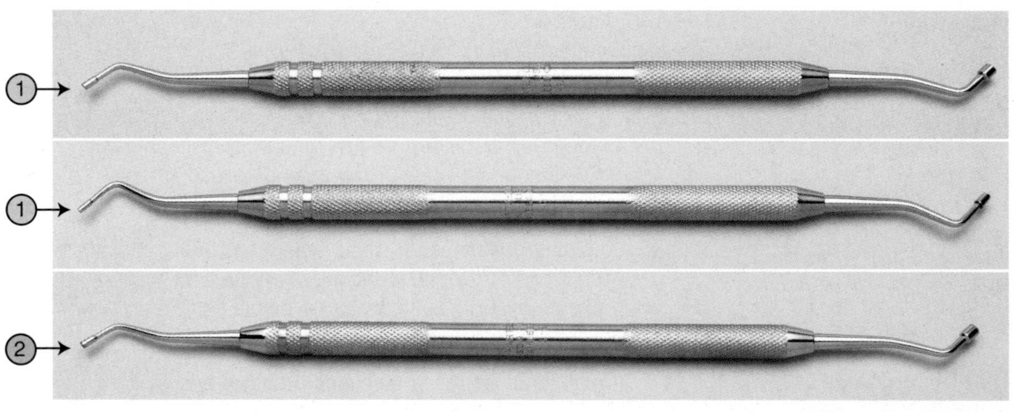
1
1
2

INSTRUMENT

Condenser (Plugger)—Smooth and Serrated 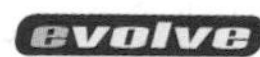

FUNCTIONS

To pack and condense amalgam into cavity preparation
To pack and condense other restorative materials
To pack and condense temporary filling material

CHARACTERISTICS

① Smooth ends (large and small pictured)
② Serrated ends
Round, flat, or diamond shaped
Single or double ended

- Double ended—One small end, one large end

Back action condenser available with right-angle working ends—Accommodates difficult areas
Range of sizes available

PRACTICE NOTE

Smooth and Serrated Condensers are used on amalgam, composite, and temporary filling tray setups.

Ⓢ Smooth and Serrated Condensers must be cleaned, bagged individually or bagged/wrapped in a tray setup, and then sterilized. A chemical/steam indicator device should be included in the wrapping.

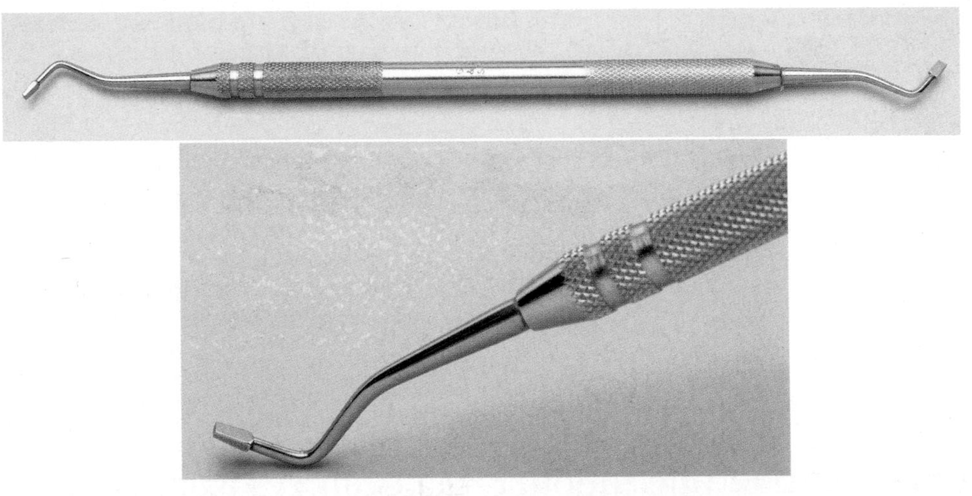

INSTRUMENT

Interproximal Condenser

FUNCTIONS To pack and condense amalgam into interproximal areas of cavity preparation
To pack and condense other restorative materials

CHARACTERISTICS Ends shaped to fit mesial or distal areas of cavity preparation
Smooth or serrated ends
Range of sizes available

PRACTICE NOTE Interproximal Condenser is used on amalgam, composite, and temporary filling tray setups.

S Interproximal Condenser must be cleaned, bagged individually or bagged/wrapped in a tray setup, and then sterilized. A chemical/steam indicator device should be included in the wrapping.

168

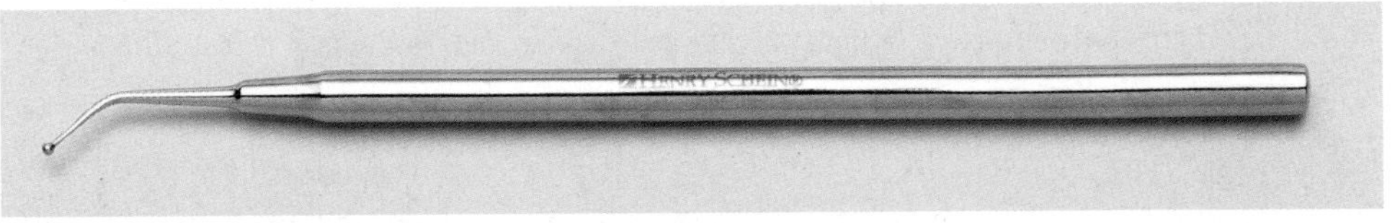

INSTRUMENT

Liner Applicator evolve

FUNCTION To place calcium hydroxide or glass ionomer in cavity preparation

CHARACTERISTICS Short or long handle
Single or double ended

PRACTICE NOTES Liner Applicator is used on amalgam, composite, crown and bridge, and temporary filling tray setups.
Also referred to as a Dycal instrument

Ⓢ Liner Applicator must be cleaned, bagged individually or bagged/wrapped in a tray setup, and then sterilized. A chemical/steam indicator device should be included in the wrapping.

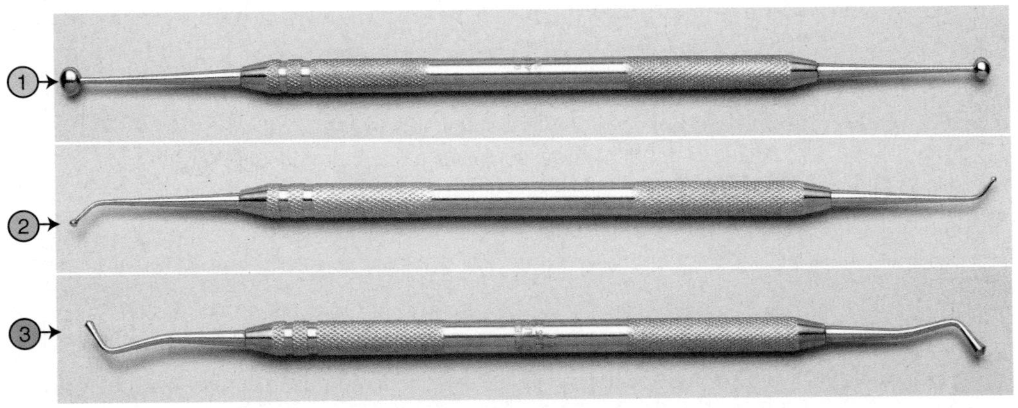
1
2
3

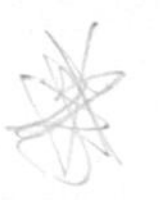

INSTRUMENT

Burnishers—Football, Ball, and Acorn evolve

FUNCTIONS

To smooth amalgam after condensing
To contour matrix band before placement
To perform initial carving of amalgam
To burnish other restorative material
To burnish temporary filling material

CHARACTERISTICS

① Football Burnisher
② Ball Burnisher
③ Acorn Burnisher
Single or double ended

PRACTICE NOTES

Football, Ball, and Acorn Burnishers are used on amalgam, composite, and temporary filling tray setups.

S Football, Ball, and Acorn Burnishers must be cleaned, bagged individually or bagged/wrapped in a tray setup, and then sterilized. A chemical/steam indicator device should be included in the wrapping.

172

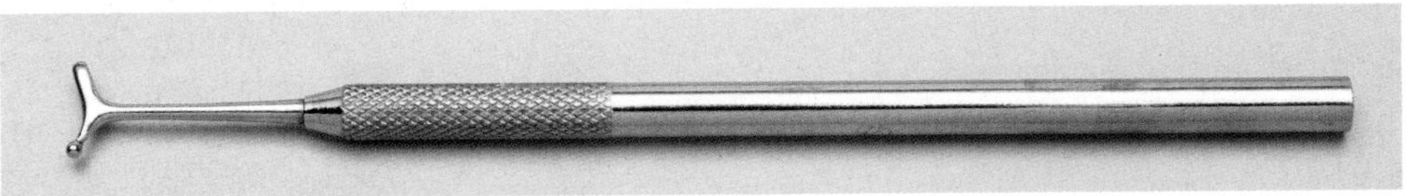

INSTRUMENT

T-Ball Burnisher

FUNCTIONS

To smooth amalgam after condensing
To contour matrix band before placement
To begin carving of amalgam
To burnish other restorative materials
To burnish temporary filling material

CHARACTERISTIC

Single ended

PRACTICE NOTE

T-Ball Burnisher is used on amalgam, composite, and temporary filling tray setups.

Ⓢ T-Ball Burnisher must be cleaned, bagged individually or bagged/wrapped in a tray setup, and then sterilized. A chemical/steam indicator device should be included in the wrapping.

174

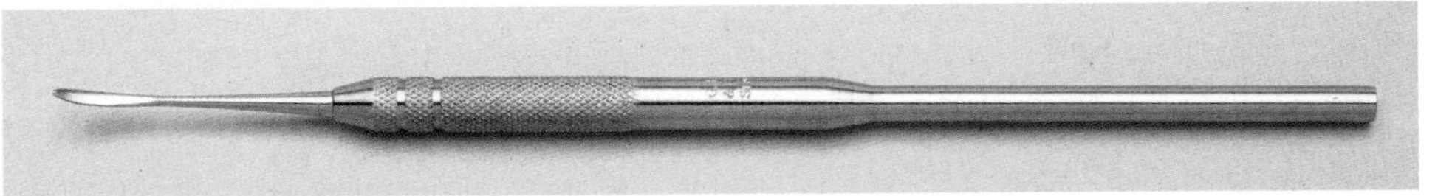

Beavertail Burnisher

INSTRUMENT

FUNCTIONS

To smooth amalgam after condensing
To perform initial carving of amalgam
To invert dental dam (refer to dental dam tray setup in Chapter 7)
To burnish other restorative materials
To burnish temporary filling material

CHARACTERISTIC

Single or double ended

PRACTICE NOTE

Beavertail Burnisher is used on amalgam, temporary filling, and dental dam tray setups.

Beavertail Burnisher must be cleaned, bagged individually or bagged/wrapped in a tray setup, and then sterilized. A chemical/steam indicator device should be included in the wrapping.

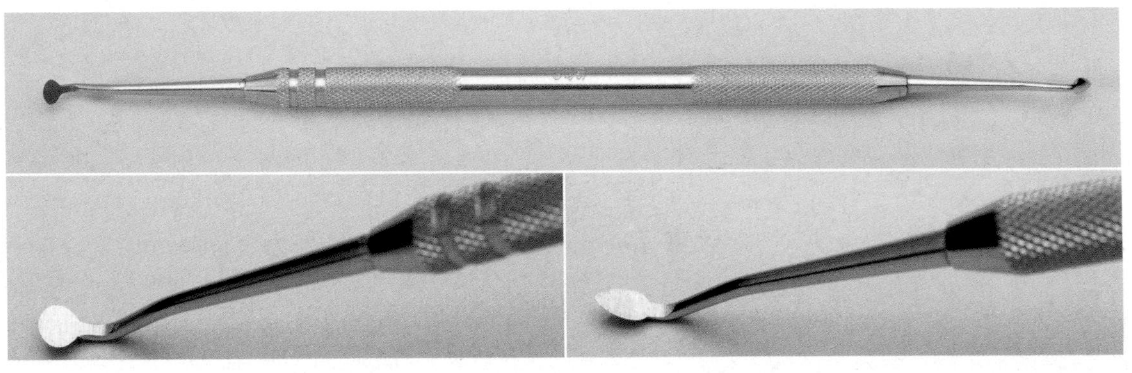

INSTRUMENT

Tanner Carver

FUNCTIONS

To carve occlusal anatomy into amalgam restorations
To carve occlusal anatomy in other restorative and temporary filling materials

CHARACTERISTICS

Double ended—Two ends shaped differently
Ends shaped differently from those of discoid-cleoid carver

PRACTICE NOTE

Tanner Carver is used on amalgam and temporary filling tray setups.

Ⓢ Tanner Carver must be cleaned, bagged individually or bagged/wrapped in a tray setup, and then sterilized. A chemical/steam indicator device should be included in the wrapping.

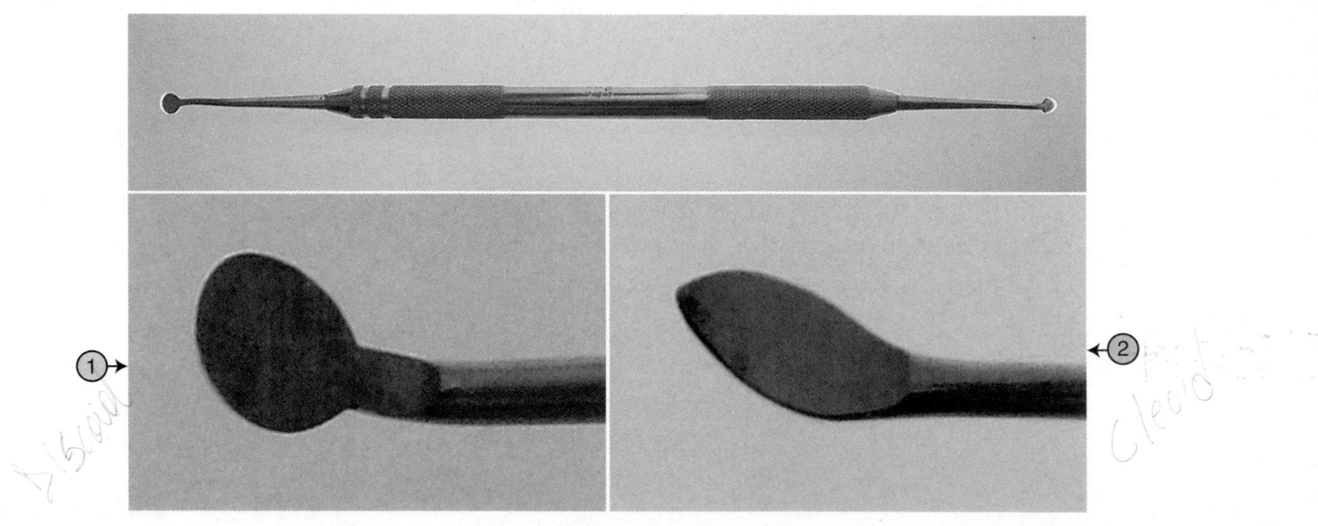
1
2

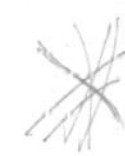

INSTRUMENT

Discoid-Cleoid Carver

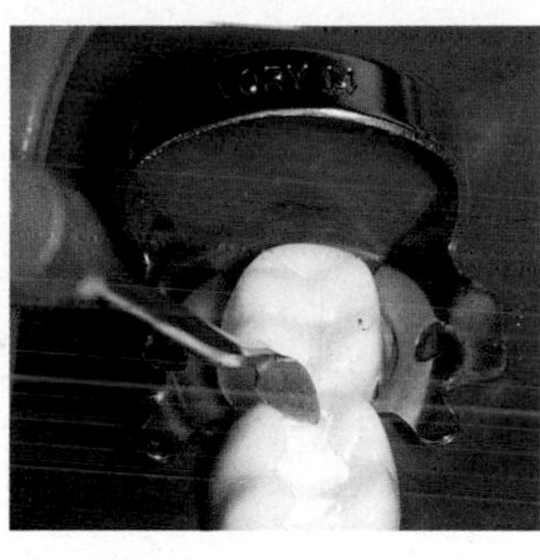

FUNCTIONS To carve occlusal anatomy into amalgam restorations
To carve occlusal anatomy in other restorative and temporary filling materials

CHARACTERISTICS Double ended—Two ends shaped differently:
① Discoid end—Disc shaped
② Cleoid end—Pointed
Ends shaped differently from those of Tanner carver

PRACTICE NOTE Discoid-Cleoid Carver is used on amalgam and temporary filling tray setups.

Ⓢ Discoid-Cleoid Carver must be cleaned, bagged individually or bagged/wrapped in a tray setup, and then sterilized. A chemical/steam indicator device should be included in the wrapping

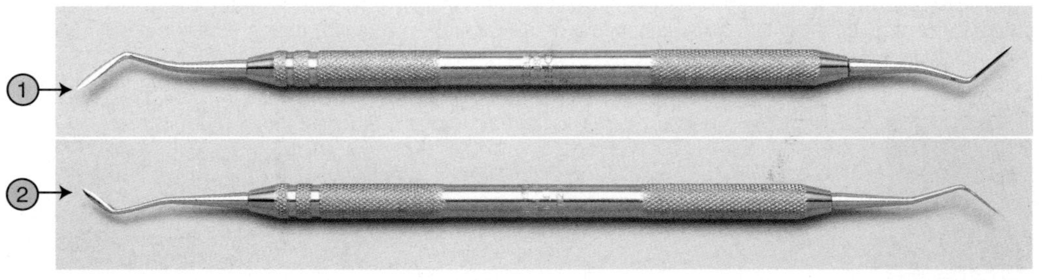
1
2

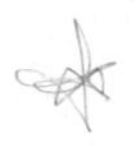

INSTRUMENT

Hollenback and Half-Hollenback Carvers

FUNCTIONS

To contour and carve occlusal and interproximal anatomy in amalgam restorations
To contour and carve occlusal and interproximal anatomy in other restorative and temporary filling materials

CHARACTERISTICS

① Hollenback
② Half-Hollenback—Half the size of Hollenback carver
Double ended—Working ends protrude at different angles

PRACTICE NOTE

Hollenback and Half-Hollenback Carvers are used on amalgam, composite, and temporary filling tray setups.

Ⓢ Hollenback and Half-Hollenback Carvers must be cleaned, bagged individually or bagged/wrapped in a tray setup, and then sterilized. A chemical/steam indicator device should be included in the wrapping.

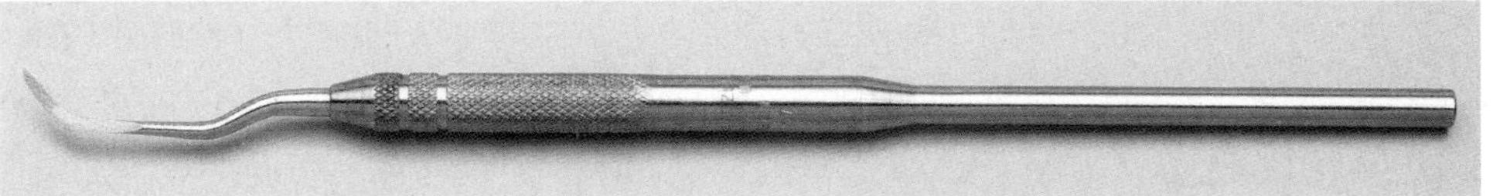

INSTRUMENT

Gold Carving Knife

FUNCTIONS

To trim interproximal amalgam restoration, recreating contour of proximal wall(s)
To trim interproximal restorations with other restorative materials, recreating contour of proximal wall(s)
To remove flash composite material from interproximal areas

CHARACTERISTICS

Single or double ended
Variety of designs

PRACTICE NOTE

Gold Carving Knife is used on amalgam and composite restorative tray setups.

Ⓢ Gold Carving Knife must be cleaned, bagged individually or bagged/wrapped in a tray setup, and then sterilized. A chemical/steam indicator device should be included in the wrapping.

184

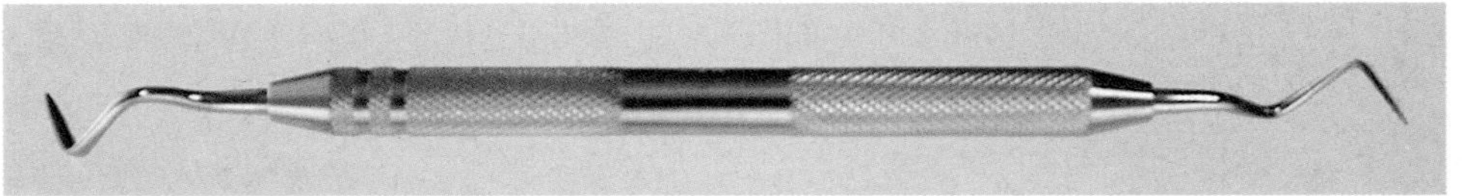

INSTRUMENT

Interproximal Carving Knife

FUNCTIONS

To trim interproximal amalgam restoration, recreating contour of proximal wall
To trim interproximal restorations with other restorative materials, recreating contour of proximal wall(s)
To remove flash composite material from interproximal areas

CHARACTERISTICS

Single or double ended
Variety of designs

PRACTICE NOTE

Interproximal Carving Knife is used on amalgam and composite restorative tray setups.

Ⓢ Interproximal Carving Knife must be cleaned, bagged individually or bagged/wrapped in a tray setup, and then sterilized. A chemical/steam indicator device should be included in the wrapping.

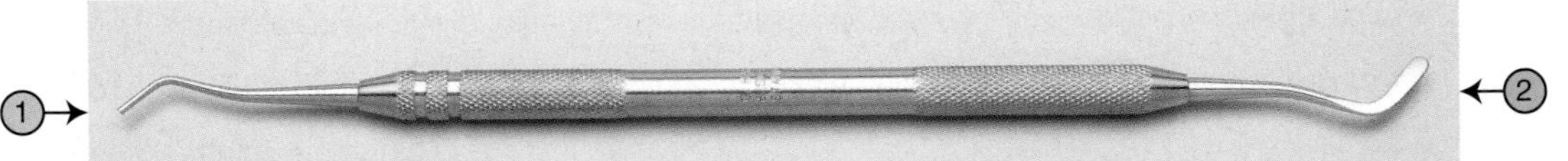
1
2

INSTRUMENT

Woodson

FUNCTION

To carry and place temporary restorative material for cavity preparation—Paddle end
To condense restorative material—Plugger end

CHARACTERISTICS

Double ended
Range of sizes available
- ① Plugger end available in variety of sizes
- ② Paddle end available in different angles, sizes

PRACTICE NOTE

Woodson is used on amalgam, composite, crown and bridge, temporary filling, and provisional crown tray setups.

Ⓢ Woodson must be cleaned, bagged individually or bagged/wrapped in a tray setup, and then sterilized. A chemical/steam indicator device should be included in the wrapping.

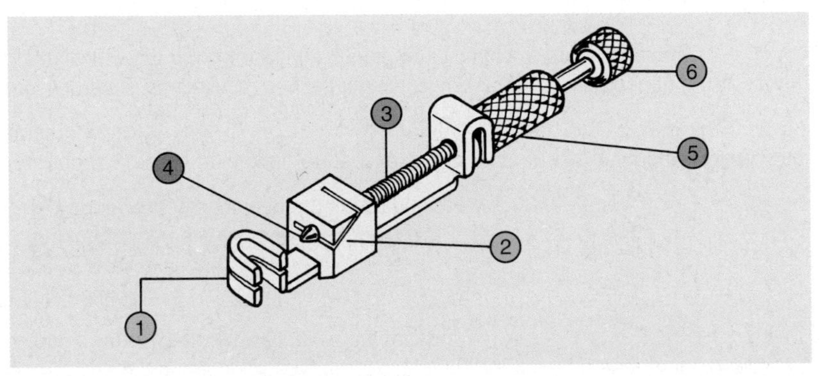
6
3
5
4
2
1

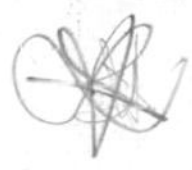

INSTRUMENT Tofflemire/Matrix Band Retainer evolve

FUNCTION To maintain stability of matrix band during condensation of restorative material for class II preparation

CHARACTERISTICS Parts:

① Guide slots: Straight slot; right and left slots for right or left quadrant
② Diagonal slot: Slides up and down on spindle; matrix band is placed in slot and spindle secures band in place; open slots are placed toward gingiva
③ Spindle: Holds matrix band in retainer
④ Spindle pin: Stabilizes band in holder
⑤ Inner knob: Adjusts size or loop of matrix band to fit around tooth and loosens band for removal
⑥ Outer knob: Positioned at end of spindle that tightens or loosens matrix band in retainer

PRACTICE NOTE Tofflemire is used on restorative tray setups.

Ⓢ Tofflemire must be cleaned, bagged individually or bagged/wrapped in a tray setup, and then sterilized. A chemical/steam indicator device should be included in the wrapping.

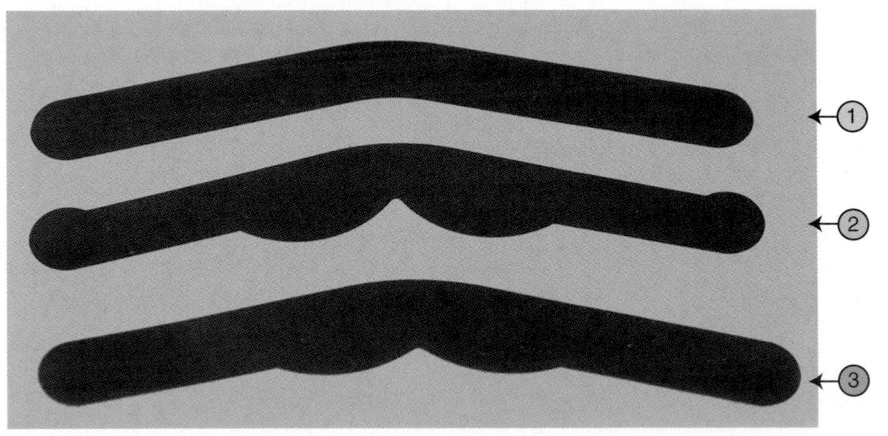
1
2
3

INSTRUMENT

Matrix Bands evolve

FUNCTION To replace missing proximal wall or walls of cavity preparation for condensation of restorative material for class II preparations

CHARACTERISTICS Variety of sizes, shapes, and thicknesses

Bands designed for specific teeth:

① Universal band—For all posterior teeth except larger teeth

② Premolar band—For premolars

③ Molar band—For larger molars

Variety of pediatric bands available for primary teeth

PRACTICE NOTE Matrix Bands are used on amalgam, composite, build-up, and temporary filling tray setups.

Ⓢ Matrix Bands should be disposed of in a Sharps container, or local and state regulations should be followed. Single use only.

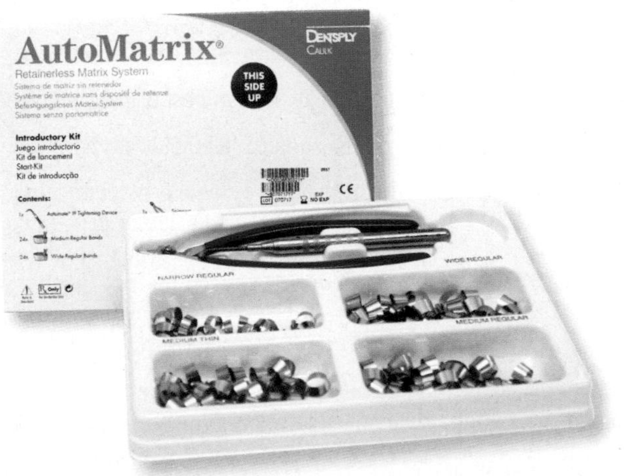
AutoMatrix®
Retainerless Matrix System
Sistema de matriz sin retenedor
Système de matrice sans dispositif de retenue
Befestigungsloses Matrix-System
Sistema senza portamatrice
Introductory Kit
Juego introductorio
Kit de lancement
Start-Kit
Kit de introducção
Contents:
DENTSPLY
CAULK
THIS SIDE UP
NARROW REGULAR
WIDE REGULAR
MEDIUM THIN
MEDIUM REGULAR

INSTRUMENT

Matrix Band System

FUNCTION

To replace missing proximal wall or walls of cavity preparation for condensation of restorative material for class II preparations.

CHARACTERISTICS

Variety of matrix band systems (pictured: AutoMatrix)
Variety of sizes and shapes
Bands designed for specific teeth:

- Universal—Posterior teeth
- Molar—Larger molars
- Premolar
- Pediatric—Primary teeth

PRACTICE NOTES

Tightening wrench is used to place, tighten, and loosen bands.
Removing Pliers are used to remove bands.
Matrix Bands are used on amalgam, composite, build-up, and temporary filling tray setups.

S Matrix Bands should be disposed of in the garbage or local and state regulations should be followed. Single use only. Tightening Wrench and Removing Pliers must be cleaned, bagged individually or bagged/wrapped in a tray setup, and then sterilized. A chemical/steam indicator device should be included in the wrapping.

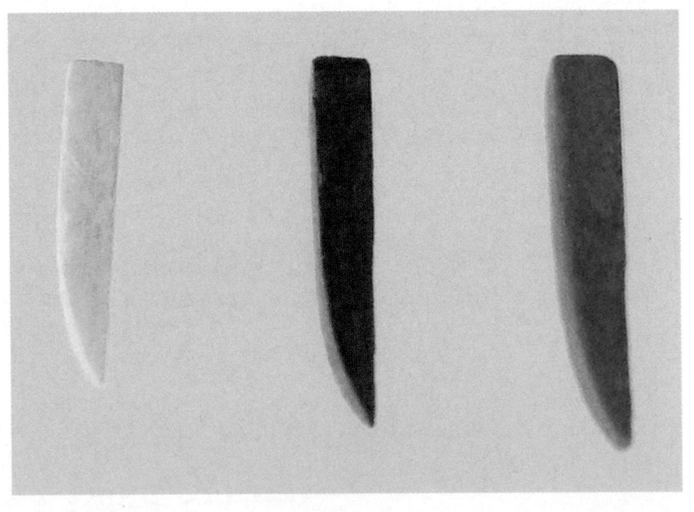

INSTRUMENT

Wooden Wedges

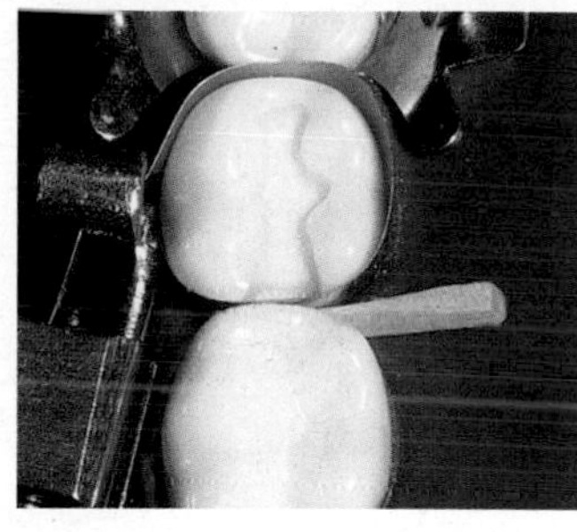

FUNCTION To hold matrix band in place along gingival margin of class II, class III, or class IV preparation

CHARACTERISTICS Wood or plastic
Triangular, round, or anatomical shapes (shown in picture)
Variety of sizes and shapes available to accommodate embrasure area

PRACTICE NOTES Wedges are placed in gingival embrasure area usually on the lingual.
Wedges are always set up with all types of matrix band systems for Class II, Class III, and/or Class IV restorations.

Wooden Wedges should be disposed of in the garbage. Single use only.

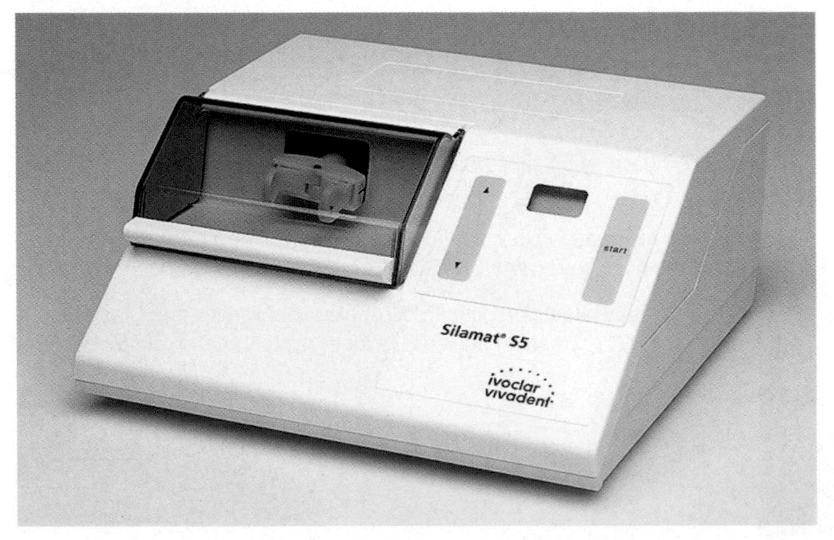
start
Silamat® S5
ivoclar
vivadent

INSTRUMENT

Amalgamator

FUNCTIONS

To mix alloy and mercury into amalgam in a capsule
To mix other types of restorative materials in a capsule
To mix precapsulated permanent and temporary cements

CHARACTERISTICS

Preloaded amalgam capsules contain alloy, mercury, and pestle to aid mixing.

- Various types of capsules are available; they are activated manually by twisting or pushing or using a capsule activator.

Thin membrane separates materials until mixing occurs.

PRACTICE NOTES

The process of mixing is called amalgamation or trituration.
The mixing time recommended by the manufacturer should be used.

Capsules must be disposed of in the garbage or state regulations must be followed. Single use only. Excess amalgam must be disposed of as amalgam waste material. Refer to local and state regulations for disposal. Amalgamator should be handled with overgloves or disinfected according to the manufacturer's recommendation.

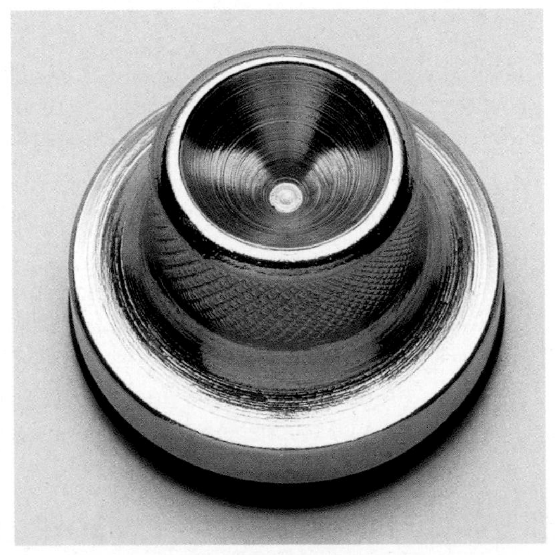

INSTRUMENT

Amalgam Well

FUNCTIONS To hold amalgam before it is placed in preparation
To hold amalgam while loading amalgam carrier

CHARACTERISTIC Metal (shown in picture), plastic, or glass

PRACTICE NOTE Amalgam Well is used on the amalgam tray setup.

S Amalgam Well must be cleaned, bagged individually or bagged/wrapped in a tray setup, and then sterilized. A chemical/steam indicator device should be included in the wrapping. Excess amalgam must be disposed of as amalgam waste material. Refer to local and state regulations for disposal.

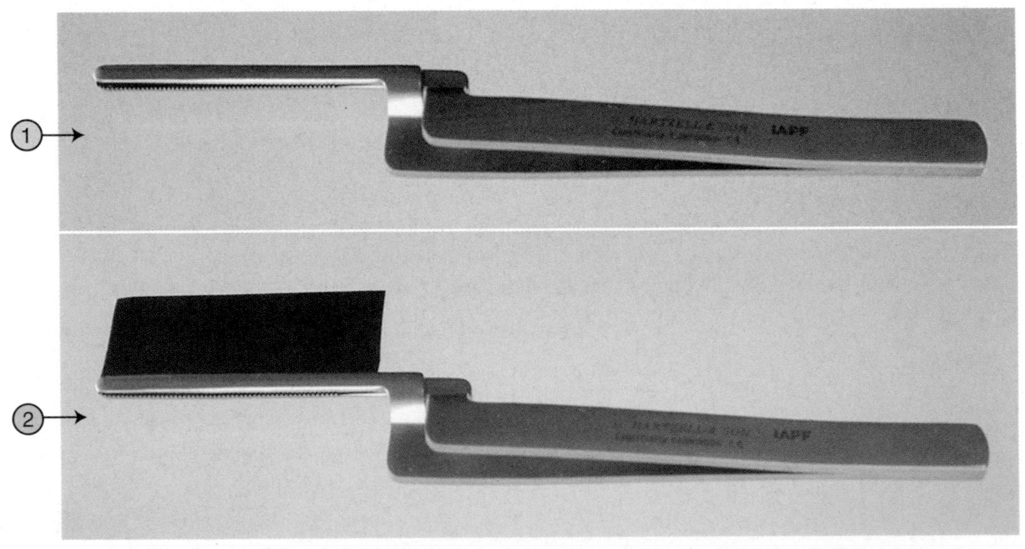
1
2

INSTRUMENT

Articulating Paper Holder evolve

FUNCTIONS

To hold articulating paper in place
To check centric and lateral occlusion

CHARACTERISTICS

① Articulating Paper Holder
② Articulating Paper Holder with blue articulating paper
Articulating paper—blue or red
Paper variety—from thin to thick
Disposable articulating paper holder available (see sealant tray setup in Chapter 13)

PRACTICE NOTE

Articulating Paper Holder and Articulating Paper are used on all restorative tray setups, including, but not limited to, amalgam, composite, fixed and removable prosthodontics, provisional crown, endodontics, orthodontic retainer delivery, and temporary filling tray setups.

Ⓢ Articulating Paper Holder (metal type) must be cleaned, bagged individually or bagged/wrapped in a tray setup, and then sterilized. A chemical/steam indicator device should be included in the wrapping. Articulating Paper Holder that is disposable should be disposed of in the garbage. Single use only. Articulating Paper should be disposed of in the garbage. Single use only.

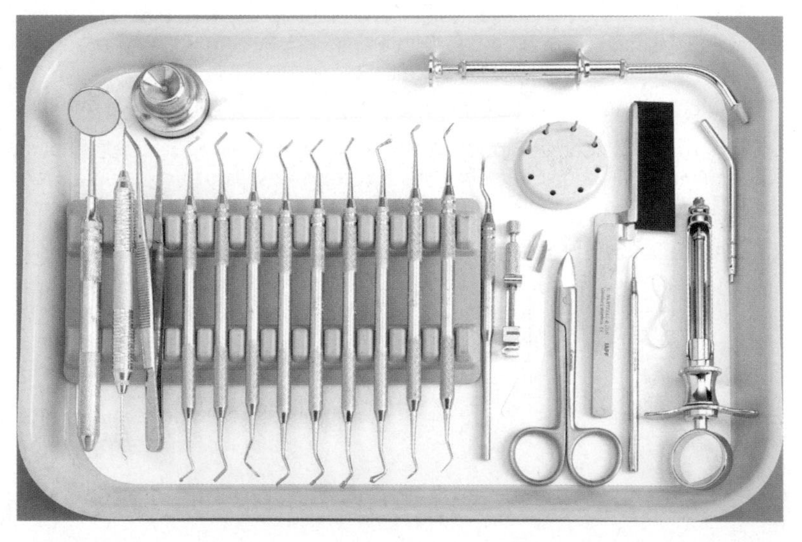

TRAY SETUP

Amalgam

TOP ROW (FROM LEFT TO RIGHT)

Amalgam well, high-volume evacuation (HVE) tip, burs in bur block, amalgam carrier-plunger style (very top of tray)

BOTTOM ROW (FROM LEFT TO RIGHT)

Mouth mirror, explorer, cotton forceps (pliers), spoon excavator, enamel hatchet, mesial gingival margin trimmer, distal gingival margin trimmer, small condenser, large condenser, acorn burnisher, Tanner carver, Half-Hollenback carver, gold carving knife, Tofflemire, wooden wedges, crown and bridge scissors, articulating paper holder and articulating paper, liner applicator, dental floss, anesthetic aspirating syringe, air/water syringe tip

S Refer to each individual picture for correct procedure for instrument sterilization or disposal of instrument and/or material.

Refer to other chapters for additional instruments on this tray setup that are not included in this chapter.

CHAPTER 9

Composite Restorative Instruments

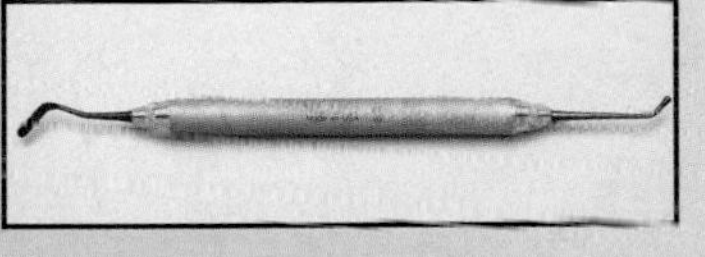

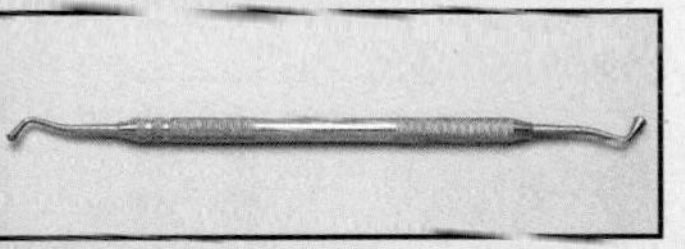

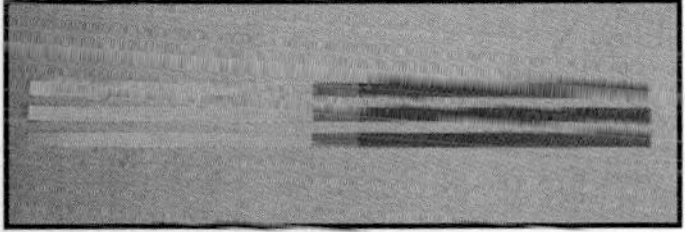

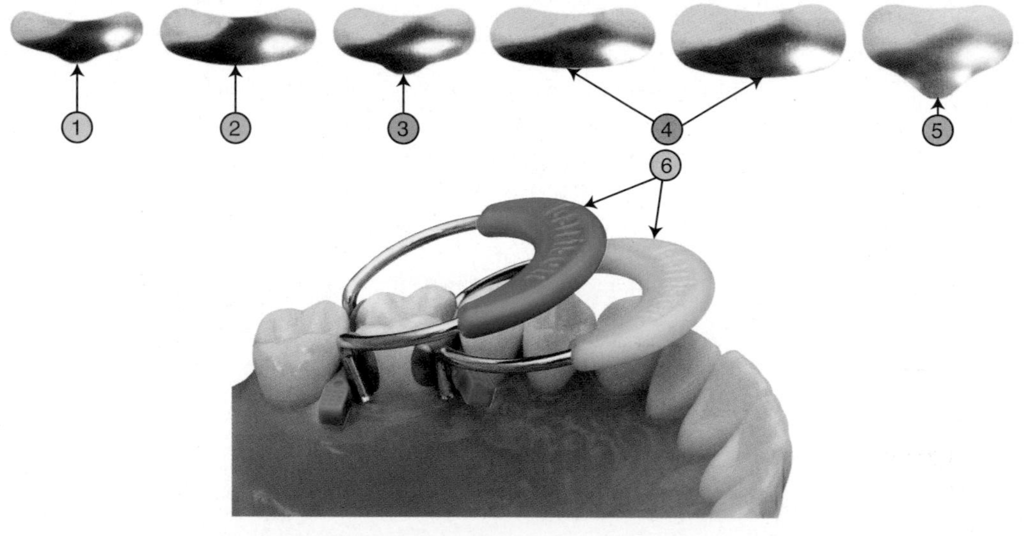

1
2
3
4
5
6

INSTRUMENT

Sectional Matrix System

FUNCTION To replace missing proximal wall of cavity preparation for placement of composite material or other restorative materials for class II restorations

CHARACTERISTICS Variety of sizes and shapes to accommodate restoration:

① Pediatric band—Primary molar
② Small band—Premolar, small molar
③ Extended small band—Premolar, molar, with deep cervical restoration
④ Standard band—Molar restoration
⑤ Large band—Deep cervical restoration
⑥ Tension rings—Different sizes to accommodate restoration

Placed on tooth with forceps (see Chapter 7, page 145)

PRACTICE NOTES Sectional Bands are used on amalgam, composite, build-up, and temporary filling tray setups.
Classes III and IV composite restorations use a Clear Mylar Matrix strip—refer to composite tray setup.

S Sectional Bands should be disposed of in the garbage or state regulations should be followed. Single use only. Tension Rings and forceps must be cleaned, bagged individually or bagged/wrapped in a tray setup, and then sterilized. A chemical/steam indicator device should be included in the wrapping. Hinged instruments should be processed open and unlocked.

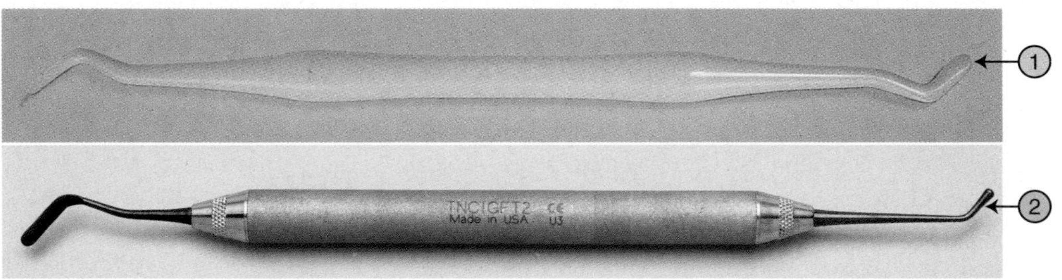
1
2
TNCIGFT2
Made in USA
U3

INSTRUMENT

Composite Placement Instrument evolve

FUNCTION

To carry composite material for cavity preparation
To place and condense composite material in cavity preparation
To carve composite material in cavity preparation

CHARACTERISTICS

Double ended
Different angles on ends
Ends shaped differently, one to accommodate initial placement of material (paddle end) and the other end to condense, contour, and carve material
Metal or plastic:
- ① Plastic composite instrument—Plastic that can be sterilized
- ② Metal composite instrument—Titanium nitride coating

Variety of sizes, shapes, and angles available

PRACTICE NOTE

Composite Placement Instrument is used on composite tray setups.

Ⓢ Composite Placement Instrument must be cleaned, bagged individually or bagged/wrapped in a tray setup, and then sterilized. A chemical/steam indicator device should be included in the wrapping.

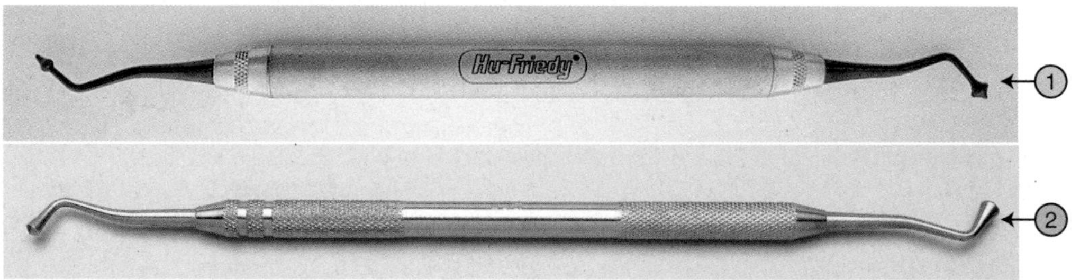
Hu-Friedy
1
2

INSTRUMENT

Composite Burnisher

FUNCTIONS To form occlusal anatomy in composite restorations
To achieve final contouring of anatomy, pits, fissures, and grooves

CHARACTERISTICS Double ended—Different angle on either end

① Composite Burnisher:
Titanium nitride coating—Creates hard, smooth, nonstick surface that resists scratching, sticking, or discoloration of composite material

② Acorn burnisher for composite restorations:
Gold titanium nitride coating—Creates hard, smooth, nonstick surface that resists scratching, sticking, or discoloration of composite material

PRACTICE NOTE Composite Burnisher is used on composite tray setups.

Ⓢ Composite Burnisher must be cleaned, bagged individually or bagged/wrapped in a tray setup, and then sterilized. A chemical/steam indicator device should be included in the wrapping.

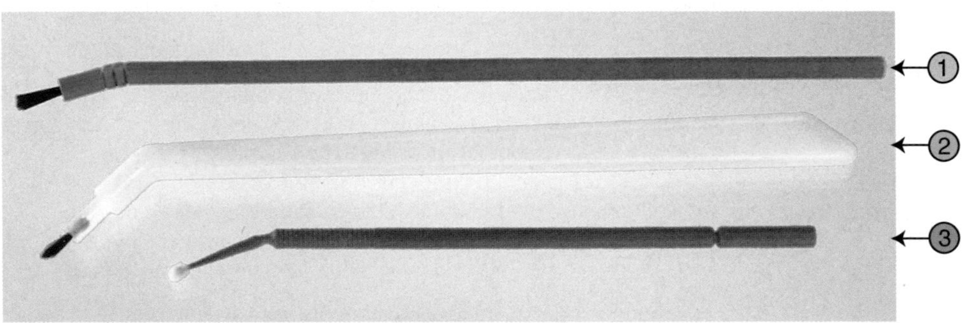
1
2
3

INSTRUMENT

Applicator evolve

FUNCTION To apply conditioning, primer, and bonding material to cavity preparation

CHARACTERISTICS Types:

① Disposable one-piece applicator—Several colors available for application of different materials; working end bends; various styles, sizes

② Two-piece applicator—Available with plastic handle that can be sterilized and removable, disposable tip

③ Microbrush applicator—Disposable, various styles, sizes

PRACTICE NOTE Applicators are used on composite sealant tray setups and any procedure involving etching, primers, and bonding materials.

S Plastic handle must be cleaned, bagged individually or bagged/wrapped in a tray setup, and then sterilized. A chemical/steam indicator device should be included in the wrapping. Disposable Applicator should be disposed of in the garbage.

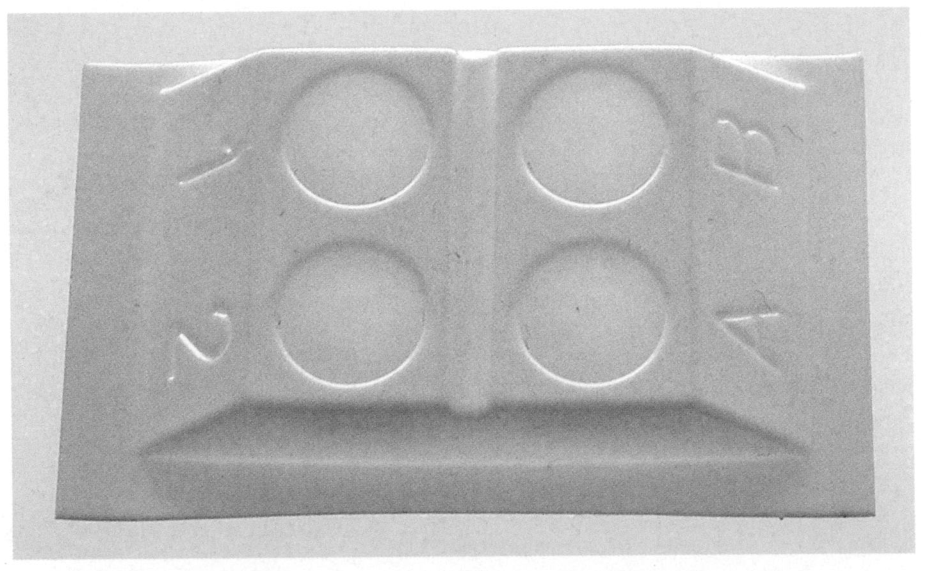

INSTRUMENT

Well for Composite Material

FUNCTION To hold material: etchant, bonding, and composite

CHARACTERISTICS Disposable (pictured) or autoclavable
Labels on each well—Designate different materials
Variety of styles and colors available

PRACTICE NOTE Wells are also used on a sealant tray setup and any procedure involving etching and primers.

S Disposable Wells should be disposed of in the garbage. Reusable wells must be cleaned, bagged individually or bagged/wrapped in a tray setup, and then sterilized. A chemical/steam indicator device should be included in the wrapping.

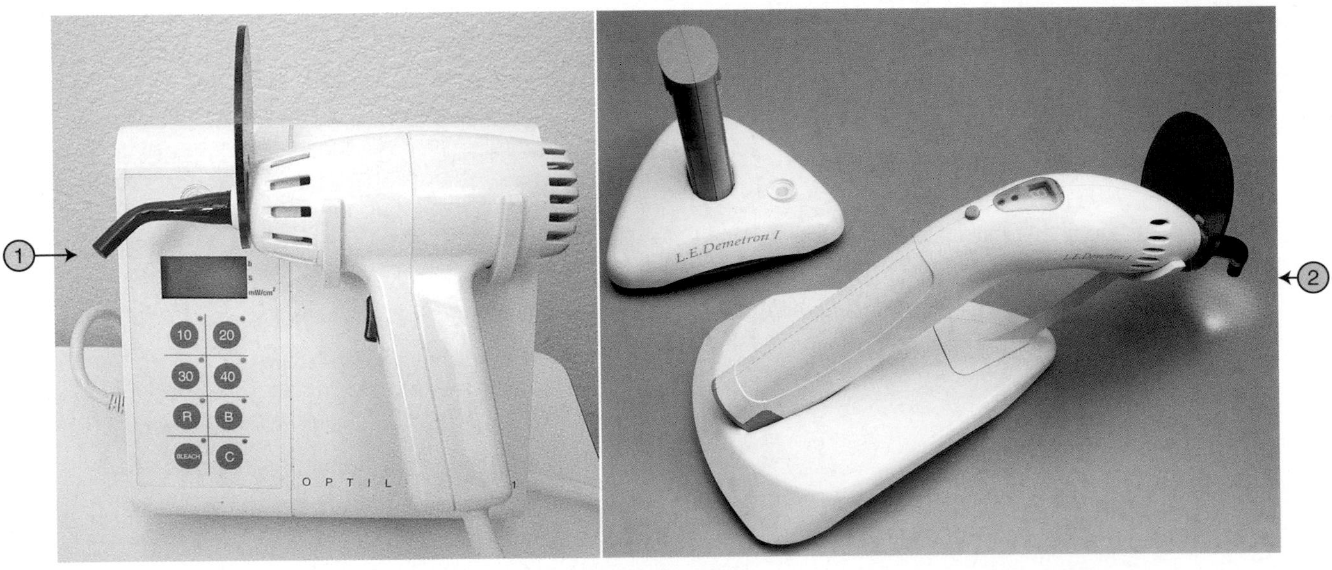
1
h
s
mW/cm²
10
20
30
40
R
B
BLEACH
C
O P T I L
L.E.Demetron I
L.E.Demetron I
2

INSTRUMENT

Curing Light—Electronic and Battery Operated evolve

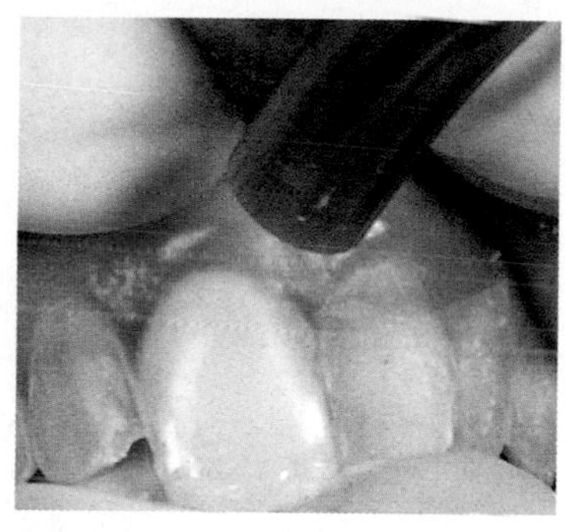

FUNCTION To harden light cured materials: bonding, composite, sealants, build-up material

CHARACTERISTICS Various styles available:

① Electric

② Battery operated—Includes battery charger with extra battery

PRACTICE NOTES Material must be cured in increments of 2 mm or less to ensure complete setting.

Refer to manufacturer's recommendation for curing time.

A testing device should be used to check the accuracy of the curing light.

Ⓢ Protective sleeves are available for the Curing Lights. Disinfect the wand and/or light using disinfection solution according to the manufacturer's recommendation.

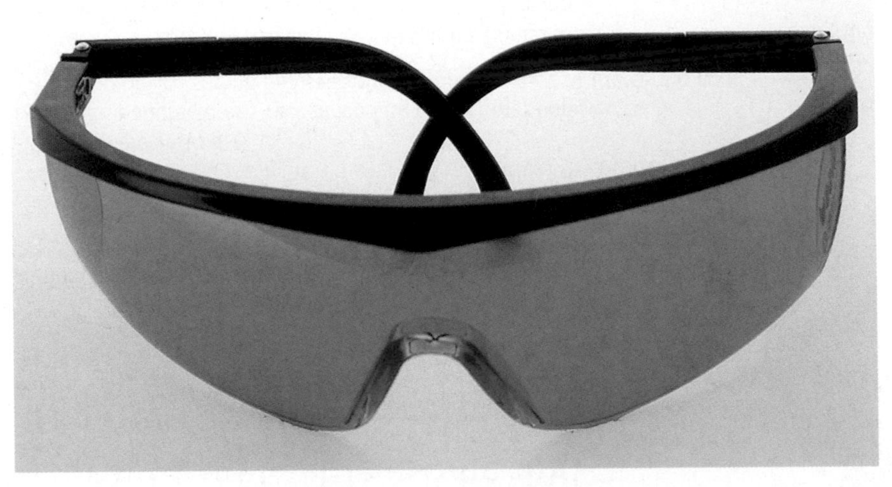

INSTRUMENT

Protective Shield for Curing Light

FUNCTION To protect operator's and assistant's eyes during curing stage of light-cured material

CHARACTERISTICS Orange color— Blocks harmful light to operator's and assistant's eyes
Protective shields also available on curing light and/or paddle shield

PRACTICE NOTE Protective Shield must be used with all curing lights.

(S) Protective Shield, paddle type, glasses, etc. must be disinfected according to the manufacturer's recommendation.

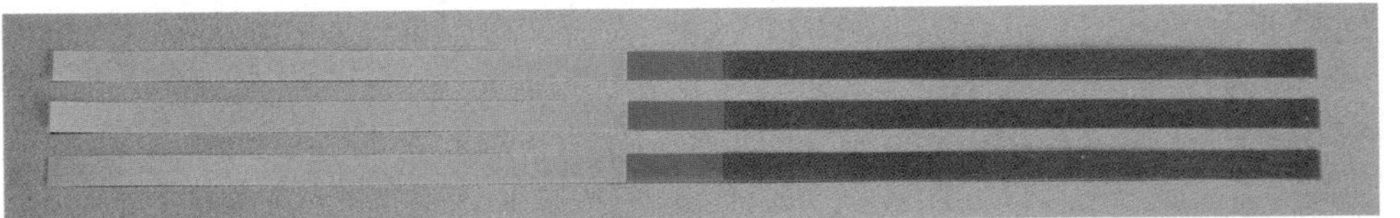

INSTRUMENT

Finishing Strip evolve

FUNCTION To finish and smooth interproximal surface of restoration

CHARACTERISTICS Abrasive textures available: synthetic or sandpaper, material
Different grit consistencies

PRACTICE NOTES Synthetic finishing strip—No abrasive material in center of strip to avoid removal of tooth structure while inserting the finishing strip interproximally.
Finishing Strip is used on composite and amalgam tray setups.

S Finishing Strip should be disposed of in garbage. Single use only.

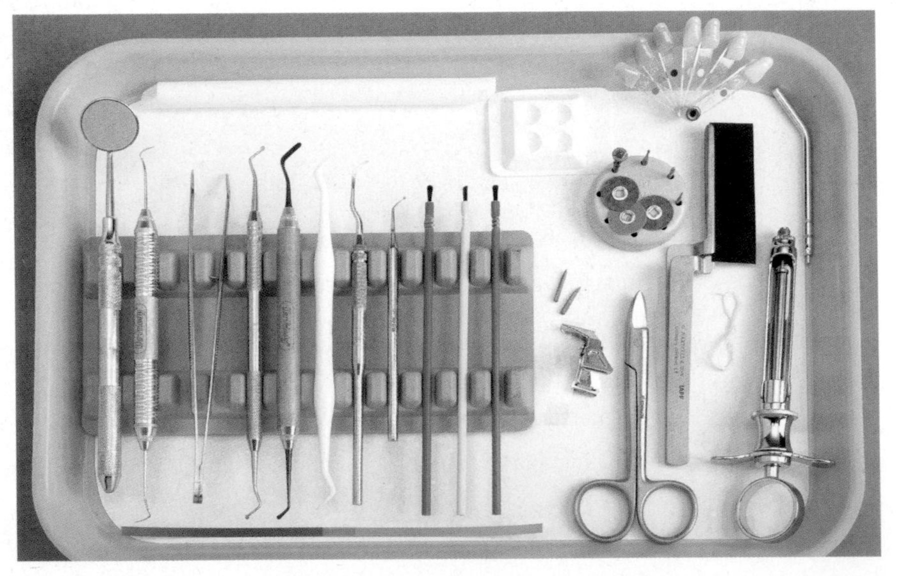

TRAY SETUP

Composite Procedure—Class III and Class IV Composite Restorative

TOP ROW (FROM LEFT TO RIGHT)

High-volume evacuator (HVE) tip, well for composite material, burs and mandrel/discs in bur block, shade guide

BOTTOM ROW (FROM LEFT TO RIGHT)

Mouth mirror, explorer, cotton forceps (pliers), spoon excavator, composite placement instrument—titanium nitride coating, composite placement instrument—plastic, gold carving knife, liner applicator, three different colors of applicator brushes, wooden wedges, clear Mylar matrix strip and clamp to hold matrix, crown and bridge scissors, articulating paper holder and articulating paper, dental floss, anesthetic aspirating syringe, air/water syringe tip

Refer to each picture for correct procedure for instrument sterilization or disposal of material.

Refer to other chapters for additional instruments on this tray setup that are not included in this chapter.

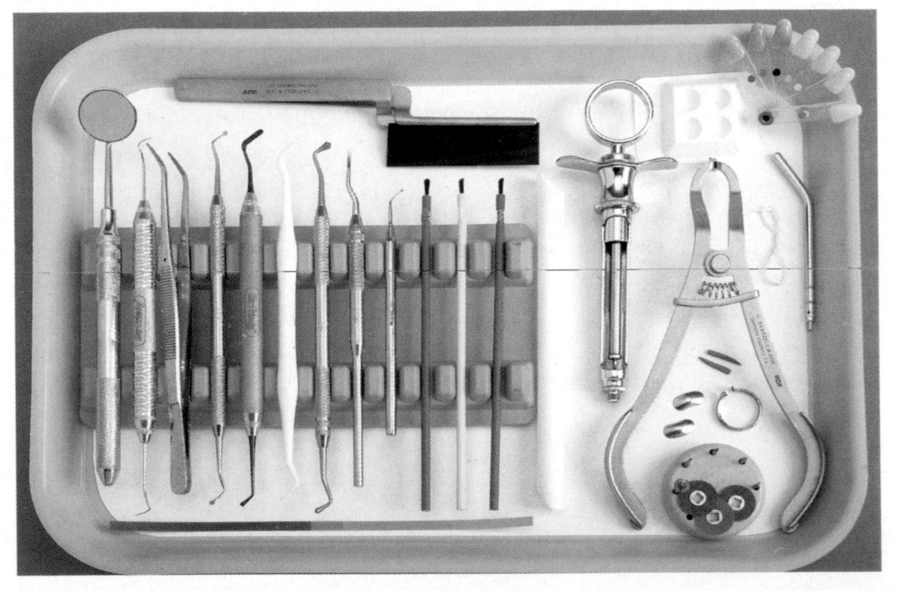

TRAY SETUP

Composite Procedure—Class I, Class II, and Class V Composite Restorative

TOP ROW (FROM LEFT TO RIGHT)

Articulating paper holder and articulating paper, well for composite material, shade guide

BOTTOM ROW (FROM LEFT TO RIGHT)

Mouth mirror, explorer, cotton forceps (pliers), spoon excavator, composite placement instrument—titanium nitride coating, composite placement instrument– plastic, composite burnisher–gold titanium nitride coating gold carving knife, liner applicator, three different colors of applicator brushes, high-volume (velocity) evacuation (HVE) tip, anesthetic syringe, forceps for tension rings, (under the forceps: matrix band, wooden wedges, tension rings, burs, and mandrel/discs in bur block), dental floss, and air/water syringe tip

BOTTOM OF TRAY

Finishing strip

S Refer to each picture for correct procedure for instrument sterilization or disposal of material.

Refer to other chapters for additional instruments on this tray setup that are not included in this chapter.

CHAPTER 10

Crown and Bridge Restorative Instruments

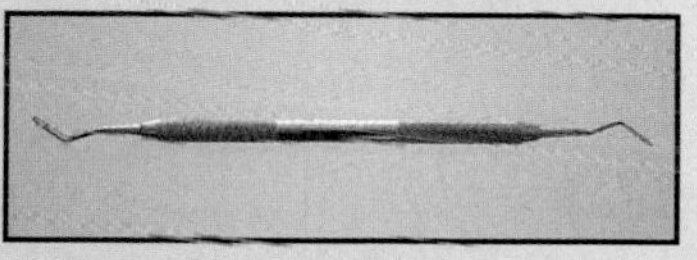

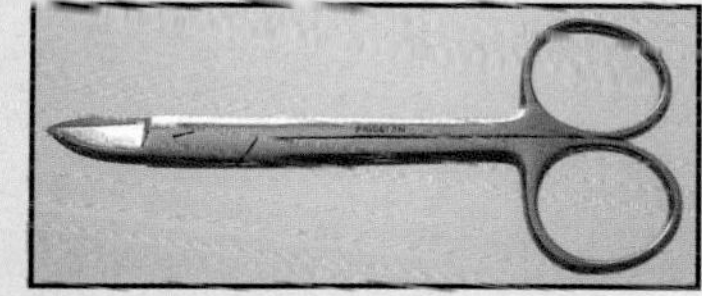

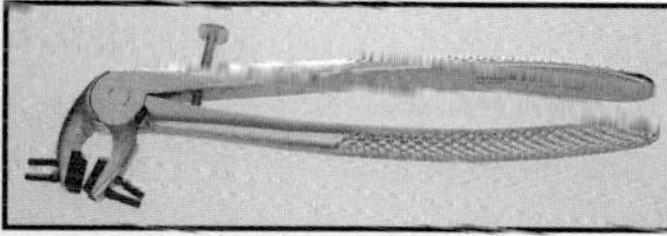

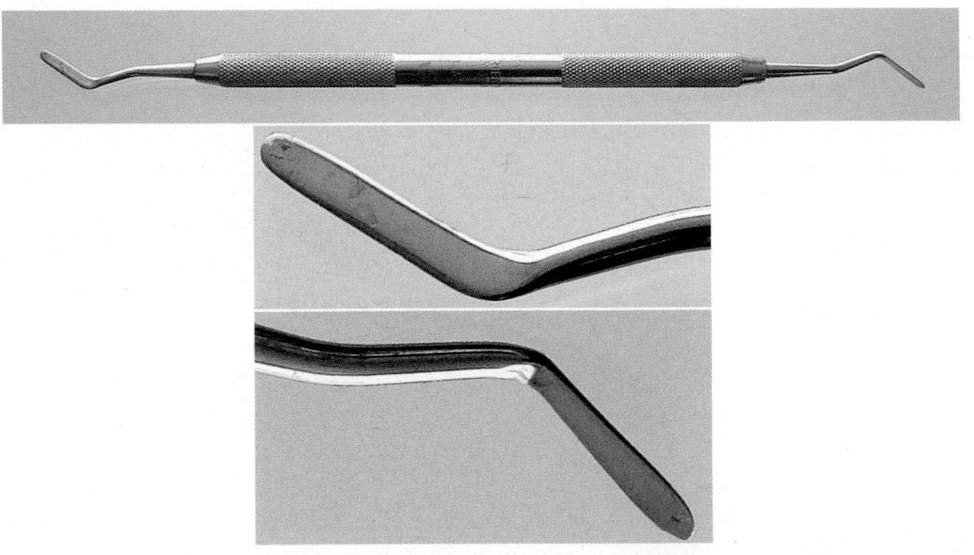

INSTRUMENT

Gingival Retraction Cord Instrument

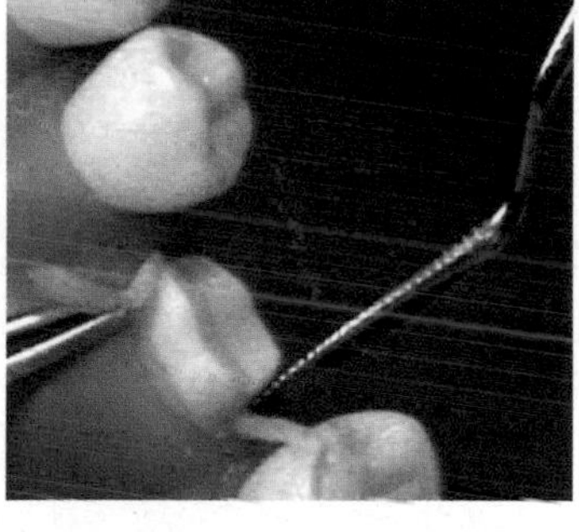

FUNCTION To place gingival retraction cord in sulcus area after tooth is prepared for a crown and before final impressions are taken

CHARACTERISTICS Smooth or serrated edges
Double ended—Different angle on each end
Variety of styles

PRACTICE NOTE Gingival Retraction Cord Instrument is mainly used on crown and bridge tray setup unless gingiva needs to be retracted for a restorative procedure.

Ⓢ Gingival Retraction Cord Instrument must be cleaned, bagged individually or bagged/wrapped in a tray setup, and then sterilized. A chemical/steam indicator device should be included in the wrapping.

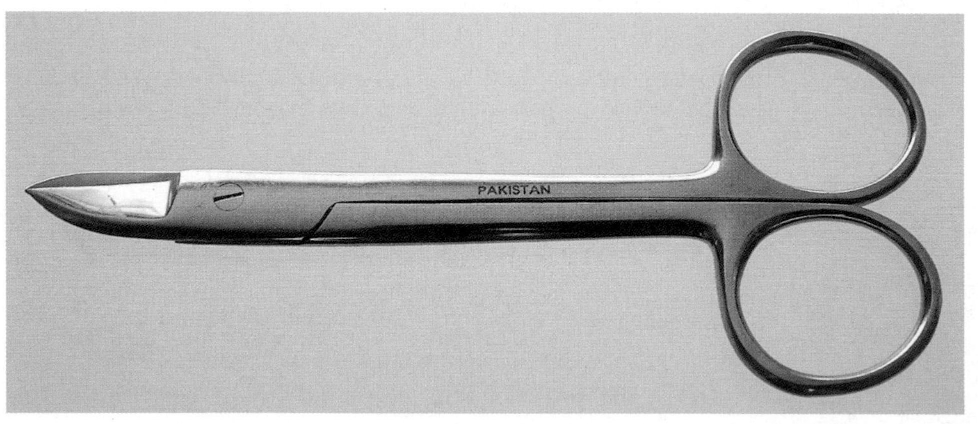
PAKISTAN

INSTRUMENT

Crown and Bridge Scissors 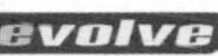

FUNCTIONS
To trim aluminum temporary crowns on gingival side
To trim custom temporary crowns
To cut gingival retraction cord
To trim matrix bands

CHARACTERISTICS
Short cutting edges—can be straight or curved, narrow or wide
Variety of sizes

PRACTICE NOTE
Crown and Bridge Scissors is used on other restorative tray setups.

S Crown and Bridge Scissors must be cleaned, bagged individually or bagged/wrapped in a tray setup, and then sterilized. A chemical/steam indicator device should be included in the wrapping. Hinged instruments should be processed open and unlocked.

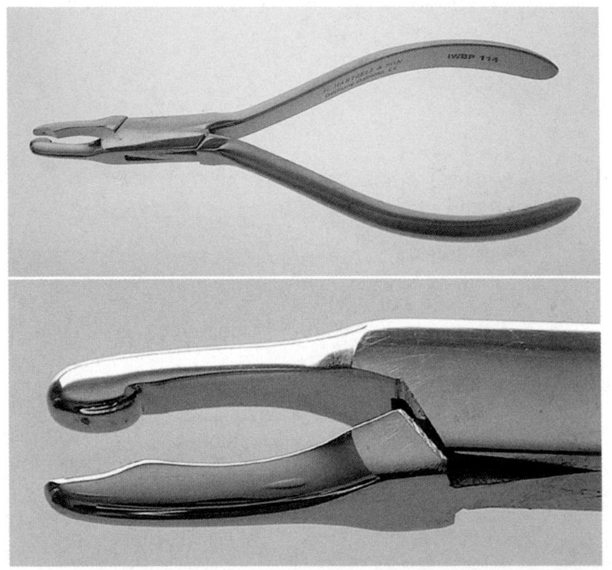
IWBP 114

INSTRUMENT

Contouring Pliers evolve

FUNCTION To crimp and contour marginal edge of temporary crown or stainless steel crown

CHARACTERISTICS Commonly used type: Johnson
Range of sizes available

PRACTICE NOTE Contouring Pliers is mainly used on crown and bridge tray setup.

Contouring Pliers must be cleaned, bagged individually or bagged/wrapped in a tray setup, and then sterilized. A chemical/steam indicator device should be included in the wrapping. Hinged instruments should be processed open and unlocked.

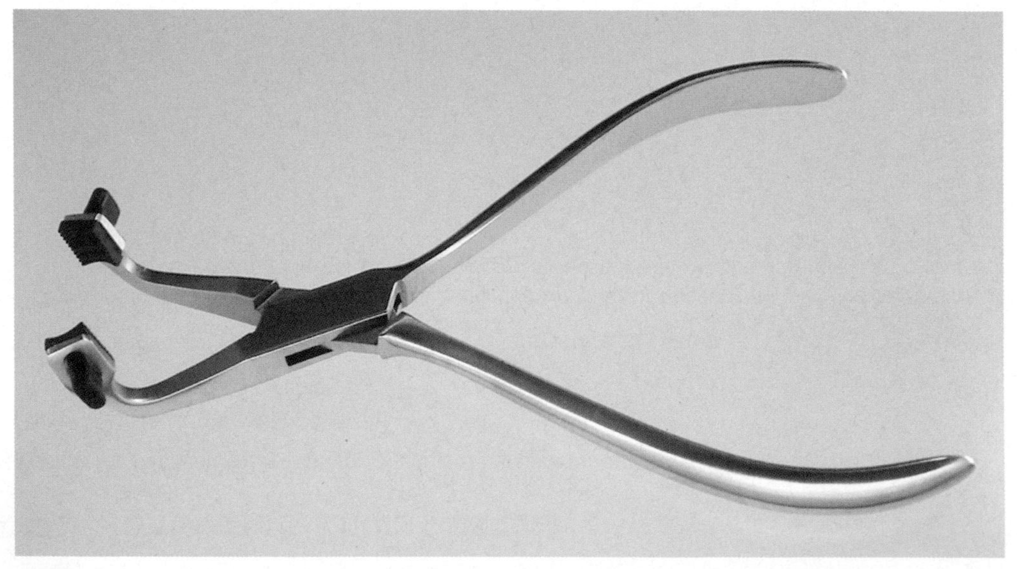

INSTRUMENT

Provisional Crown–Removing Forceps

FUNCTION To remove provisional crown from tooth

CHARACTERISTIC Range of sizes available

PRACTICE NOTE Provisional Crown–Removing Forceps is mainly used on crown and bridge tray setup.

Provisional Crown–Removing Forceps must be cleaned, bagged individually or bagged/wrapped in a tray setup, and then sterilized. A chemical/steam indicator device should be included in the wrapping. Hinged instruments should be processed open and unlocked.

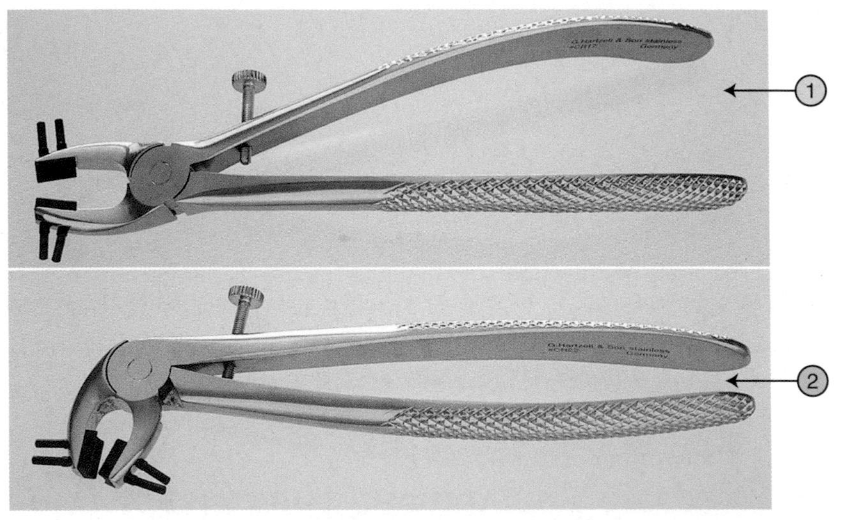
1
2

INSTRUMENT

Trial Crown Remover

FUNCTION

To remove permanent crown from tooth during try-in phase
To remove provisional crown

CHARACTERISTICS

Types:

① Maxillary Trial Crown Remover
② Mandibular Trial Crown Remover

Replaceable pads—Provide nonslipping, tight grip

PRACTICE NOTE

Trial Crown Remover is mainly used on crown and bridge tray setup.

Ⓢ Trial Crown Remover must be cleaned, bagged individually or bagged/wrapped in a tray setup, and then sterilized. A chemical/steam indicator device should be included in the wrapping. Hinged instruments should be processed open and unlocked.

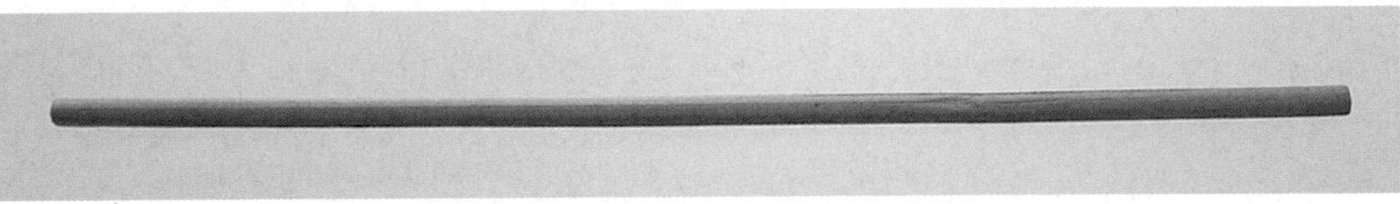

INSTRUMENT

Wooden Bite Stick evolve

FUNCTION To seat permanent crown while patient bites in centric occlusion

CHARACTERISTICS Soft wood
Range of sizes available

PRACTICE NOTE Wooden Bite Stick is mainly used on crown and bridge tray setup.

S Wooden Bite Stick must be cleaned, bagged individually or bagged/wrapped in a tray setup, and then sterilized. A chemical/steam indicator device should be included in the wrapping or disposed of in the garbage.

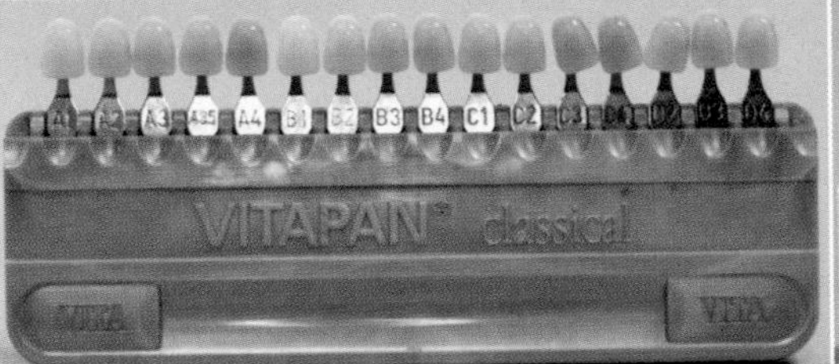
VITAPAN® classical
VITA
VITA
A3
B3
B4
C1
C2

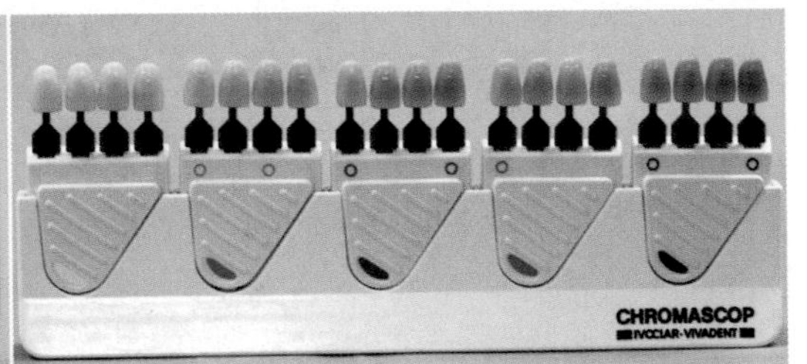
CHROMASCOP
IVOCLAR·VIVADENT

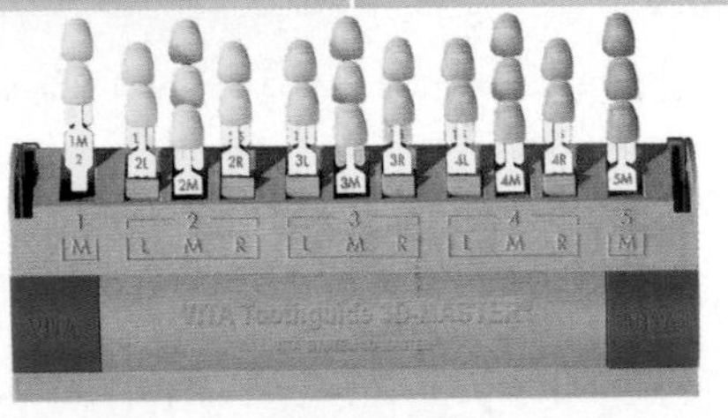
1M
2L
2M
2R
3L
3M
3R
4M
4R
5M
1
2
3
4
5
M
L M R
L M R
L M R
M

INSTRUMENT

Shade Guides/Digital Color Imaging

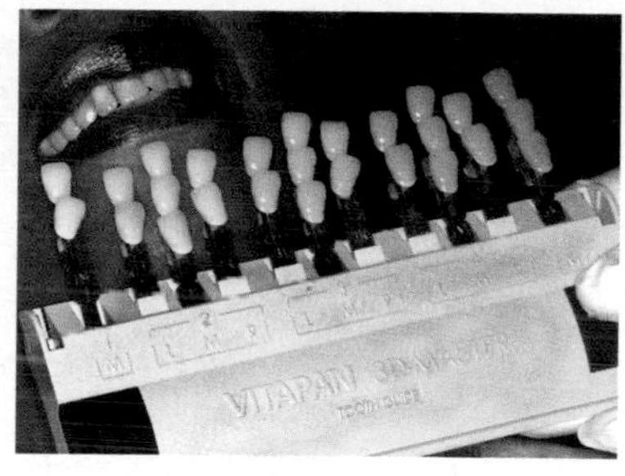

FUNCTIONS

To select a shade for permanent fixed restorations
Example: crowns, veneers, bridges
To select a shade for removable appliances
Example: partials, dentures

CHARACTERISTICS

Many different shade guides are available. Samples shown: VITAPAN Classical and CHROMASCOP *(top)*
Many different digital or computerized shade guides available. Sample shown: VITA Toothguide 3D-MASTER *(bottom)*

PRACTICE NOTE

Each tooth may have different shades: one for the gingival third, one for the body or middle third, and one shade for the incisal edge (usually needed for anteriors)

Ⓢ Shade Guides must be disinfected according to the manufacturer's recommendation.

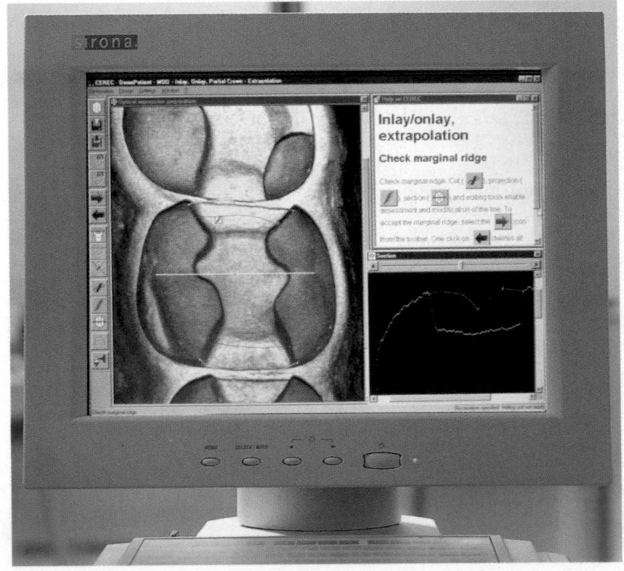
sirona
Inlay/onlay,
extrapolation
Check marginal ridge

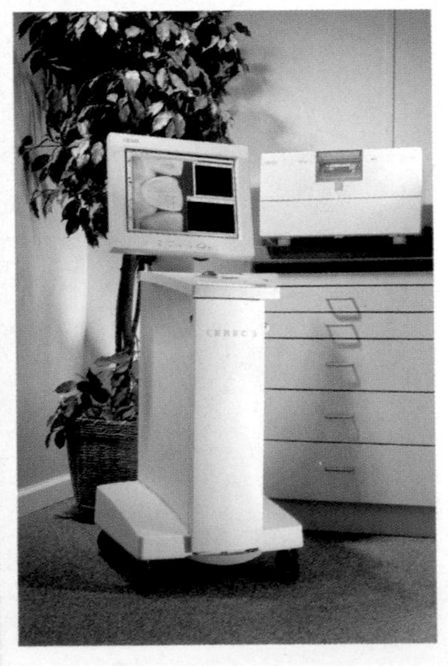
CEREC 3

INSTRUMENT

Cerec Machine evolve

FUNCTION To outline crown with an intraoral wand that connects to a computer
To construct the anatomy, gingival margins, occlusal and contact parts of the crown on the computer
To send the information to the unit to construct the crown

CHARACTERISTICS Crown is made of porcelain.

PRACTICE NOTE The Cerec machine allows the patient to have one appointment for preparing and seating a crown.

S Barriers should be used for the intraoral wand. Barriers or overgloves should be used for manipulating the computer on the Cerec machine. Otherwise, refer to the manufacturer's recommendation for disinfecting.

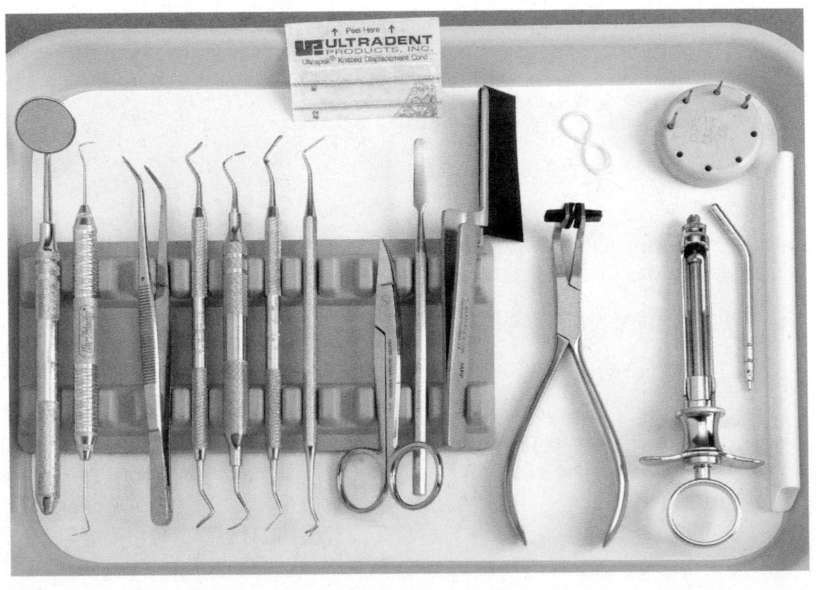
↑ Peel Here ↑
ULTRADENT
PRODUCTS, INC.
Ultrapak® Knitted Displacement Cord

TRAY SETUP

Crown and Bridge Preparation

TOP ROW (FROM LEFT TO RIGHT)

Gingival retraction cord, dental floss, burs in bur block

BOTTOM ROW (FROM LEFT TO RIGHT)

Mouth mirror, explorer, cotton forceps (pliers), spoon excavator, curette, gingival retraction cord instrument, Woodson, crown and bridge scissors, flexible cement mixing spatula, articulating paper holder and articulating paper, provisional crown-removing forceps, anesthetic aspirating syringe, air/water syringe tip, high-volume evacuation (HVE) tip

S Refer to each picture for correct procedure for instrument sterilization or disposal of material.

Refer to other chapters for additional instruments on this tray setup that are not included in this chapter.

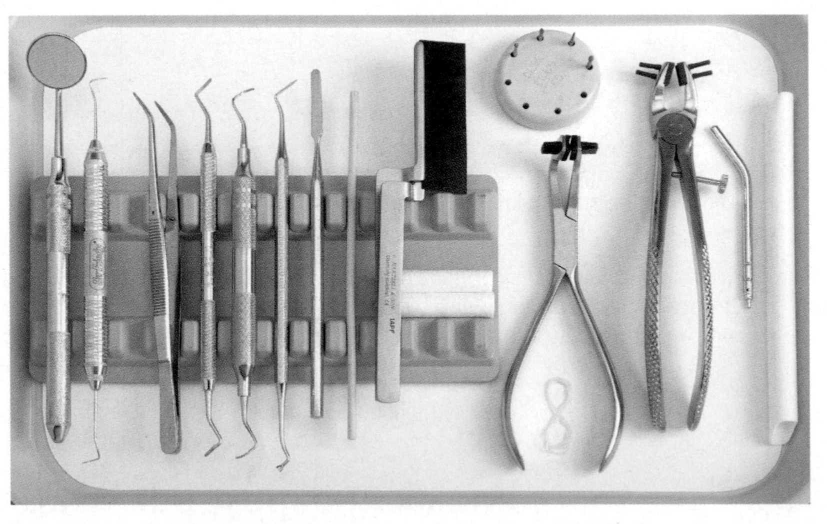

TRAY SETUP

Crown and Bridge Cementation

TOP ROW (FROM LEFT TO RIGHT)
Burs in bur block

BOTTOM ROW (FROM LEFT TO RIGHT)
Mouth mirror, explorer, cotton forceps (pliers), spoon excavator, curette, Woodson, flexible cement mixing spatula, wooden bite stick, articulating paper holder and articulating paper, cotton rolls, provisional crown–removing forceps, dental floss (under provisional crown-removing forceps), trial crown remover-maxillary, air/water syringe tip, high-volume evacuation (HVE) tip

Ⓢ Refer to each picture for correct procedure for instrument sterilization or disposal of material.

Refer to other chapters for additional instruments on this tray setup that are not included in this chapter.

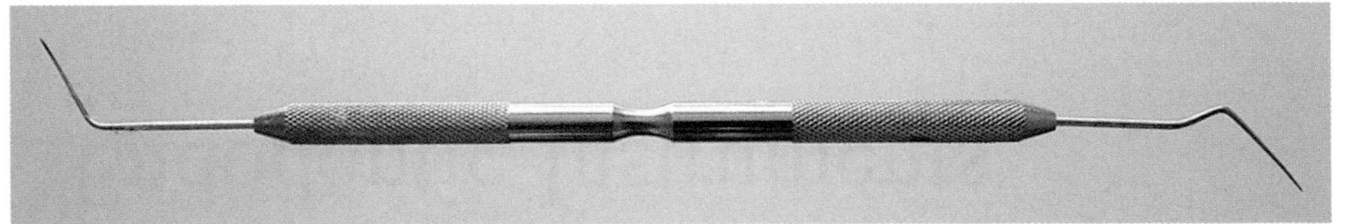

INSTRUMENT

Endodontic Explorer

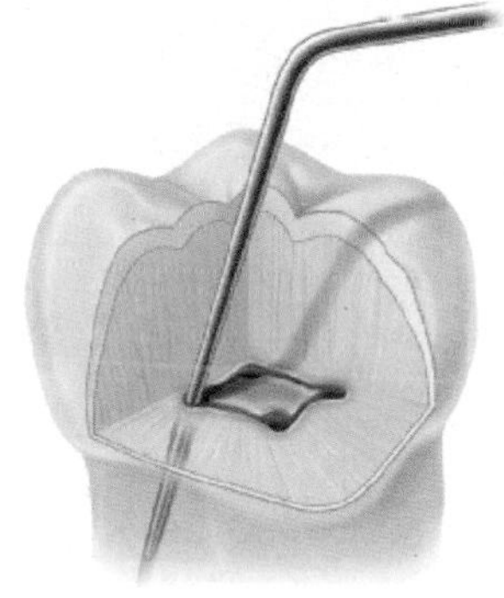

FUNCTION To locate opening of small canal orifices for endodontic procedure

CHARACTERISTICS Double ended
Working end—Longer than regular Explorer to reach opening of canals

PRACTICE NOTES Endodontic Explorer is used exclusively on endodontic tray setups

S Endodontic Explorer must be cleaned, bagged individually or bagged/wrapped in a tray setup, and then sterilized. A chemical/steam indicator device should be included in the wrapping.

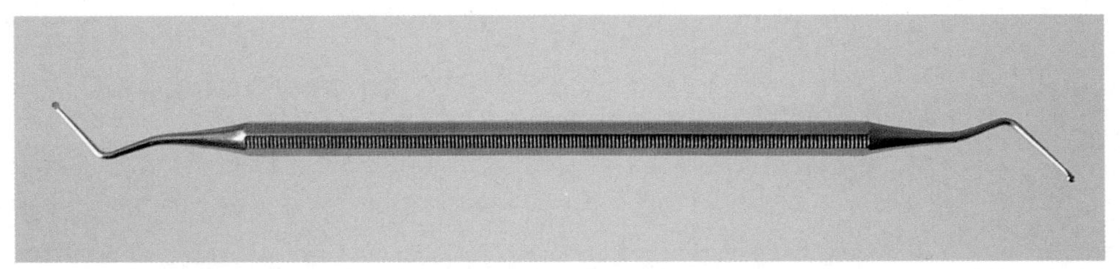

INSTRUMENT

Endodontic Long-Shank Spoon Excavator

FUNCTION To curet inside of tooth to base of pulp chamber

CHARACTERISTICS Long shank to reach deep into cavity preparation
Double ended
Range of sizes available

PRACTICE NOTE Endodontic Long-Shank Spoon is used exclusively on endodontic tray setups

Ⓢ Endodontic Long-Shank Spoon Excavator must be cleaned, bagged individually or bagged/wrapped in a tray setup, and then sterilized. A chemical/steam indicator device should be included in the wrapping.

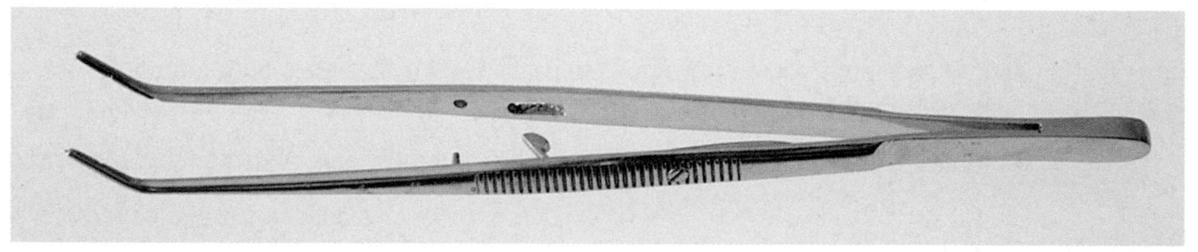

INSTRUMENT

Endodontic Locking Forceps (Pliers)

FUNCTION To grasp and lock material for transfer into and out of oral cavity

CHARACTERISTIC Similar to regular cotton forceps except for locking mechanism to secure material on the working end of the forceps (pliers)

PRACTICE NOTE Endodontic Locking Forceps is used on endodontic tray setup and could also be used on restorative tray setups.

S Endodontic Locking Forceps must be cleaned, bagged individually or bagged/wrapped in a tray setup, and then sterilized. A chemical/steam indicator device should be included in the wrapping. Hinged instruments should be processed open and unlocked.

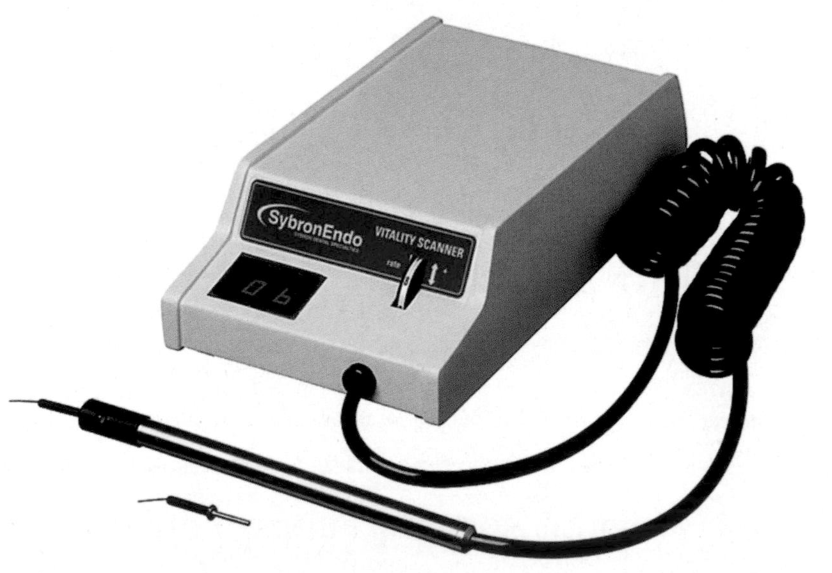
SybronEndo
VITALITY SCANNER
rate
0 b

INSTRUMENT

Vitalometer/Pulp Tester evolve

FUNCTION To test vitality of pulp in teeth

CHARACTERISTICS Two types—Electronic, digital (digital readout)
Electric or battery operated

PRACTICE NOTES The tester sends an impulse of electric current to the pulp, causing a reaction.
The current is increased by small increments until the patient indicates feeling a sensation.
Toothpaste is applied to the tip of the electrode to conduct electricity.
The tip is placed on the coronal part (facial or lingual) of a natural tooth.
Each root/pulp on the tooth is tested.
Vitalometer is used exclusively with endodontic tray setups.

S Vitalometer tip must be cleaned, bagged individually or bagged/wrapped in a tray setup, and then sterilized. A chemical/steam indicator device should be included in the wrapping. Barriers should be used on the unit and/or the manufacturer's recommendation for sterilization of Vitalometer tip and disinfection of unit should be followed.

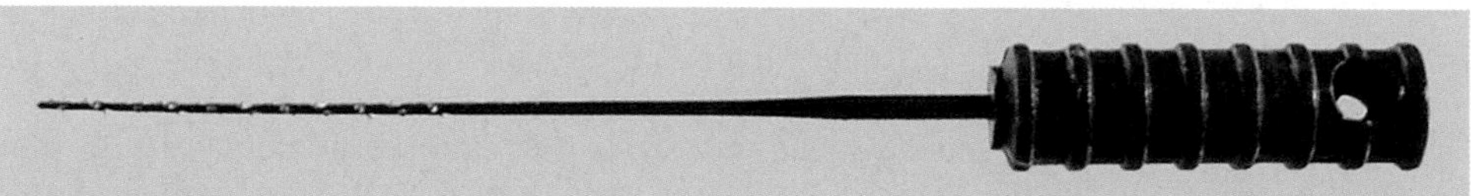

INSTRUMENT

Broach

FUNCTION To remove pulp tissue from canal(s)

CHARACTERISTICS Working end—Barbed wire protrusions on shaft grab and remove vital or nonvital pulp fibers
Handles—Color coded according to size
Range of sizes—Diameter increases with size
Discarded after each use

PRACTICE NOTE Broach is used exclusively on endodontic tray setups.

S Endodontic Broach must be disposed of in a Sharps container. For single use only.

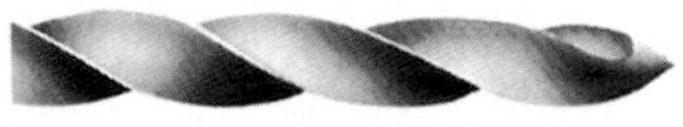

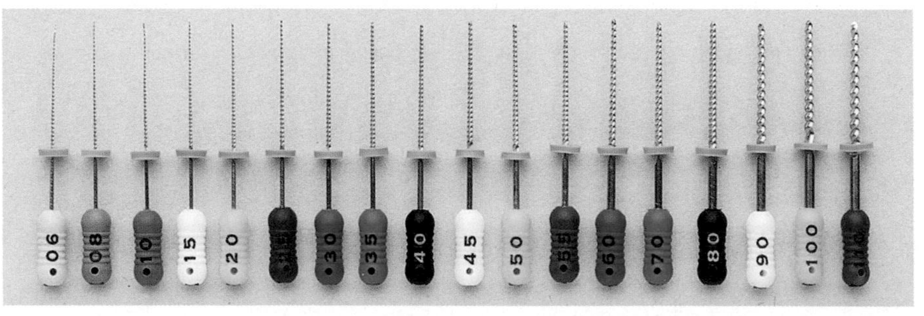
06
08
10
15
20
30
35
40
45
50
60
70
80
90
100

INSTRUMENT

Endodontic File—K Type evolve

FUNCTION To clean inside walls of canal
To contour inner walls of canal

CHARACTERISTICS Twisted design—More twists per millimeter than reamer
Used with push-pull motion
Handles—Color coded according to size
Range of sizes—To accommodate width of canal; diameter increases with size
Available in different lengths
Examples: 21 mm, 25 mm, 31 mm

PRACTICE NOTE Endodontic File—K Type is used exclusively on endodontic tray setups.

S Endodontic File—K Type must be cleaned, bagged individually or bagged/wrapped in a tray setup, and then sterilized. A chemical/steam indicator device should be included in the wrapping, or used file must be disposed of in a Sharps container. Rubber stopper on the file should be disposed of in the garbage.

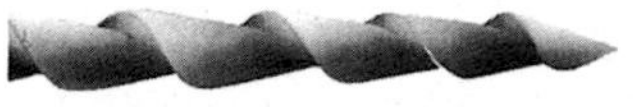

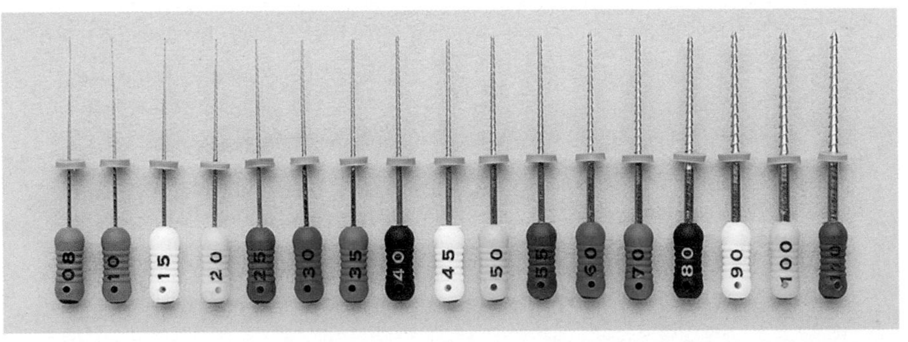
08
10
15
20
25
30
35
40
45
50
55
60
70
80
90
100

INSTRUMENT

Endodontic File—Hedstrom

FUNCTIONS

To clean inside walls of canal
To enlarge and smooth inner walls of canal

CHARACTERISTICS

Triangular cutting edge
Handles —Color coded according to size
Range of sizes—To accommodate width of canal; diameter increases with size
Available in different lengths

Examples: 21 mm, 25 mm, 31 mm

PRACTICE NOTE

Endodontic File—Hedstrom is used exclusively on endodontic tray setups.

Ⓢ Endodontic File—Hedstrom must be cleaned, bagged individually or bagged/wrapped in a tray setup, and then sterilized. A chemical/steam indicator device should be included in the wrapping, or used file must be disposed of in a Sharps container. Rubber stopper on the file should be disposed of in the garbage.

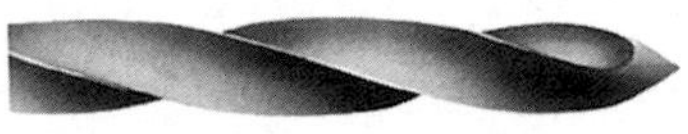

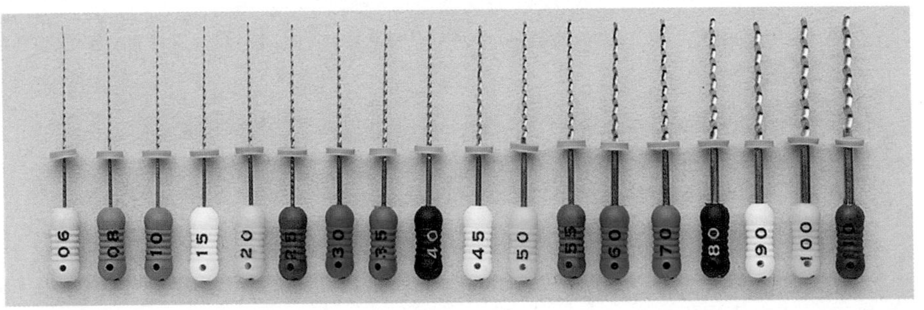

INSTRUMENT

Reamer

FUNCTIONS

To cut and smooth dentinal walls of canal
To enlarge inner walls of canal

CHARACTERISTICS

Twisted triangular cutting edge (similar to K-type file, but cutting edge is farther apart and has fewer twists per millimeter)
Used with twisting motion
Handles—Color coded according to size
Range of sizes—To accommodate width of canal; diameter increases with size
Available in different lengths
Examples: 21 mm, 25 mm, 31 mm

PRACTICE NOTES

Reamer is used exclusively on endodontic tray setups.

(S) Reamer must be cleaned, bagged individually or bagged/wrapped in a tray setup, and then sterilized.
A chemical/steam indicator device should be included in the wrapping, or used reamer must be disposed of in a Sharps container. Rubber stopper on the file should be disposed of in the garbage.

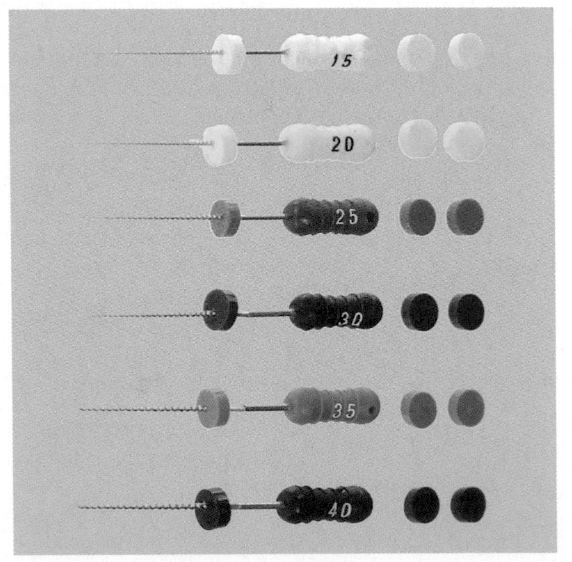
15
20
25
30
35
40

INSTRUMENT

Endodontic Stoppers

FUNCTION To place onto the intracanal instrument such as a file or reamer to help determine length of canal

CHARACTERISTICS Files or reamers are measured from stopper to apex of root to determine length of canal. (Radiographs also help determine length.)

Stoppers are made from rubber, silicone, or plastic.

PRACTICE NOTES Endodontic Stoppers are color coded to correspond to a particular file or reamer or a single color of stopper is used for all files or reamers.

Endodontic Stoppers are used exclusively on endodontic tray setups.

S Endodontic Stoppers should be disposed of in the garbage.

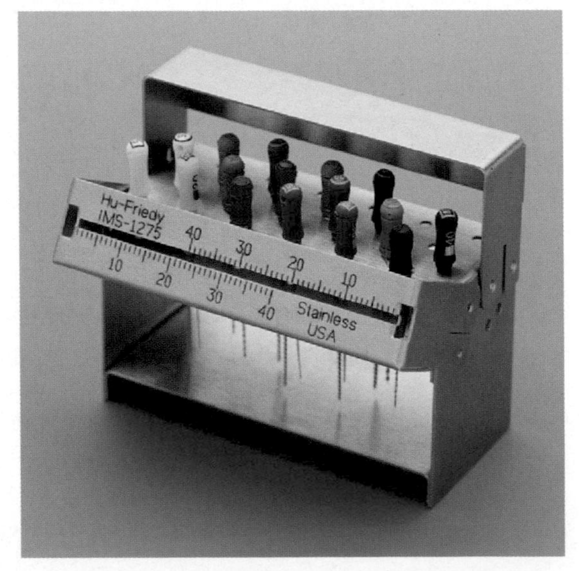

Hu-Friedy
IMS-1275
Stainless
USA

INSTRUMENT

Endodontic Stand

FUNCTIONS To hold endodontic files and reamers

To measure endodontic files and reamers with millimeter ruler etched in container; may be measured from right or left side of stand

CHARACTERISTICS Container closes with endodontic files and reamers for sterilization processes.

PRACTICE NOTE Endodontic Stand is used exclusively with endodontic tray setups.

S File or Reamer in Endodontic Stand and Endodontic Stand must be cleaned, bagged individually or bagged/wrapped in a tray setup, and then sterilized. A chemical/steam indicator device should be included in the wrapping, or used file or reamer must be disposed of in a Sharps container. Rubber Stopper on the file should be disposed of in the garbage.

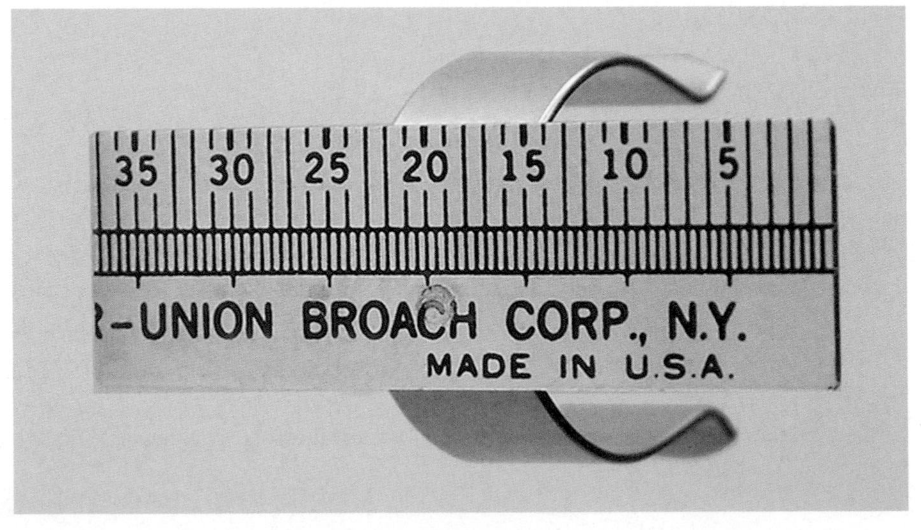
35 30 25 20 15 10 5
R-UNION BROACH CORP., N.Y.
MADE IN U.S.A.

INSTRUMENT

Endodontic Millimeter Ruler

FUNCTION To measure files, reamers, other instruments, and materials in millimeter increments

CHARACTERISTIC Variety of designs

PRACTICE NOTE Endodontic Millimeter Ruler could be used in other areas of dentistry other than on endodontic tray setups.

S Endodontic Millimeter Ruler must be cleaned, bagged individually or bagged/wrapped in a tray setup, and then sterilized. A chemical/steam indicator device should be included in the wrapping.

272

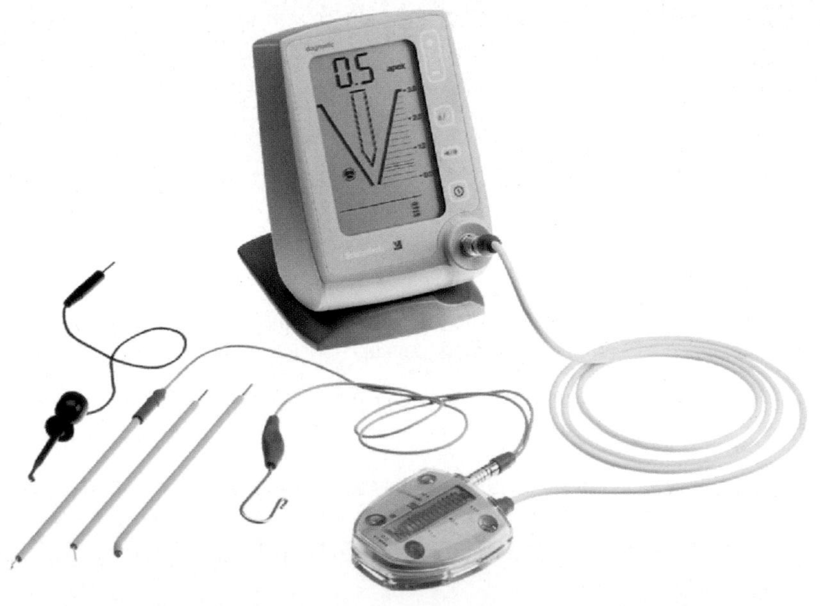

INSTRUMENT

Electronic Apex Locator

FUNCTION To electronically measure length of canal to apex of tooth

CHARACTERISTICS Attaches to file or reamer and is placed in canal using dry or wet environment
Length readout—Tone or digital

PRACTICE NOTE Electronic Apex Locator is used exclusively with endodontic tray setups.

Ⓢ Electronic Apex Locator device that enters patient's mouth must be cleaned, bagged individually or bagged/wrapped in a tray setup, and then sterilized. A chemical/steam indicator device should be included in the wrapping. Barriers should be used on the unit and/or the manufacturer's recommendation for sterilization should be followed.

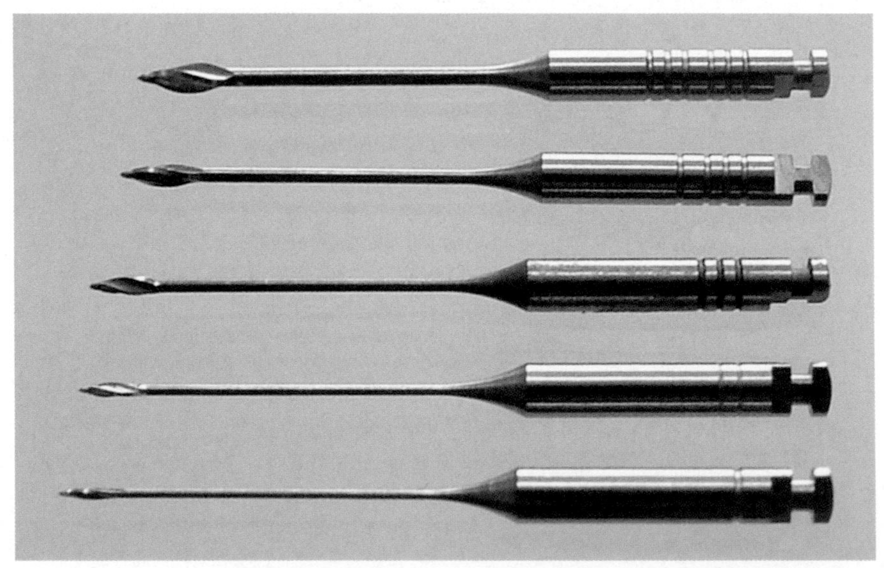

INSTRUMENT

Gates Glidden Bur or Drill

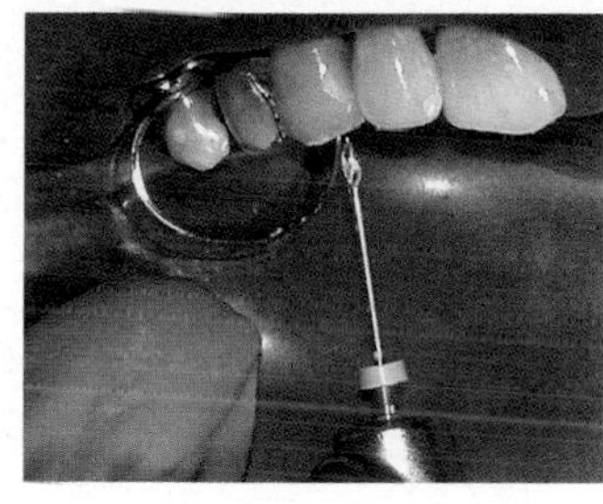

FUNCTIONS
To enlarge walls of pulp chamber
To open canal orifice

CHARACTERISTICS
Long-shank bur
Elliptical or flame-shaped cutting edge
Latch type—Used with slow-speed contra-angle handpiece (air driven or electric)
Range of sizes—Size identified by number of grooves on shank
Two lengths—Shorter for posterior teeth, longer for anterior teeth

PRACTICE NOTE
Gates Glidden Burs are used exclusively on endodontic tray setups.

Ⓢ Gates Glidden Bur or Drill must be cleaned, bagged individually or bagged/wrapped in a tray setup, and then sterilized. A chemical/steam indicator device should be included in the wrapping, or used Gates Glidden Bur must be disposed of in a Sharps container.

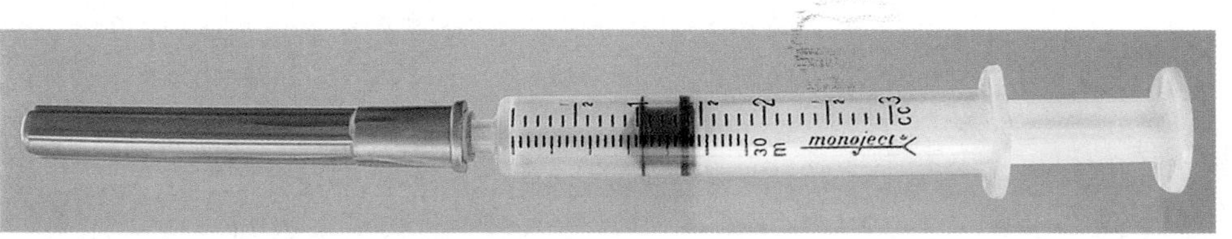
1
2
3
cc
30
m
monoject

INSTRUMENT

Endodontic Irrigating Syringe

FUNCTION To carry and dispense irrigating solution into canal for cleansing during debridement of canal

CHARACTERISTICS Disposable
Two sizes—3 cc (pictured) and 12 cc

PRACTICE NOTE Endodontic Irrigating Syringe could be used in other areas of dentistry other than on endodontic tray setups.

Ⓢ Endodontic Irrigating Syringe should be disposed of in a Sharps container. For single use only.

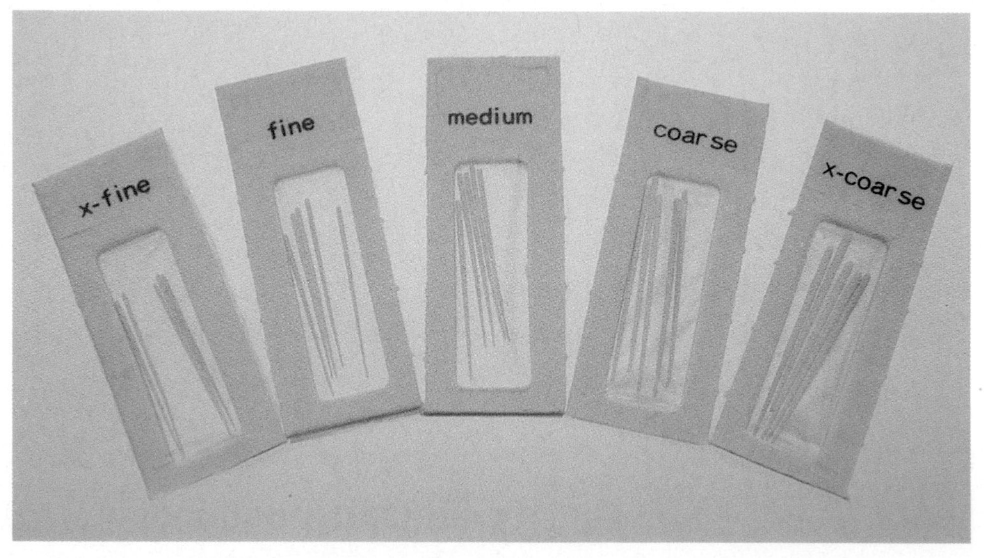
x-fine
fine
medium
coarse
x-coarse

INSTRUMENT

Sterile Absorbent Paper Points

FUNCTION To dry pulp chambers of canal—New points inserted repeatedly until pulp chamber is completely dry

CHARACTERISTICS Size of point corresponds to width of canal
Range of sizes available

PRACTICE NOTE The length of the paper point is measured to ensure that it corresponds to the length of the canal.
Paper Points are used exclusively on endodontic tray setups.

S Sterile Absorbent Paper Points should be disposed of in the garbage.

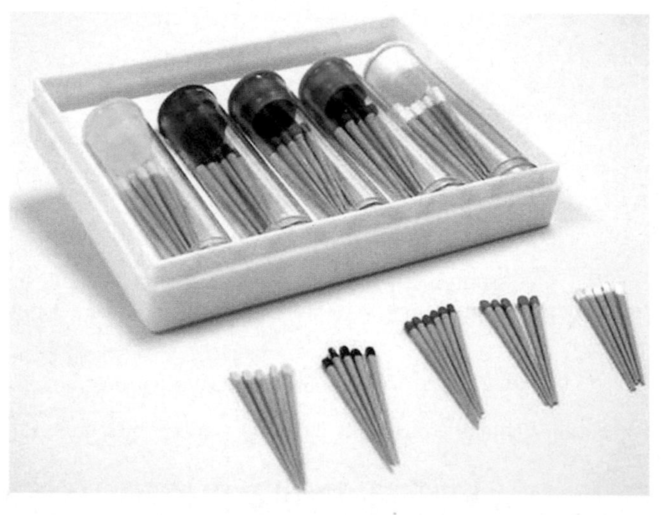

INSTRUMENT

Gutta-Percha evolve

FUNCTION To fill pulp chamber after completion of canal preparation (called *obturation*)

CHARACTERISTICS Solid at room temperature; becomes soft and pliable when heated
May be heated in a cartridge and then dispensed into canal
Range of sizes—To correspond to size of canal

PRACTICE NOTES Endodontic Sealer, a cement material, is used with gutta-percha for final sealing of the canal.
Gutta-Percha is used exclusively on an endodontic tray setup.

Gutta-Percha should be disposed of in the garbage.

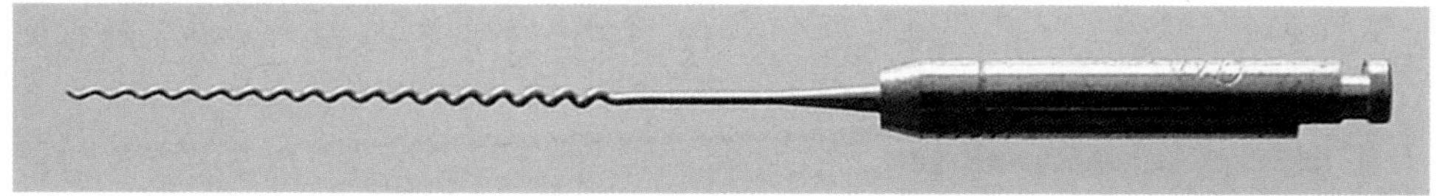

INSTRUMENT

Lentulo Spiral evolve

FUNCTION To place endodontic sealer or cement in canal for final seal before placement of gutta-percha

CHARACTERISTIC Latch type Shank—Used with slow-speed contra-angle handpiece (air driven or electric)

PRACTICE NOTE Lentulo Spiral is used exclusively on endodontic tray setups.

S Lentulo Spiral must be cleaned, bagged individually or bagged/wrapped in a tray setup, and then sterilized. A chemical/steam indicator device should be included in the wrapping, or used Lentulo Spiral must be disposed of in a Sharps container.

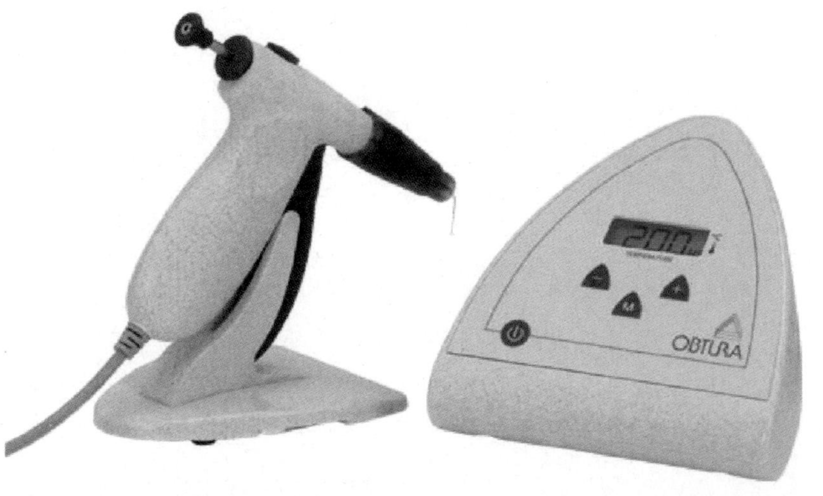
200
M
OBTURA

INSTRUMENT

Gutta-Percha Warming Unit evolve

FUNCTIONS To heat gutta-percha outside the mouth before use
To inject heated gutta-percha in thermoplastic state into prepared canals

CHARACTERISTICS Gutta-percha pellets—Used to load unit
Delivery system—Needle attaches to gun delivering gutta-percha into canal

PRACTICE NOTES Temperature of the gutta-percha in the unit can be adjusted to control the viscosity of the material.
Gutta-Percha Warming Unit is used exclusively with endodontic tray setups.

S Gutta-Percha Warming Unit Needle attached to the Gutta-Percha Warming Unit gun must be cleaned, bagged individually or bagged/wrapped in a tray setup, and then sterilized. A chemical/steam indicator device should be included in the wrapping. Needle must be disposed of in a Sharps container. Gutta-Percha Warming Unit must be disinfected according to the manufacturer's recommendation.

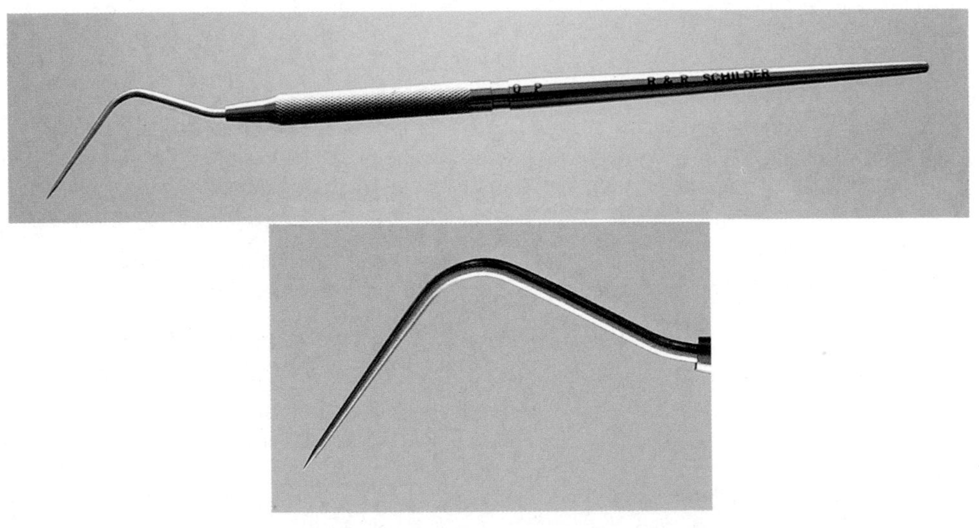
0 P
R & R SCHILDER

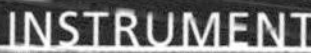

Endodontic Spreader

FUNCTIONS

To help condense gutta-percha laterally in canal
To use for final filling of canal

CHARACTERISTICS

Pointed tip
Working end—Has rings in millimeter increments
Two handle styles—Conventional (pictured), finger spreader
Range of sizes—To correspond to size of canal

PRACTICE NOTE

Endodontic Spreader is used exclusively on endodontic tray setups.

Ⓢ Endodontic Spreader must be cleaned, bagged individually or bagged/wrapped in a tray setup, and then sterilized. A chemical/steam indicator device should be included in the wrapping.

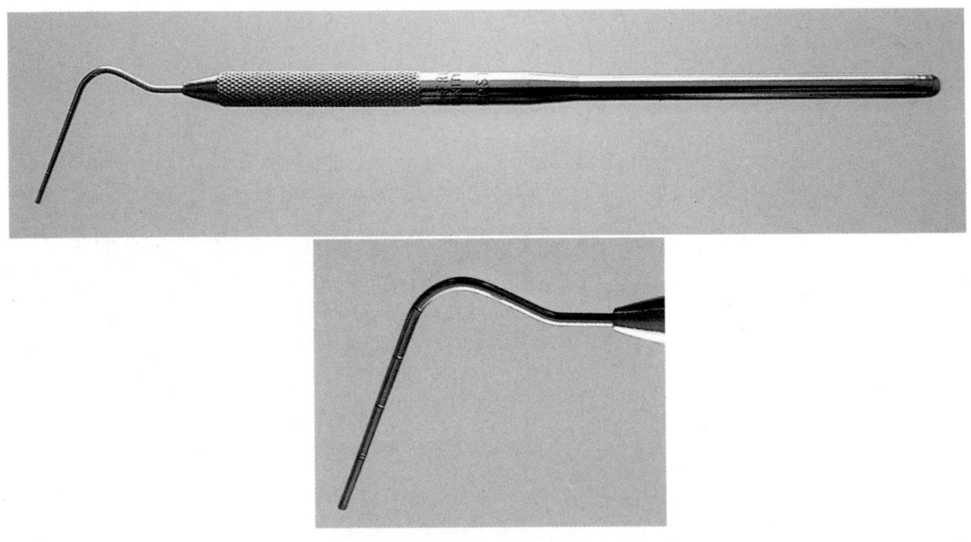

INSTRUMENT

Endodontic Plugger

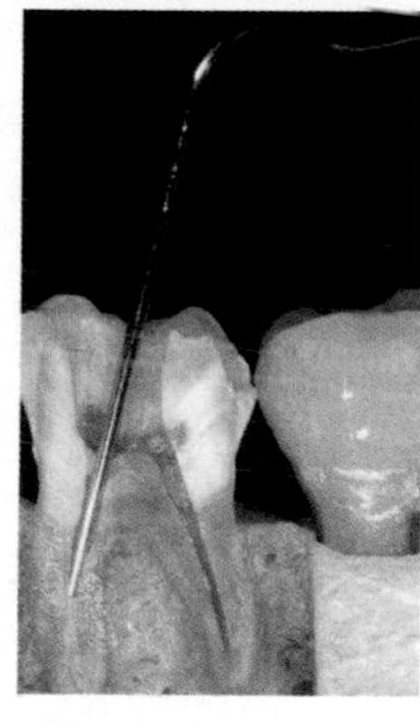

FUNCTIONS

To help condense gutta-percha vertically in canal
To use for final filling of canal

CHARACTERISTICS

Flat tip
Working end—Has rings in millimeter increments
Two handle styles—Conventional (pictured), finger spreader
Range of sizes—To correspond to size of canal

PRACTICE NOTE

Endodontic Plugger is used exclusively on endodontic tray setups.

Ⓢ Endodontic Plugger must be cleaned, bagged individually or bagged/wrapped in a tray setup, and then sterilized. A chemical/steam indicator device should be included in the wrapping.

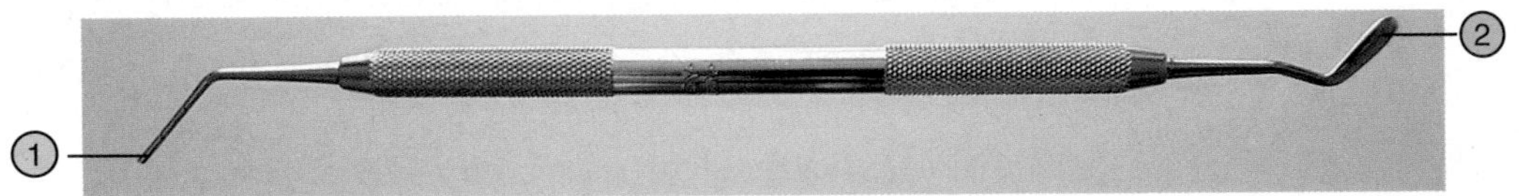
1
2

INSTRUMENT

Glick Instrument

FUNCTIONS

To condense gutta-percha into endodontically prepared teeth using plugger end
To sever excess gutta-percha after plugger end is heated
To carry and place material into tooth using paddle end

CHARACTERISTICS

Double ended:
- ① Plugger end—May have rings in millimeter increments
- ② Paddle end

PRACTICE NOTE

Glick Instrument is used exclusively on endodontic tray setups.

Ⓢ Glick Instrument must be cleaned, bagged individually or bagged/wrapped in a tray setup, and then sterilized. A chemical/steam indicator device should be included in the wrapping.

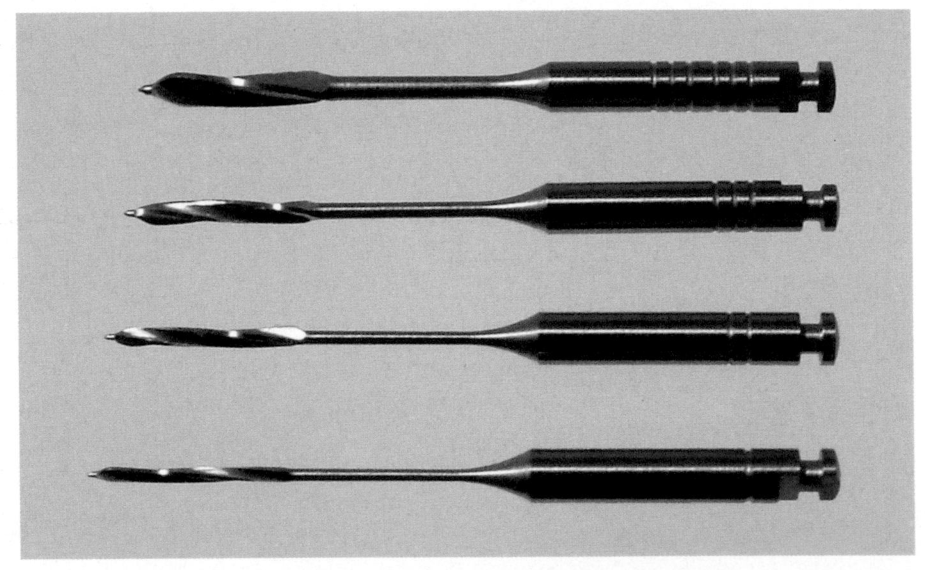

INSTRUMENT

Peso File

FUNCTIONS To prepare canal for endodontic post
To remove portion of gutta-percha sealed in canal to make room for endodontic post

CHARACTERISTICS Parallel cutting edges
Latch type Shank—Used with slow-speed contra-angle handpiece (air driven or electric)
Range of sizes—Size identified by number of grooves on shank

PRACTICE NOTE Peso File is used exclusively on endodontic tray setups.

Ⓢ Peso File must be cleaned, bagged individually or bagged/wrapped in a tray setup, and then sterilized. A chemical/steam indicator device should be included in the wrapping, or used Peso File must be disposed of in a Sharps container.

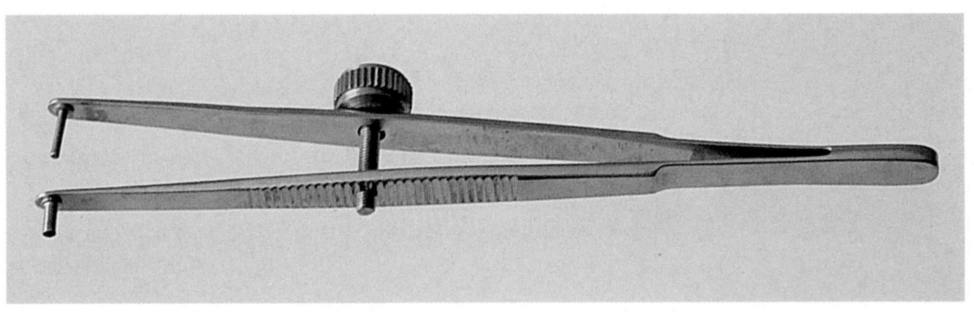

INSTRUMENT

Micro Retro Amalgam Carrier

FUNCTION To carry amalgam to surgical site of apicoectomy

CHARACTERISTICS Very small—To accommodate retro fills for apicoectomy

Surgical apicoectomy procedure is performed, if needed, after an endodontic procedure is completed.

PRACTICE NOTE Micro Retro Amalgam Carrier is used with a surgical tray setup for an apicoectomy.

Ⓢ Micro Retro Amalgam Carrier must be cleaned, bagged individually or bagged/wrapped in a tray setup, and then sterilized. A chemical/steam indicator device should be included in the wrapping.

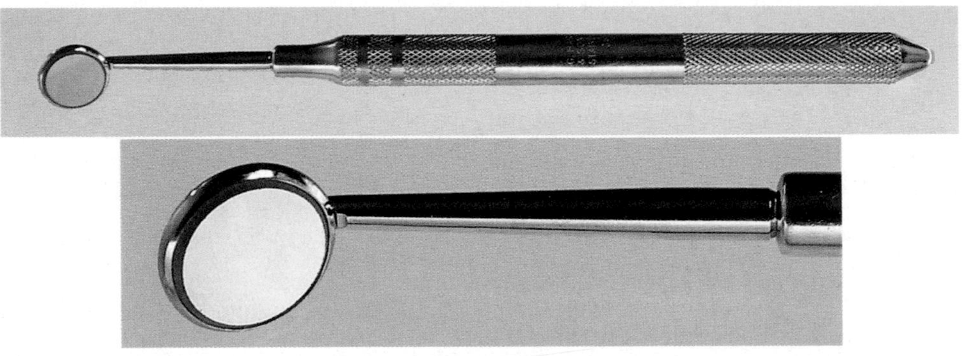

INSTRUMENT

Micro Retro Mouth Mirror

FUNCTION To view surgical site of apicoectomy retro fill

CHARACTERISTICS Very small—To accommodate retro fills for apicoectomy
Smaller sizes available

PRACTICE NOTE Micro Retro Mouth Mirror is used with a surgical tray setup for an apicoectomy.

Ⓢ Micro Retro Mouth Mirror must be cleaned, bagged individually or bagged/wrapped in a tray setup, and then sterilized. A chemical/steam indicator device should be included in the wrapping.

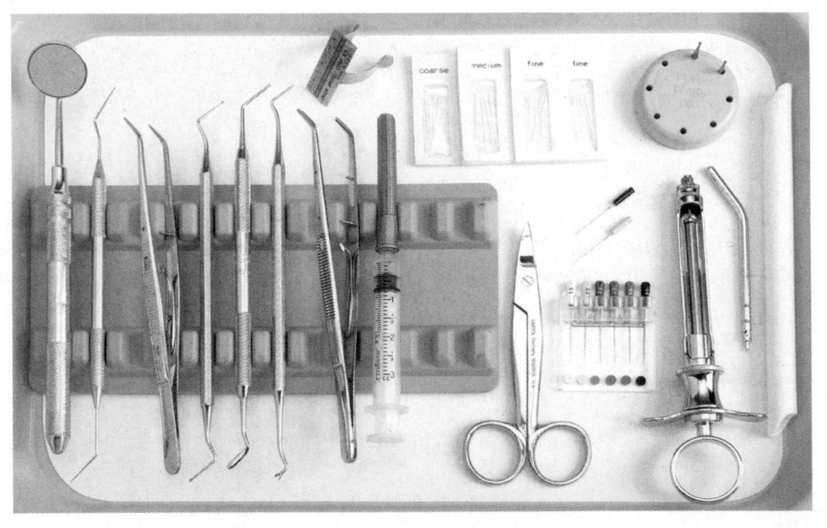

coarse
medium
fine
fine

TRAY SETUP

Opening a Tooth for Endodontic Therapy

TOP ROW (FROM LEFT TO RIGHT)

Millimeter ruler with finger ring, coarse, medium, fine absorbent sterile paper points, burs in bur block

BOTTOM ROW (FROM LEFT TO RIGHT)

Mouth mirror, endodontic explorer, endodontic locking forceps, endodontic long-shank spoon excavator, Glick instrument, Woodson, endodontic locking forceps (extra), irrigating disposable syringe, scissors, broaches, endodontic file K-Type with color-coded rubber stops, anesthetic aspirating syringe, air/water syringe tip, high-volume evacuation (HVE) tip

S Refer to each picture for correct procedure for instrument sterilization or disposal of instrument or material.

Refer to other chapters for additional instruments on this tray setup that are not included in this chapter.

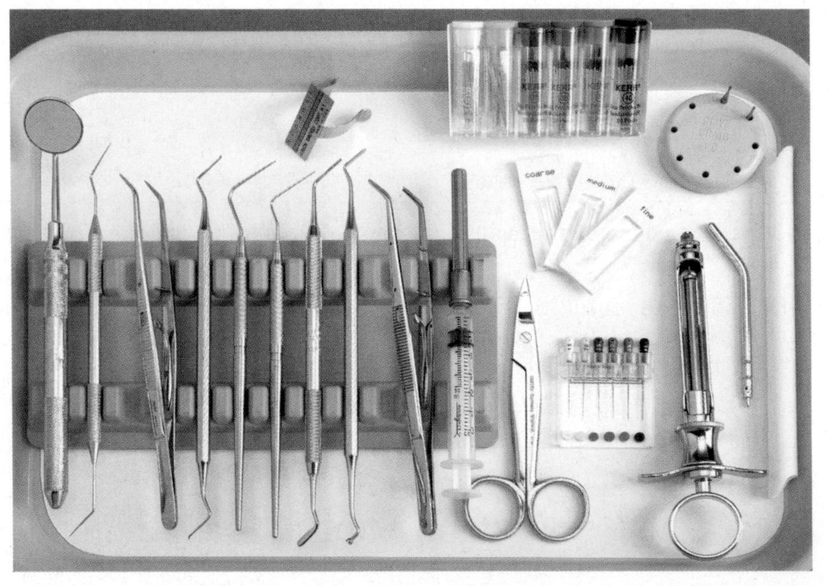
KERR
KERR
KERR
KERR
coarse
medium
fine

TRAY SETUP

Sealing a Tooth for Endodontic Therapy

TOP ROW (FROM LEFT TO RIGHT)

Millimeter ruler with finger ring, gutta-percha in vials—assorted sizes, coarse, medium, fine absorbent sterile paper points, burs in bur block

BOTTOM ROW (FROM LEFT TO RIGHT)

Mouth mirror, endodontic explorer, endodontic locking forceps, endodontic long-shank spoon excavator, endodontic spreader, endodontic plugger, Glick instrument, Woodson, endodontic locking cotton forceps (extra), irrigating disposable syringe, scissors, endodontic file K-Type with color-coded rubber stops, anesthetic aspirating syringe, air/water syringe tip, high-volume evacuation (HVE) tip

S Refer to each picture for correct procedure for instrument sterilization or disposal of instrument or material.

Refer to other chapters for additional instruments on this tray setup that are not included in this chapter.

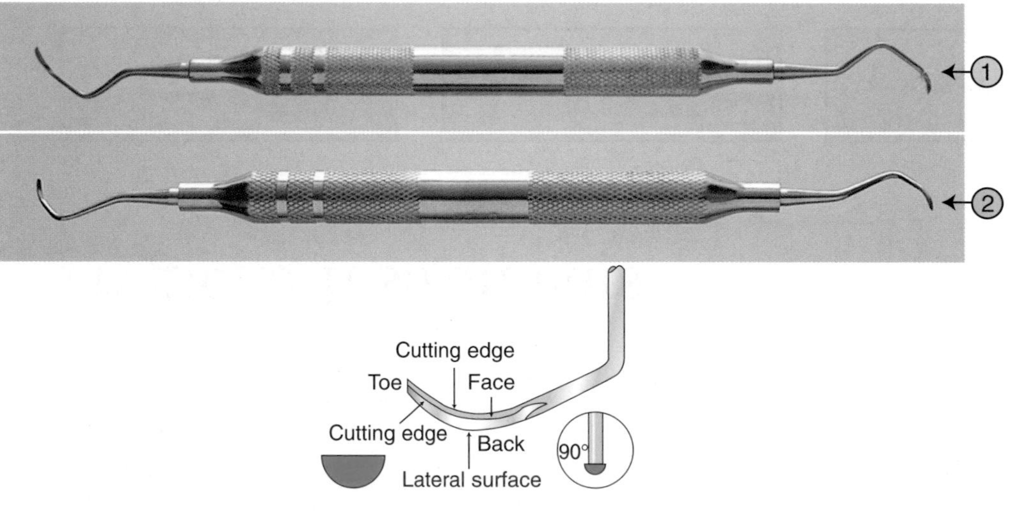
1
2
Cutting edge
Toe
Face
Cutting edge
Back
Lateral surface
90°

INSTRUMENT

Universal Curettes (Curet)

FUNCTIONS

To scale and remove deposits and stains from teeth
To scale supragingival and subgingival surfaces
To remove soft tissue lining of periodontal pocket and root planning

CHARACTERISTICS

Blade—Two cutting edges, rounded toe; rounded back; at 90-degree angle to lower shank
Flexible or rigid shank; length varies to accommodate clinical crown of tooth
Single or double ended
Range of sizes
Curette named by designer:

1. Barnhart 1/2
2. Ratcliff 3/0

PRACTICE NOTE

Universal Curettes are used on hygiene, periodontal, and operative tray setups.

Ⓢ Universal Curettes must be cleaned, bagged individually or bagged/wrapped in a tray setup, and then sterilized. A chemical/steam indicator device should be included in the wrapping.

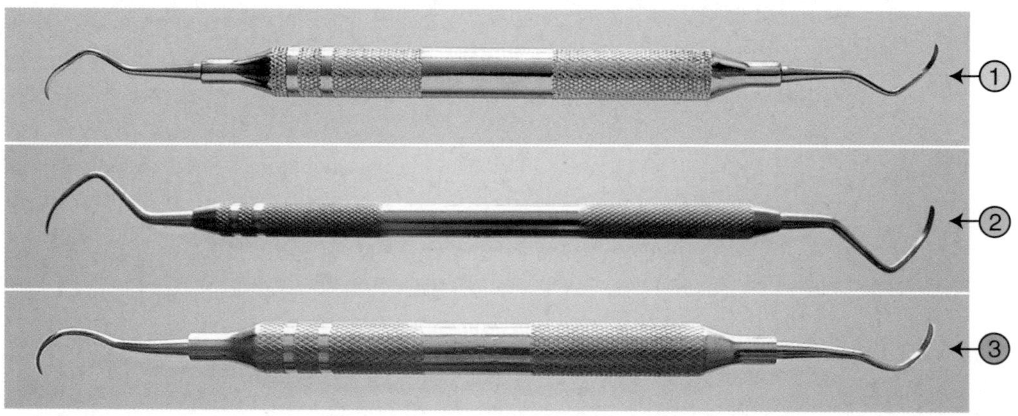
1
2
3

INSTRUMENT

Universal Curettes (Curet)

FUNCTIONS

To scale and remove deposits and stains from teeth
To scale supragingival and subgingival surfaces
To remove soft tissue lining of periodontal pocket and root planning

CHARACTERISTICS

Blade—Two cutting edges, rounded toe; rounded back; at 90-degree angle to lower shank
Flexible or rigid shank; length varies to accommodate clinical crown of tooth
Single or double ended
Range of sizes
Curette named by designer:

① UC/Rule $^{5}/_{6}$
② Loma Linda $^{11}/_{12}$
③ McCall $^{17}/_{18}$

PRACTICE NOTE

Universal Curettes are used on hygiene, periodontal, and operative tray setups.

Ⓢ Universal Curettes must be cleaned, bagged individually or bagged/wrapped in a tray setup, and then sterilized. A chemical/steam indicator device should be included in the wrapping.

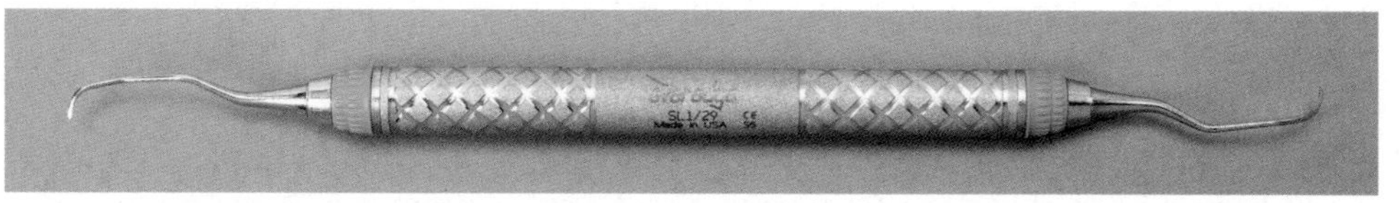
SL1/29
Made in USA

INSTRUMENT

Langer Universal Curettes

FUNCTIONS

To scale and remove deposits and stains from teeth
To scale supragingival and subgingival surfaces
To remove soft tissue lining of periodontal pocket and root planning

CHARACTERISTICS

Blade—Two cutting edges, with face at 90-degree angle to lower shank
Design function with three bends in the shank, improving posterior access
Langer Universal Curettes designed with the shank design of a Gracey combined with a Universal blade
Single or double ended
Range of sizes

PRACTICE NOTE

Langer Universal Curettes are used on hygiene and periodontal tray setups.

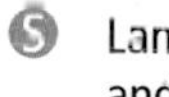

Langer Universal Curettes must be cleaned, bagged individually or bagged/wrapped in a tray setup, and then sterilized. A chemical/steam indicator device should be included in the wrapping.

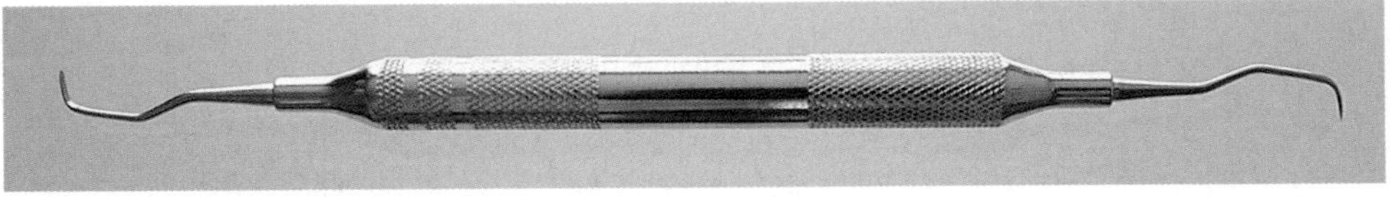

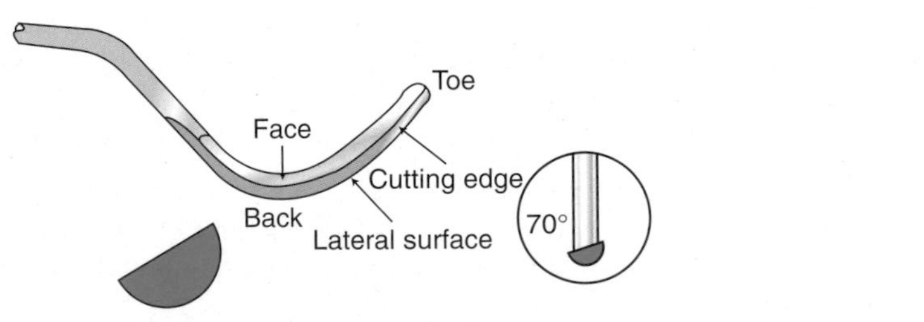
Toe
Face
Cutting edge
Back
Lateral surface
70°

INSTRUMENT

Area-Specific Curettes—Anterior evolve

FUNCTIONS

To scale and remove deposits from subgingival surfaces of anterior teeth
To use for root planning, periodontal debridement, and soft tissue curettage

CHARACTERISTICS

Two cutting edges (only lower cutting edge is used)
Blade—Rounded back and toe; at 70-degree angle to lower shank; types—standard, rigid, extra rigid
Curvature of blade designed to adapt to specific teeth and surfaces
Range of sizes available: 1/2, 3/4, 5/6
Curette named by designer: Gracey, Kramer-Nevins, Turgeon

PRACTICE NOTE

Area-Specific Curettes—Anterior are used on hygiene and periodontal tray setups.

S Area-Specific Curettes must be cleaned, bagged individually or bagged/wrapped in a tray setup, and then sterilized. A chemical/steam indicator device should be included in the wrapping.

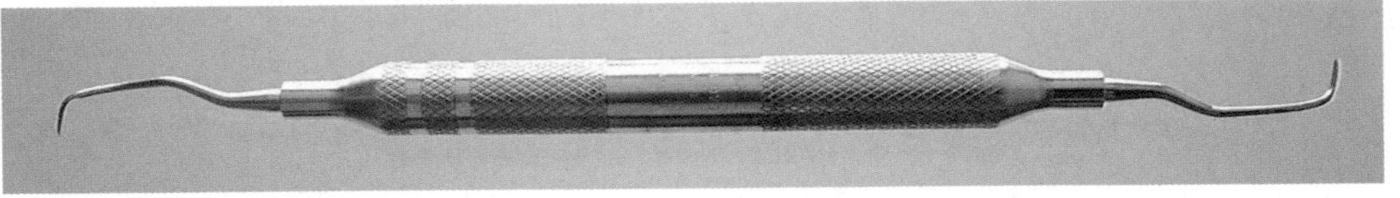

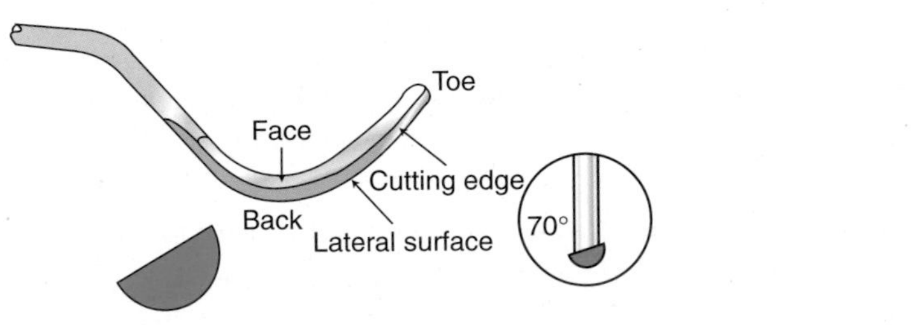

Toe
Face
Cutting edge
Back
Lateral surface
70°

INSTRUMENT

Area-Specific Curettes—Posterior evolve

FUNCTIONS

To scale and remove deposits from subgingival surfaces of posterior teeth
To use for root planning, periodontal debridement, and soft tissue curettage

CHARACTERISTICS

Two cutting edges (only lower cutting edge is used)
Blade—Rounded back and toe; at 70-degree angle to lower shank; types—Standard, rigid, extra rigid
Curvature of blade designed to adapt to specific teeth and surfaces
Range of size, shape, and bends in shank
Two bends in shank

Examples: 7/8, 9/10

Three bends in shank

Examples: 11/12, 13/14, 15/16, 17/18

Curette named by designer: Gracey, Kramer-Nevins, Turgeon

PRACTICE NOTE

Area-Specific Curettes—Posterior are used on hygiene and periodontal tray setups.

Area-Specific Curettes must be cleaned, bagged individually or bagged/wrapped in a tray setup, and then sterilized. A chemical/steam indicator device should be included in the wrapping.

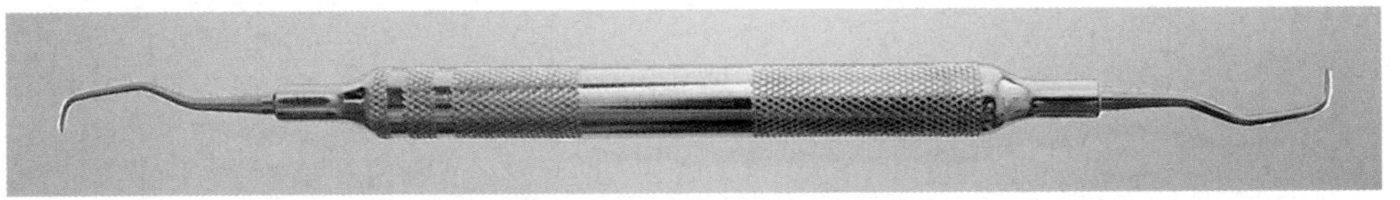

INSTRUMENT

Extended Area-Specific Curettes—Anterior

FUNCTION To scale and remove deposits in deep periodontal pockets 5 mm or deeper

CHARACTERISTICS
Two cutting edges (only lower cutting edge is used)
Blade at 70-degree angle to lower shank; types—Standard, rigid, extra rigid
Curvature of blade designed to adapt to anteriors
Terminal shank redesigned—3 mm longer than standard Area-Specific Curette
Manufacturer's trademark name usually follows 1/2, 3/4, 5/6 numbering system
Range of sizes—Commonly used types: 3/4, 5/6
Double-ended curettes packaged in sets
Curettes named by designer: Gracey 1/2

PRACTICE NOTE Extended Area-Specific Curettes—Anterior are used on hygiene and periodontal tray setups.

Ⓢ Extended Area-Specific Curettes must be cleaned, bagged individually or bagged/wrapped in a tray setup, and then sterilized. A chemical/steam indicator device should be included in the wrapping.

316

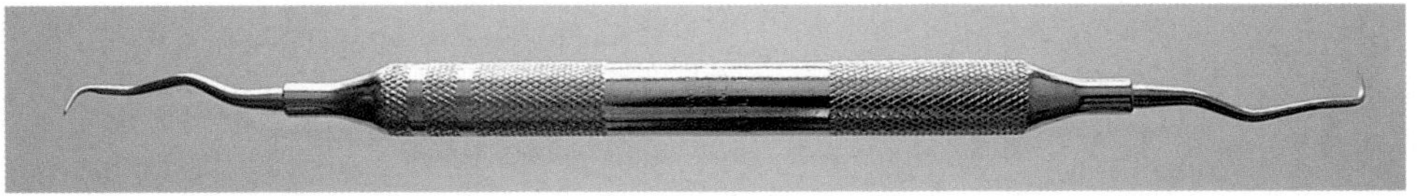

INSTRUMENT

Extended Area-Specific Curettes—Posterior

FUNCTION To scale and remove deposits in deep periodontal pockets (5 mm or deeper)

CHARACTERISTICS Two cutting edges (only lower cutting edge is used)
Blade at 70-degree angle to lower shank; types—Standard, rigid, extra rigid
Curvature of blade designed to adapt to premolars, molars
Terminal shank redesigned—3 mm longer than standard Area-Specific Curette
Range of sizes
Commonly used types: 11/12, 13/14, 15/16, 17/18
Double-ended curettes packaged in sets
Curettes named by designer: Gracey 11/12 Rigid, Gracey 11/12

PRACTICE NOTE Extended Area-Specific Curettes—Posterior are used on hygiene and periodontal tray setups.

S Extended Area-Specific Curettes must be cleaned, bagged individually or bagged/wrapped in a tray setup, and then sterilized. A chemical/steam indicator device should be included in the wrapping.

318

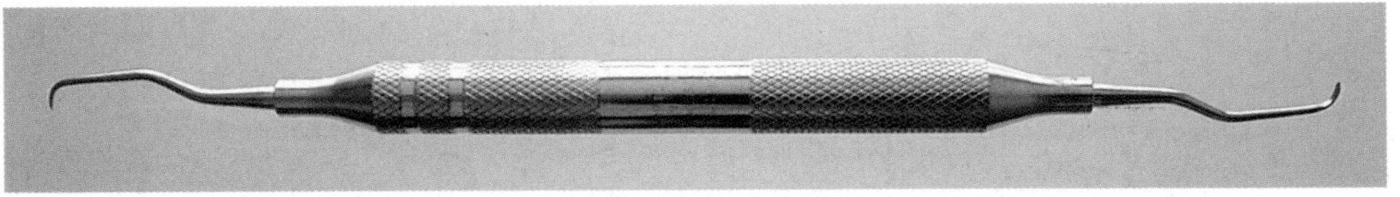

INSTRUMENT

Mini Extended Area-Specific Curettes—Anterior

FUNCTION To scale in deep periodontal pockets (5 mm)

CHARACTERISTICS
Blade redesigned to be half the length of Extended Area-Specific Curette
Designed for narrow roots, pockets, or furcations
Two cutting edges (only lower cutting edge is used)
Blade at 70-degree angle to lower shank; types—Standard, rigid, extra rigid
Curvature of blade designed to adapt to anteriors
Range of sizes
Manufacturer's trademark name usually follows 1/2, 3/4, 5/6 numbering system
Curettes named by designer: Gracey 1/2

PRACTICE NOTE Mini Extended Area-Specific Curettes—Anterior are used on hygiene and periodontal tray setups.

Mini Extended Area-Specific Curettes must be cleaned, bagged individually or bagged/wrapped in a tray setup, and then sterilized. A chemical/steam indicator device should be included in the wrapping.

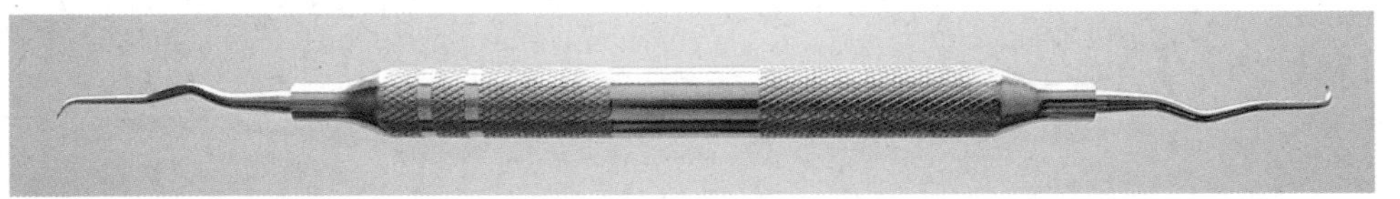

INSTRUMENT

Mini Extended Area-Specific Curettes—Posterior

FUNCTION To scale in deep periodontal pockets (5 mm)

CHARACTERISTICS Blade redesigned to be half the length of Extended Area-Specific Curette
Designed for narrow roots, pockets, or furcations
Two cutting edges (only lower cutting edge is used)
Blade at 70-degree angle to lower shank; types—Standard, rigid, extra rigid
Curvature of blade designed to adapt to premolars, molars
Range of size, shape, and bends in shank available
Two bends in shank

Examples: 7/8, 9/10

Three bends in shank

Examples: 11/12, 13/14, 15/16, 17/18

Curettes named by designer: Gracey 11/12, mini extender

PRACTICE NOTE Mini Extended Area-Specific Curettes—Posterior are used on hygiene and periodontal tray setups.

S Mini Extended Area-Specific Curettes must be cleaned, bagged Individually or bagged/wrapped in a tray setup, and then sterilized. A chemical/steam indicator device should be included in the wrapping.

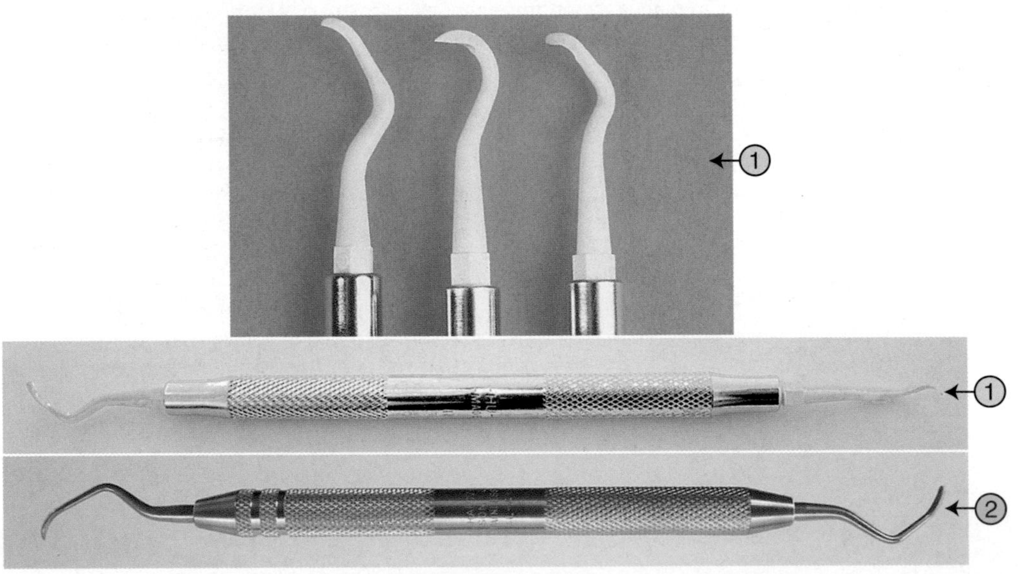
1
1
2

INSTRUMENT

Implant Scaler

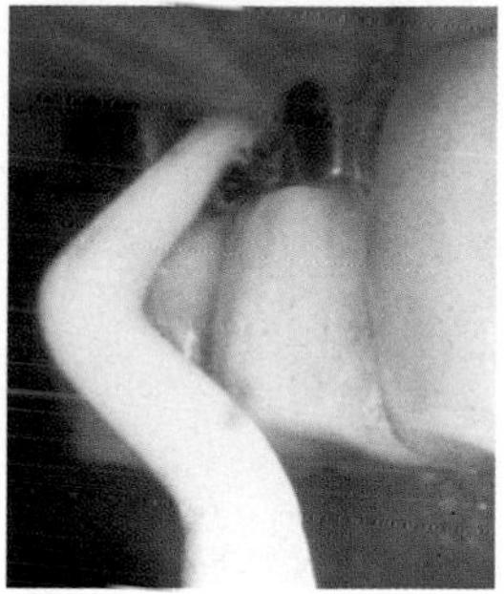

FUNCTION To remove deposits and stains from surface of implant

CHARACTERISTICS
① Disposable tips (each tip should be sterilized before use)
② Titanium-coated scaler
Different designs allow scaling without scratching of titanium implants
Some tips are made of Plasteel—a high-grade resin

PRACTICE NOTE Implants are used on hygiene and periodontal tray setups.

Ⓢ Handle and titanium-coated scaler must be cleaned, bagged individually or bagged/wrapped in a tray setup, and then sterilized. A chemical/steam indicator device should be included in the wrapping. Disposable scaler tip should be disposed of in a Sharps container.

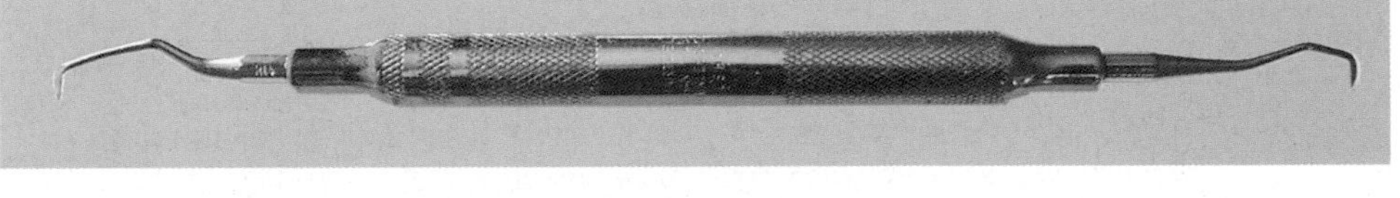

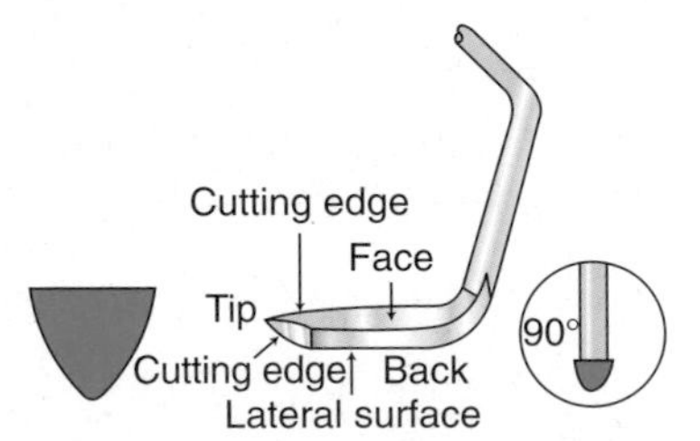
Cutting edge
Face
Tip
Cutting edge
Back
Lateral surface
90°

INSTRUMENT

Straight Sickle Scaler

FUNCTION To remove large amounts of deposits from supragingival surfaces

CHARACTERISTICS Two cutting edges on straight blade that ends in sharp point
Long, two bends in shank
Variety of sizes and angles
Single or double ended—Two ends may be shaped differently

PRACTICE NOTE Straight Sickle Scaler is used on hygiene and periodontal tray setups.

S Straight Sickle Scaler must be cleaned, bagged individually or bagged/wrapped in a tray setup, and then sterilized. A chemical/steam indicator device should be included in the wrapping.

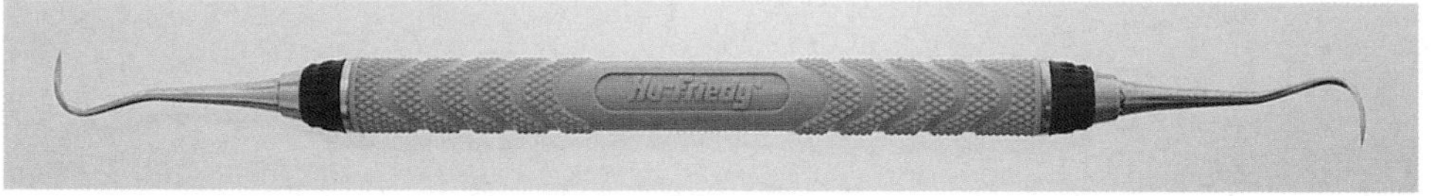
Hu-Friedy

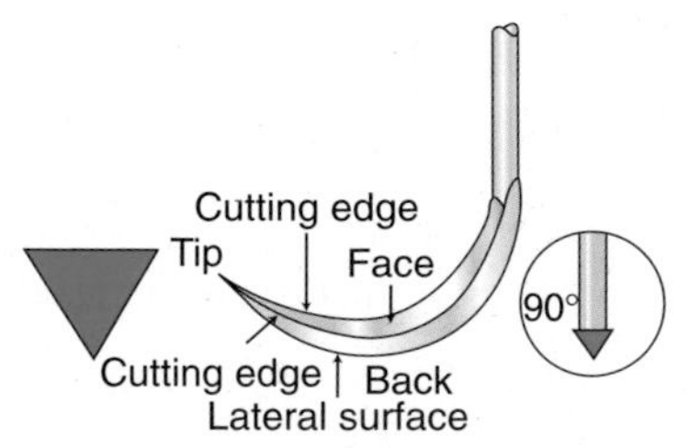
Cutting edge
Tip
Face
90°
Cutting edge
Back
Lateral surface

INSTRUMENT

Curved Sickle Scaler

FUNCTION To remove large amounts of deposits from supragingival surfaces

CHARACTERISTICS Two cutting edges on curved blade that ends in sharp point
Long, straight shank with one gentle bend
Variety of sizes and angles
Single or double ended—Two ends may be shaped differently

PRACTICE NOTE Curved Sickle Scaler is used on hygiene and periodontal tray setups.

S Curved Sickle Scaler must be cleaned, bagged individually or bagged/wrapped in a tray setup, and then sterilized. A chemical/steam indicator device should be included in the wrapping.

328

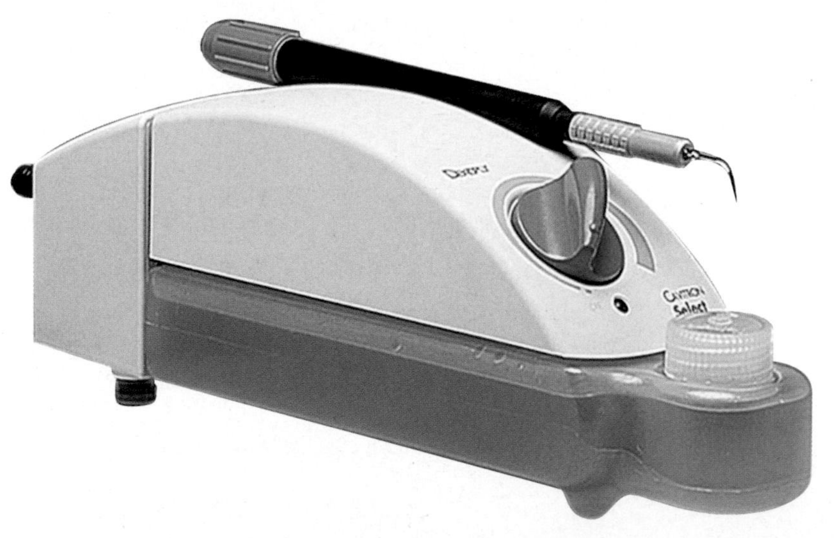

INSTRUMENT

Ultrasonic Scaling Unit (Power Scaler)

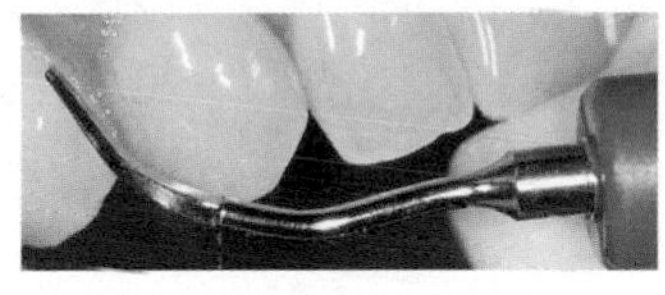

FUNCTION To use with water-cooled ultrasonic tips vibrating at high frequency

CHARACTERISTICS Ultra-high frequency sound waves convert mechanical energy into vibrations (frequency ranges from 18 to 50 kHz).

Some units have self-contained water reservoirs (pictured).

Some units have an additional air/water/sodium bicarbonate slurry polishing system to remove extrinsic stains and dental plaque.

Variety of sizes and designs are available.

PRACTICE NOTE Ultrasonic Scaling Unit/Power Scaler is used during a routine prophylaxis appointment or for other appointments for root planning.

Ⓢ Barriers should be used for Power Scaler. Refer to the manufacturer's recommendation for disinfecting the unit. Power Scaler inserts must be cleaned, bagged individually or bagged/wrapped in a tray setup, and then sterilized. A chemical/steam indicator device should be included in the wrapping.

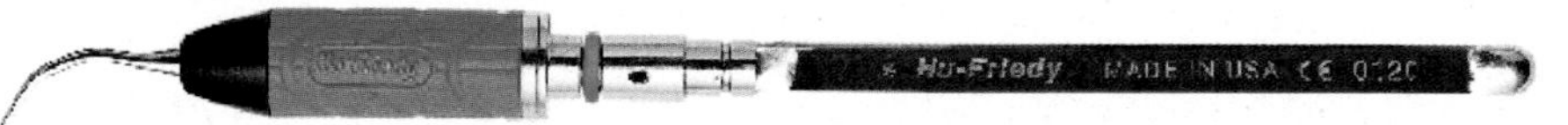
Hu-Friedy MADE IN USA CE 0120

INSTRUMENT

Ultrasonic Scaler Instrument Tip—Supragingival

FUNCTIONS

To remove supragingival calculus on teeth
To remove bacterial plaque from periodontal pockets
To remove heavy debris and stains from teeth
To remove excess cement from orthodontic bands after cementation and after band removal

CHARACTERISTICS

Ultrasonic Scaler Instrument Tip—Supragingival is inserted into the tubing on the Ultrasonic Scaling Unit
Available in different lengths (called stacks): 25 kHz or 30 kHz, depending on unit
Water-cooled inserts (water systems vary with internal or external water delivery)
Variety of shapes, sizes, and designs, depending on designated and varying grips

Example: Original Prophy
Tip style: Finely beveled internal water delivery tube

PRACTICE NOTE

Ultrasonic Scale Tip—Supragingival is used on hygiene and periodontal tray setups.
These tips are also known as ultrasonic inserts.

S Ultrasonic Scaler Tip—Supragingival must be cleaned, bagged individually or bagged/wrapped in a tray setup, and then sterilized. A chemical/steam indicator device should be included in the wrapping.

332

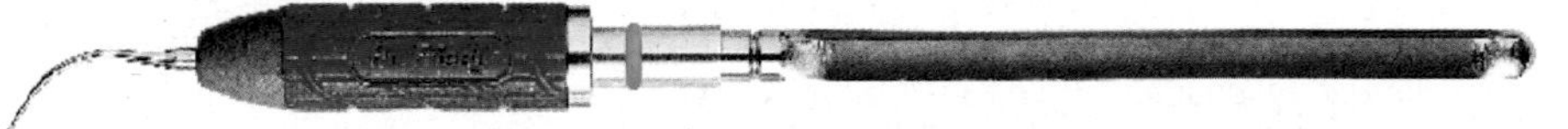

INSTRUMENT

Ultrasonic Scaler Instrument Tip—Subgingival

FUNCTIONS

To remove subgingival calculus on teeth
To remove bacterial plaque from periodontal pockets

CHARACTERISTICS

Ultrasonic Scaler Instrument Tip—Subgingival is inserted into the tubing on the Ultrasonic Scaling Unit
Available in different lengths (called stacks): 25 kHz or 30 kHz, depending on unit
Water-cooled inserts (water systems vary with internal or external water delivery)
Variety of shapes, sizes, and designs, depending on designated area and varying grips

Example: After Five design
Tip style: Finely beveled internal water delivery tube

PRACTICE NOTE

Ultrasonic Scaler Tip—Subgingival is used on hygiene and periodontal tray setups.
These tips are also known as ultrasonic inserts.

S Ultrasonic Scaler Tip—Subgingival must be cleaned, bagged individually or bagged/wrapped in a tray setup, and then sterilized. A chemical/steam indicator device should be included in the wrapping.

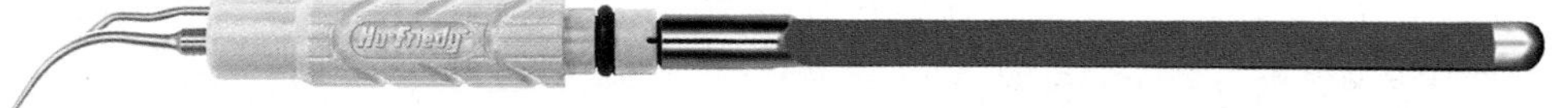
Hu-Friedy

INSTRUMENT

Ultrasonic Scaler Instrument Tip—Furcation

FUNCTION To remove bacterial plaque from furcation areas

CHARACTERISTICS Ultrasonic Scaler Instrument Tip—Furcation is inserted into the tubing on the Ultrasonic Scaling Unit
Available in different lengths (called stacks): 25 kHz or 30 kHz, depending on unit
Water-cooled inserts (water systems vary with internal or external water delivery)
Variety of shapes, sizes, and designs, depending on designated area and varying grips
Example: Furcation Plus design
Tip style: 0.8-mm ball end adapts to furcation, external water delivery tube

PRACTICE NOTE Ultrasonic Scaler Tip—Furcation is used on hygiene and periodontal tray setups.
These tips are also known as ultrasonic inserts.

S Ultrasonic Scaler Tip—Furcation must be cleaned, bagged individually or bagged/wrapped in a tray setup, and then sterilized. A chemical/steam indicator device should be included in the wrapping.

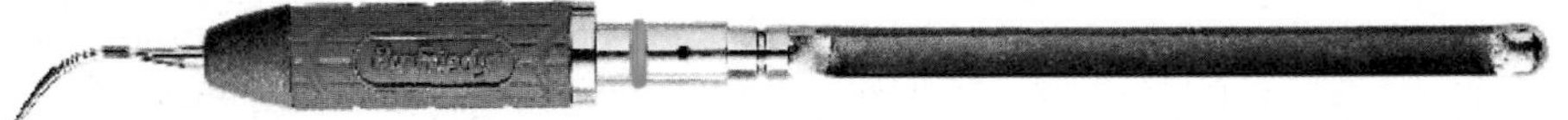
Hu-Friedy

INSTRUMENT

Ultrasonic Scaler Instrument Tip—Universal

FUNCTION To remove bacterial plaque and general deposits

CHARACTERISTICS Ultrasonic Scaler Instrument Tip—Universal is inserted into the tubing on the Ultrasonic Scaling Unit
Available in different lengths (called stacks): 25 kHz or 30 kHz, depending on unit
Water-cooled Inserts (water systems vary with internal or external water delivery)
Variety of shapes, sizes, and designs, depending on designated area and varying grips

Example: Streamline design

Tip style: Water delivered directly from base of tip, eliminating need for external water system; efficient at low settings

PRACTICE NOTES Ultrasonic Scaler Tip—Universal is used on hygiene and periodontal tray setups.
These tips are also known as ultrasonic inserts.

Ⓢ Ultrasonic Scaler Tip—Universal must be cleaned, bagged/wrapped individually or bagged/wrapped in a tray setup, and then sterilized with a chemical indicator device included in the wrapping.

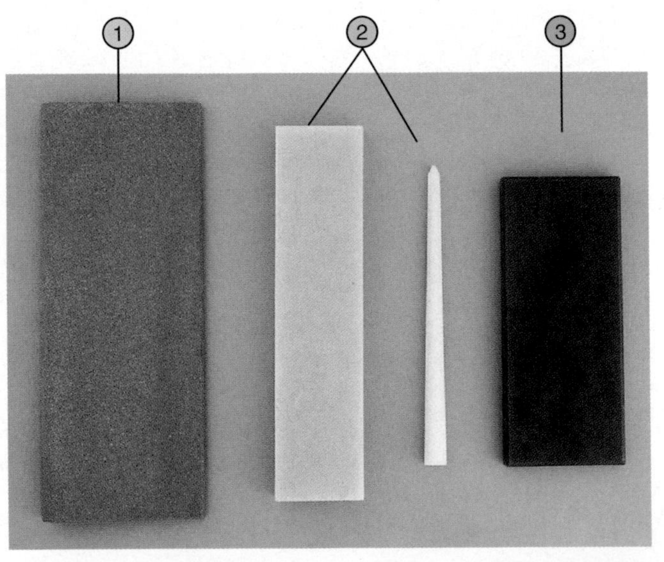
1
2
3

INSTRUMENT

Sharpening Stones evolve

FUNCTION To sharpen scalers and curettes

CHARACTERISTICS Types of Stones:

① India stones—Remove the most metal when used and should be followed with an Arkansas or ceramic stone

② Arkansas stones—Provide a polished edge (flat and cone-shaped pictured)

③ Ceramic stones—Provide a polished edge and do not require lubrication

PRACTICE NOTE Sharpening Stones are used on hygiene and periodontal tray setups.

Ⓢ Sharpening Stones must be cleaned, bagged individually or bagged/wrapped in a tray setup, and then sterilized. A chemical/steam indicator device should be included in the wrapping.

340

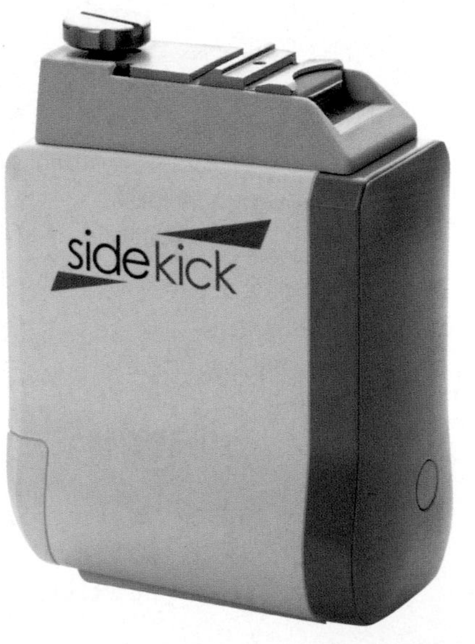

INSTRUMENT

Battery-Operated Sharpening Device

FUNCTION To sharpen scalers and curettes

CHARACTERISTICS Stone moves underneath a stainless-steel guideplate, which puts the blade at factory angles.
Sharpener has a power device with instrument guide channels and a vertical backstop to help control blade angulation.
Pictured: Sidekick Sharpener

PRACTICE NOTE Battery-Operated Sharpening Device should be used with sterile scalers and curettes, and then instruments resterilized after sharpening.

Ⓢ Barrier wrap; disinfect or sterilize certain parts of equipment according to the manufacturer's recommendation. Sterilized instruments should be used for sharpening and then must be cleaned, bagged individually or bagged/wrapped in a tray setup, and then sterilized. A chemical/steam indicator device should be included in the wrapping.

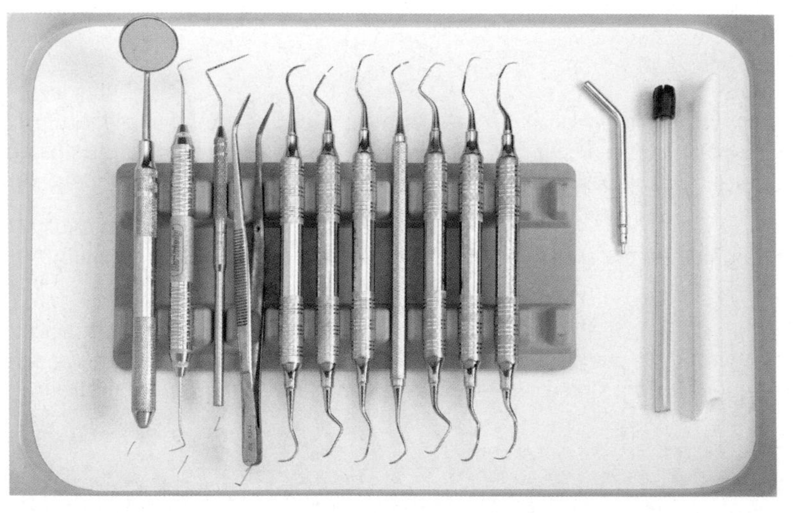

TRAY SETUP

Hygiene

FROM LEFT TO RIGHT

Mouth mirror, explorer, periodontal probe, cotton forceps, curved sickle scaler, 4L/4R universal posterior, universal Langer 1/2, Ratcliff 3/4, Gracey 7/8, Gracey 11/12, Gracey 13/14, air/water syringe tip, low-volume saliva ejector, high-volume evacuation (HVE) tip

Ⓢ Refer to each picture for correct procedure for instrument sterilization or disposal of instrument or material.

Refer to other chapters for additional instruments on this tray setup that are not included in this chapter.

344

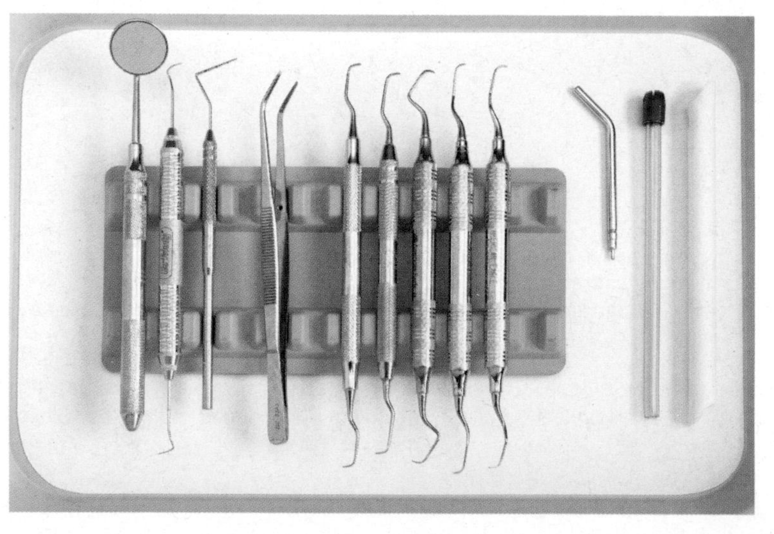

TRAY SETUP

Root Planing

FROM LEFT TO RIGHT

Mouth mirror, explorer, periodontal probe, cotton forceps, Gracey 1/2, Gracey 3/4, Gracey 7/8, Gracey 11/12, Gracey 13/14, air/water syringe tip, low-volume saliva ejector, high-volume evacuation (HVE) tip

S Refer to each individual picture for correct procedure for instrument sterilization or disposal of instrument or material.

Refer to other chapters for additional instruments on this tray setup.

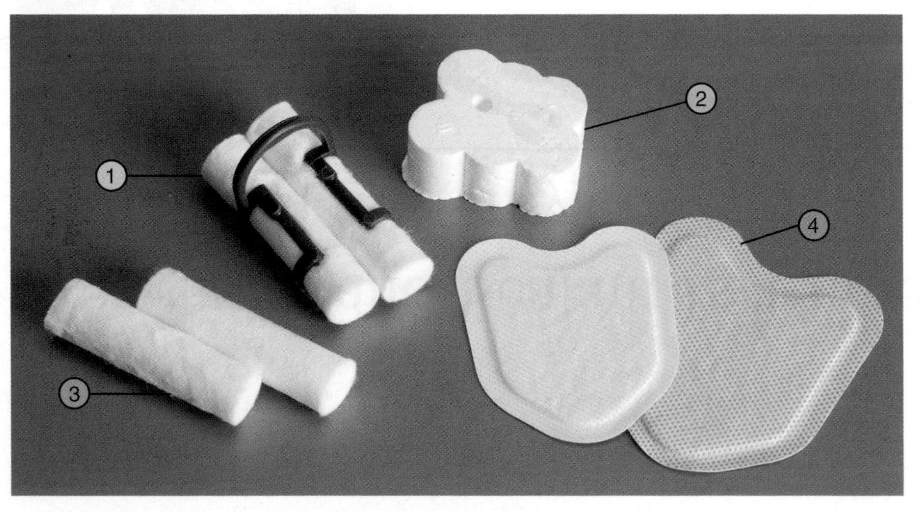
1
2
3
4

INSTRUMENT

Disposables

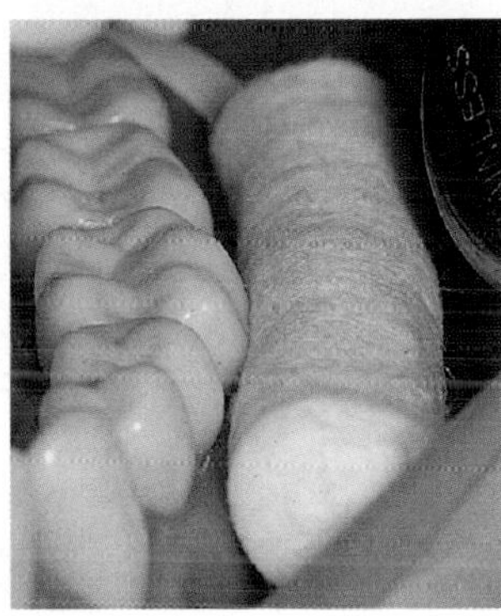

FUNCTIONS To use with all types of dental procedures
To use when area in the mouth needs to stay dry

CHARACTERISTICS

① Cotton roll holder for mandibular arch
One cotton roll is placed on the buccal side of the teeth, and the other is placed on the lingual side of the teeth.

② Disposable bite block

③ Cotton Rolls

④ Dry Aids for keeping mouth dry
Dry Aid is placed on the buccal mucosa—inside the cheek—opposite the maxillary second molar near the Stensen's duct to absorb saliva originating from the parotid gland.

PRACTICE NOTE Disposables are used on sealant and other restorative tray setups.

Ⓢ All disposables should be disposed of in the garbage. Single use only.

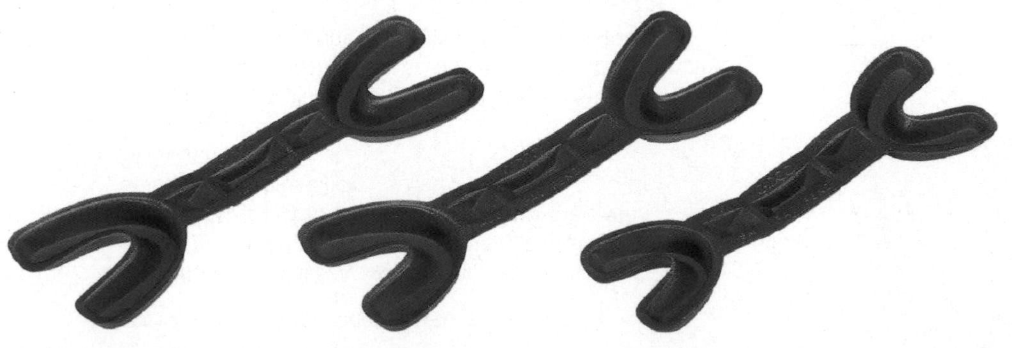

INSTRUMENT

Fluoride Trays—Disposable

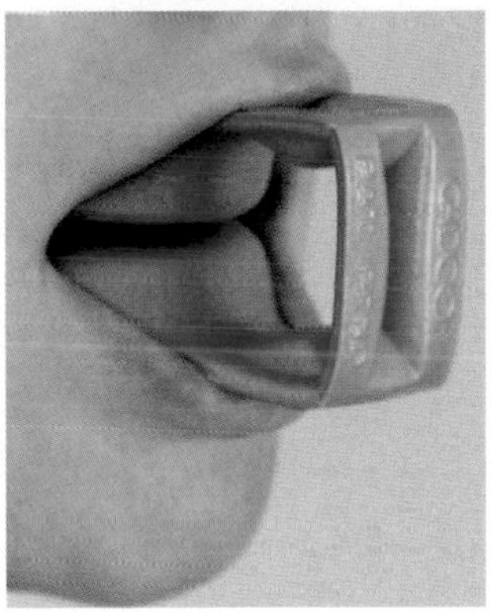

FUNCTIONS To fill trays with fluoride
To help prevent decay by mineralizing the teeth

CHARACTERISTIC Variety of disposable trays and fluoride available

PRACTICE NOTE Fluoride treatment is usually given to children at their 6-month check up appointment.
Fluoride Trays are used on fluoride tray setups.

Ⓢ Fluoride Trays should be disposed of in the garbage. Single use only.

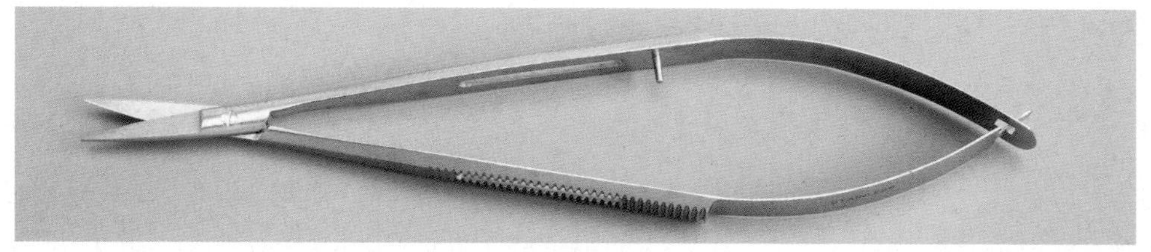

INSTRUMENT

Scissors—Short Blade

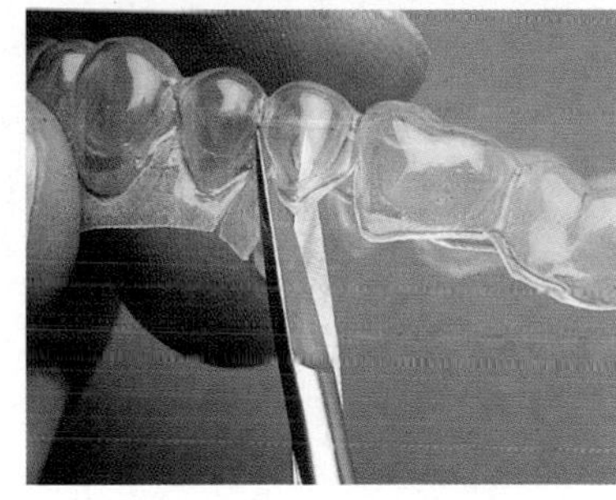

FUNCTION To precisely cut material especially for bleaching trays.

CHARACTERISTIC Fine cutting blade

PRACTICE NOTE Short blade scissors are used on bleaching tray setup and on other operative tray setups.

Ⓢ Scissors—Short Blade must be cleaned, bagged individually or bagged/wrapped in a tray setup, and then sterilized. A chemical/steam indicator device should be included in the wrapping. Hinged instruments should be processed open and unlocked.

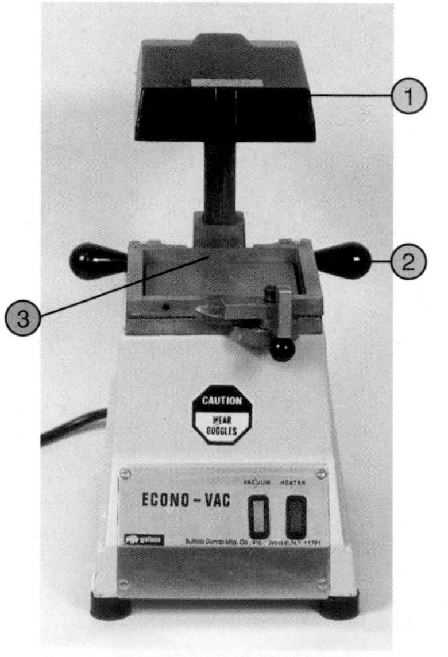
1
2
3
CAUTION
WEAR GOGGLES
ECONO - VAC
VACUUM
HEATER
Buffalo Dental Mfg. Co., Inc. Syosset, N.Y. 11791

INSTRUMENT

Vacuum Form

FUNCTIONS

To make bleaching trays, custom temporary crowns, night guards, orthodontic positioners, and mouth guards
To heat plastic square for bleaching trays
To vacuum form the plastic tray over the patient's model to make the bleaching tray

CHARACTERISTICS

① Heating element that softens the thermoplastic resin
② Handles to pull down plastic
③ Vacuum to mold plastic to tray after it is pulled down

PRACTICE NOTE

Block-out material is light cured on the facial side of the model before bleaching trays are made with the vacuum former.

Ⓢ The manufacturer's recommendation should be followed for disinfecting the Vacuum Form.

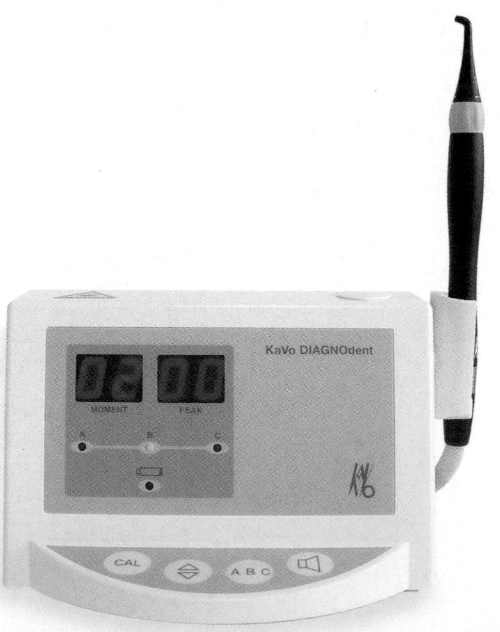
KaVo DIAGNOdent
MOMENT
PEAK
A
B
C
CAL
A B C

INSTRUMENT

Diagnodent

FUNCTION

To aid in the detection of caries within the tooth structure

To detect caries in the structure of the tooth prior to placing sealants

CHARACTERISTICS

Diagnodent accurately diagnoses occlusal caries.

Laser detects the caries in the tooth, and a digital display is seen on the screen.

PRACTICE NOTE

Diagnodent is used with sealant and occasionally restorative tray setups.

Ⓢ The manufacturer's recommendation should be followed for disinfecting Diagnodent. Barriers should be placed on wand that is used intraorally.

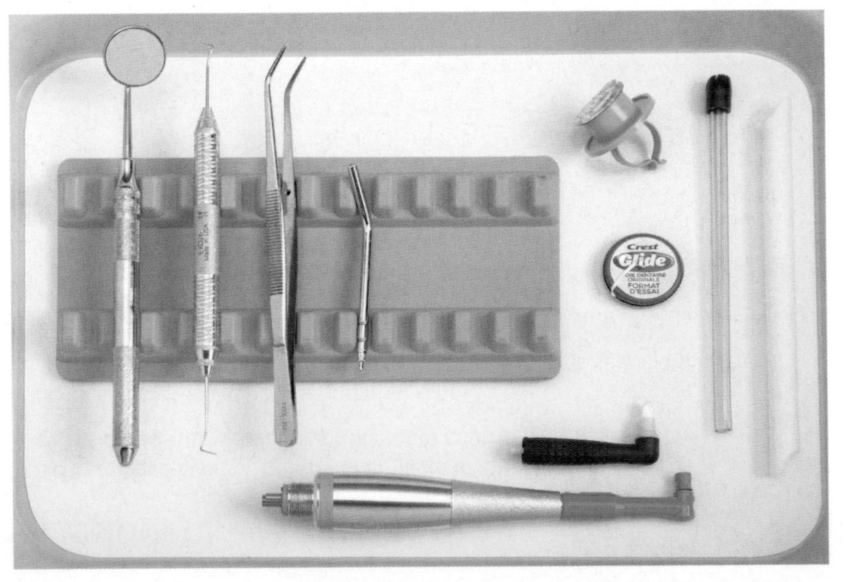
Crest
Glide
OIE DENTAIRE
ORIGINALE
FORMAT
D'ESSAI

TRAY SETUP

Prophylaxis Polishing

TOP—LEFT TO RIGHT

Mouth mirror, explorer, cotton forceps, air/water syringe tip, polishing agent without fluoride, dental floss, low-volume saliva ejector, high-volume evacuator (HVE) tip

BOTTOM—LEFT TO RIGHT

Prophy slow-speed handpiece with disposable prophy angle attachment with polishing cup, disposable prophy angle attachment with tapered brush

Ⓢ Refer to each picture for correct procedure for instrument sterilization or disposal of instrument or material.

Refer to other chapters for additional instruments on this tray setup that are not included in this chapter.

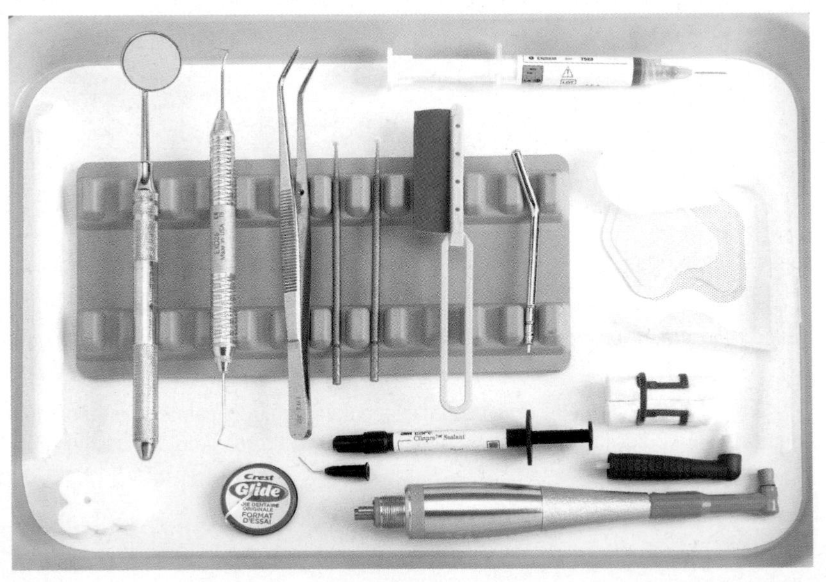
Crest
Glide
SOIE DENTAIRE ORIGINALE
FORMAT D'ESSAI
Clinpro™ Sealant

TRAY SETUP

Sealant

VERY TOP OF TRAY
Syringe with etchant

TOP ROW—LEFT TO RIGHT
High-volume evacuator tip (HVE), mouth mirror, explorer, cotton forceps, microbrushes, disposable articulating paper holder and articulating paper, air/water syringe tip, dry aids, low-volume evacuator for mandibular, cotton rolls in disposable holder

BOTTOM ROW—LEFT TO RIGHT
Disposable bite block, dental floss, sealant syringe and syringe tip, prophy slow-speed handpiece with disposable prophy angle attachment with polishing cup, disposable prophy angle attachment with tapered brush

S Refer to each picture for correct procedure for instrument sterilization or disposal of instrument or material

Refer to other chapters for additional instruments on this tray setup that are not included in this chapter.

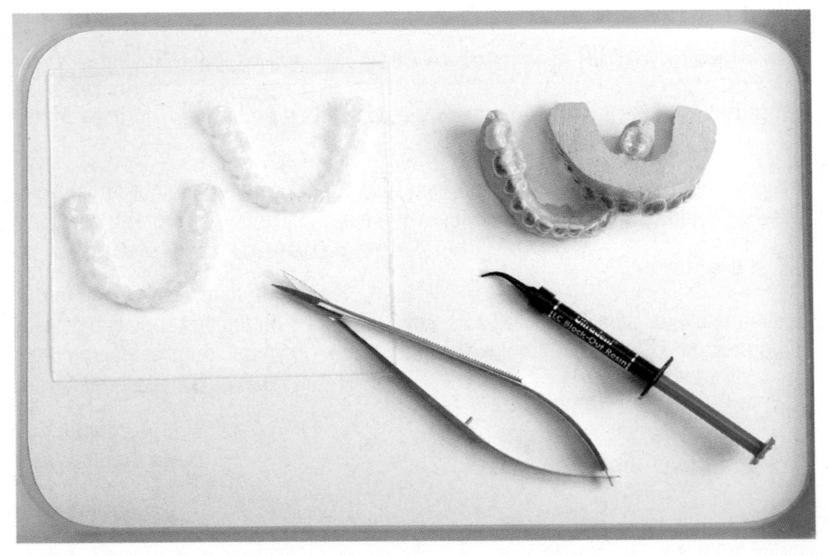
Ultradent
LC Block-Out Resin

TRAY SETUP

Bleaching

LEFT TO RIGHT

Thermoplastic resin square, bleaching trays (maxillary and mandibular), short-blade scissors, block-out material for models, bleaching trays on maxillary and mandibular models

Ⓢ Refer to each picture for correct procedure for instrument sterilization or disposal of instrument or material.

Refer to other chapters for additional instruments on this tray setup that are not included in this chapter.

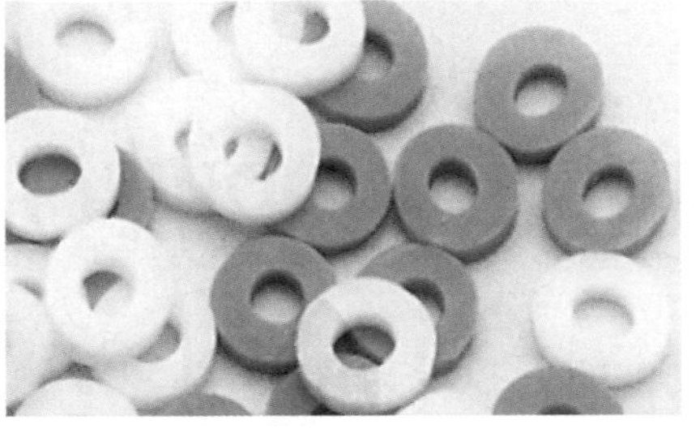

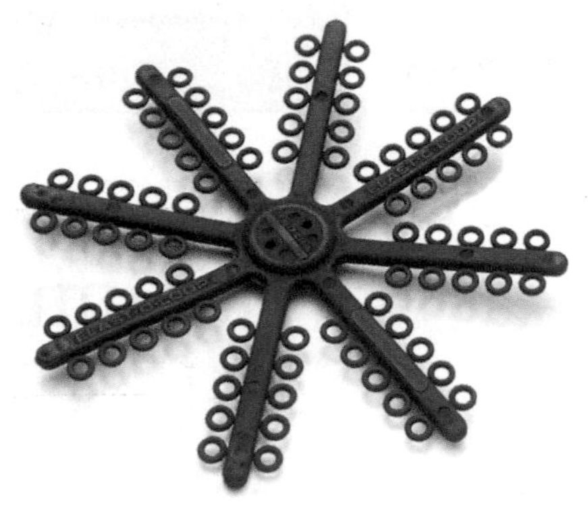

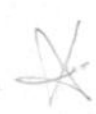

INSTRUMENT

Elastic Separators evolve

FUNCTIONS To separate teeth prior to banding a tooth for orthodontic braces
To place around contact area of tooth

CHARACTERISTIC Elastomeric separators—Various sizes for different contact areas

PRACTICE NOTE Separators are placed on orthodontic separating tray setup

Ⓢ Elastomeric Separators should be disposed of in the garbage. Single use only.

368

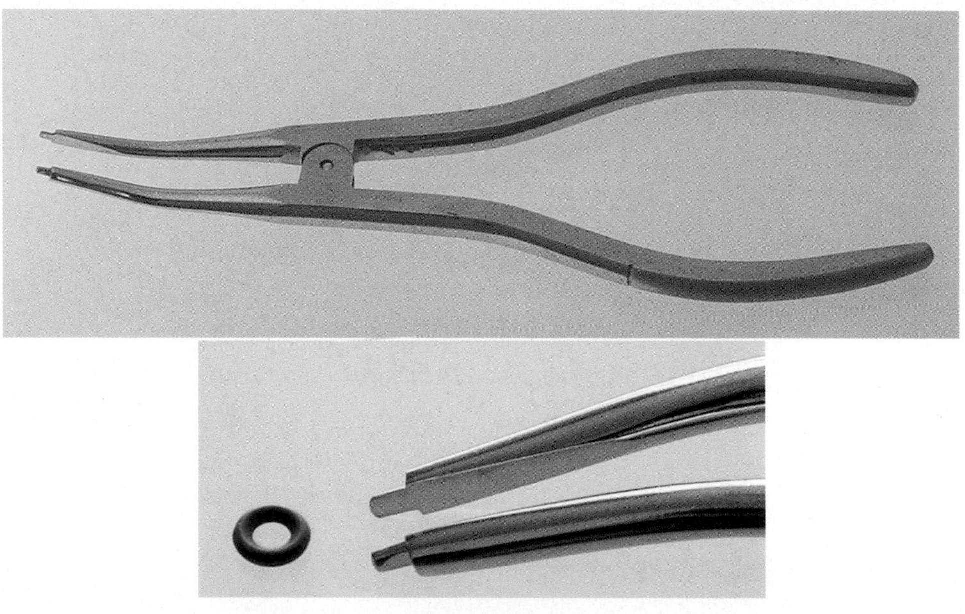

INSTRUMENT

Elastic Separating Pliers evolve

FUNCTION To grip and place separators around contact area of tooth

CHARACTERISTIC Single ended

PRACTICE NOTE Elastic Separating Pliers is only used on the orthodontic tray setup.

Ⓢ Elastic Separating Pliers must be cleaned, bagged individually or bagged/wrapped in a tray setup, and then sterilized. A chemical/steam indicator device should be included in the wrapping. Hinged instruments should be processed open and unlocked.

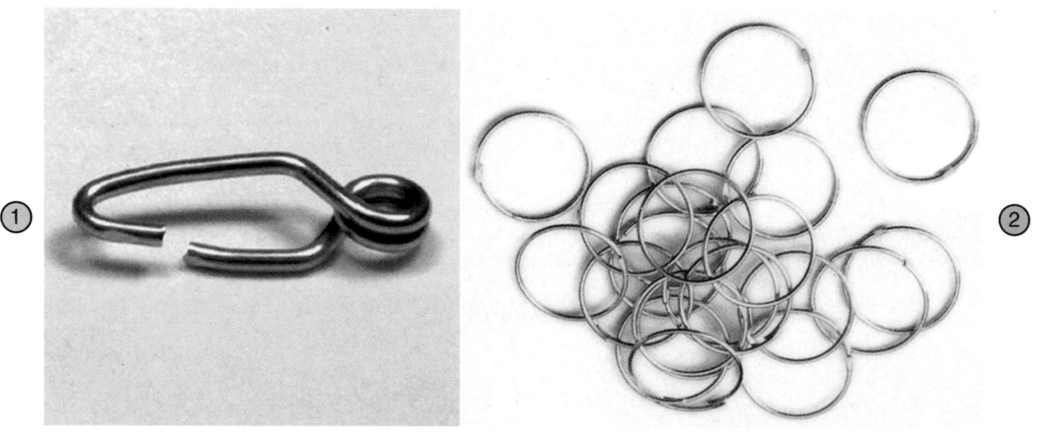
1
2

INSTRUMENT

Steel Spring Separators/Brass Wire Separators evolve

FUNCTIONS To separate teeth prior to banding a tooth for orthodontic braces
To place around contact area of tooth

CHARACTERISTICS
① Steel Spring Separators—various sizes for different size contact areas
② Brass Wire Separators—placed around contact and twisted clockwise, then cut 3 mm and tucked in order to not impinge on tissue or occlusion
Placed with orthodontic hemostat or bird beak pliers

PRACTICE NOTE Separators are placed on orthodontic separating tray setup.

Ⓢ Steel Spring Separators and Brass Wire Separators should be disposed of in a Sharps container. Single use only.

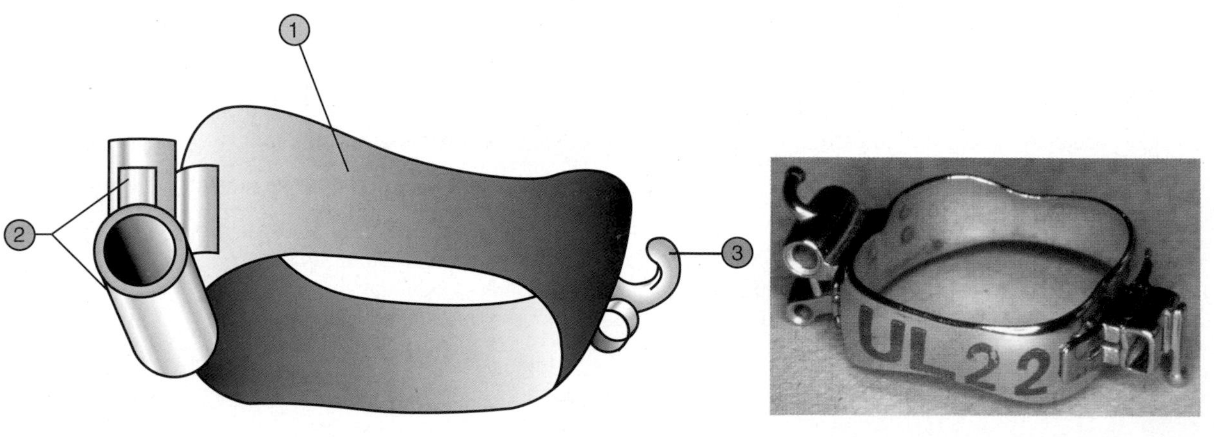
1
2
3
UL22

INSTRUMENT

Orthodontic Band with Bracket and Tubing

FUNCTIONS

To fit and cement or bond band around the middle third of the coronal part of the tooth
To hold orthodontic arch wire in place (arch wire moves the teeth)
To secure headgear in tubing on band

CHARACTERISTICS

① Band
② Tubing:
Arch wire tube (top)—holds arch wire in place
Headgear tube (bottom)—holds headgear in place
③ Brackets on band (cleats)—holds arch wire in place

PRACTICE NOTE

Orthodontic Band is used on orthodontic banding tray setup.

Ⓢ Orthodontic Band should be disposed of in a Sharps container. Single use only.

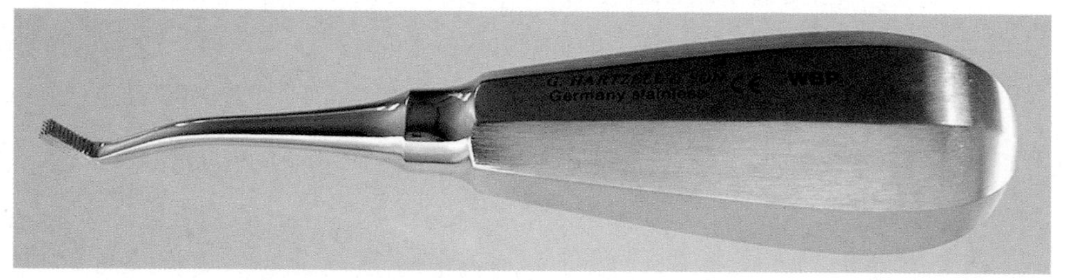
G. HARTZELL & SON
Germany stainless
WBP

INSTRUMENT

Band Pusher

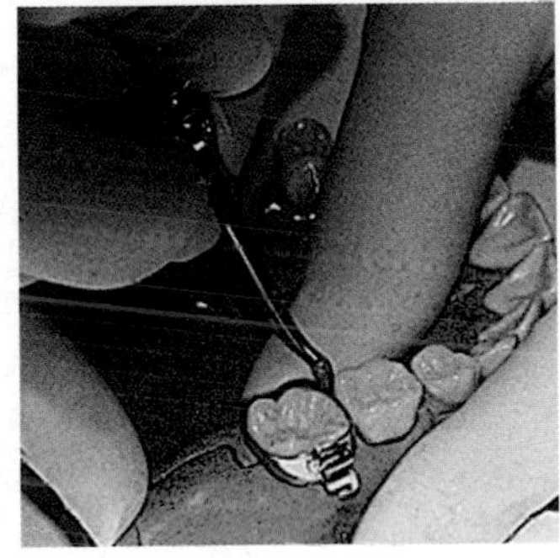

FUNCTION To push orthodontic bands into place during try-in and cementing phases

CHARACTERISTIC Single or double ended

PRACTICE NOTE Band Pusher is only used on the orthodontic tray setup.

Ⓢ Band Pusher must be cleaned, bagged individually or bagged/wrapped in a tray setup, and then sterilized. A chemical/steam indicator device should be included in the wrapping.

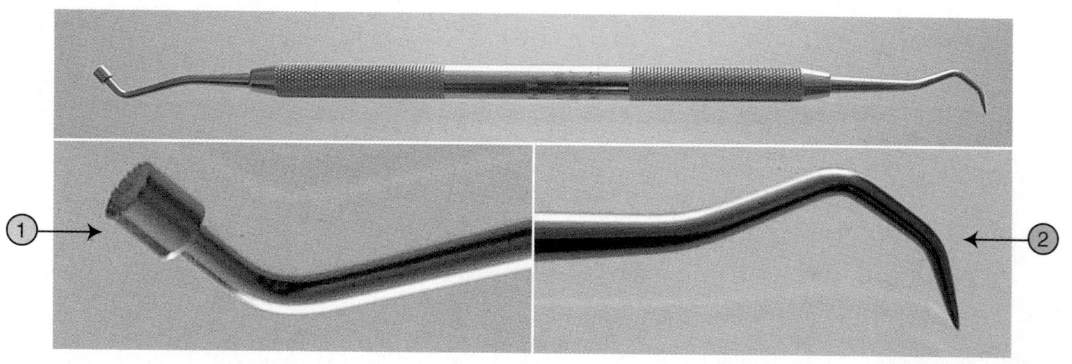
1
2

INSTRUMENT

Band Pusher or Plugger with Scaler

FUNCTIONS

To seat or place orthodontic bands during try-in and cementing phases
To remove excess material after cementation or bonding of bands

CHARACTERISTICS

Double ended:

① Band Pusher or Plugger
② Scaler

PRACTICE NOTE

Band Pusher with Scaler is only used on the orthodontic tray setup.

Ⓢ Band Pusher or Plugger with Scaler must be cleaned, bagged individually or bagged/wrapped in a tray setup, and then sterilized. A chemical/steam indicator device should be included in the wrapping.

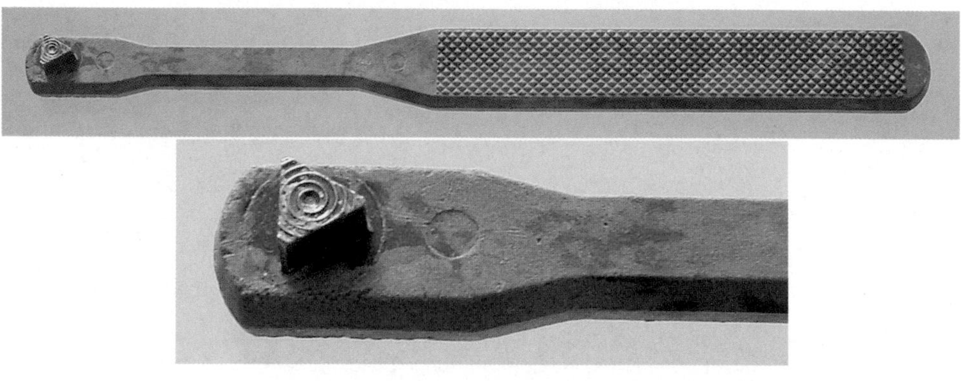

INSTRUMENT

Band Seater—Bite Stick

FUNCTION To assist seating or placing of orthodontic bands for try-in or cementing phase

CHARACTERISTICS Single ended
Available in square tip or triangle tip (pictured)

PRACTICE NOTES The patient bites down on the end of the instrument to apply pressure to seat the band.
Band Seater—Bite Stick is only used on the orthodontic tray setup.

Ⓢ Band Seater—Bite Stick must be cleaned, bagged individually or bagged/wrapped in a tray setup, and then sterilized. A chemical/steam indicator device should be included in the wrapping.

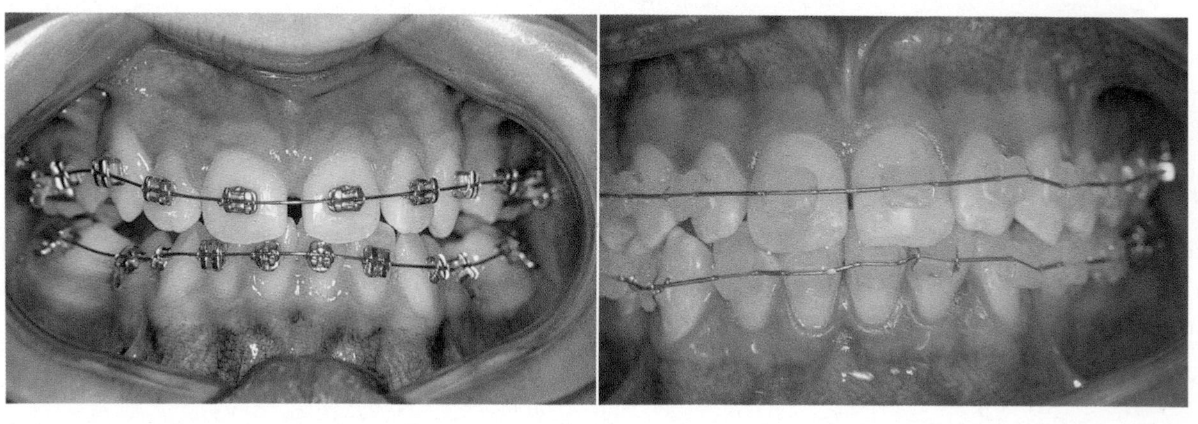

INSTRUMENT

Orthodontic Bracket

FUNCTION To hold orthodontic arch wire in place (arch wire moves the teeth)

CHARACTERISTICS Band is bonded to tooth
Brackets (cleats)—holds arch wire in place
Many different types available (pictured: stainless-steel [left] and ceramic [right] brackets)

PRACTICE NOTE Orthodontic Brackets are used on orthodontic bonding tray setup.

Orthodontic Brackets should be disposed of in a Sharps container. Single use only.

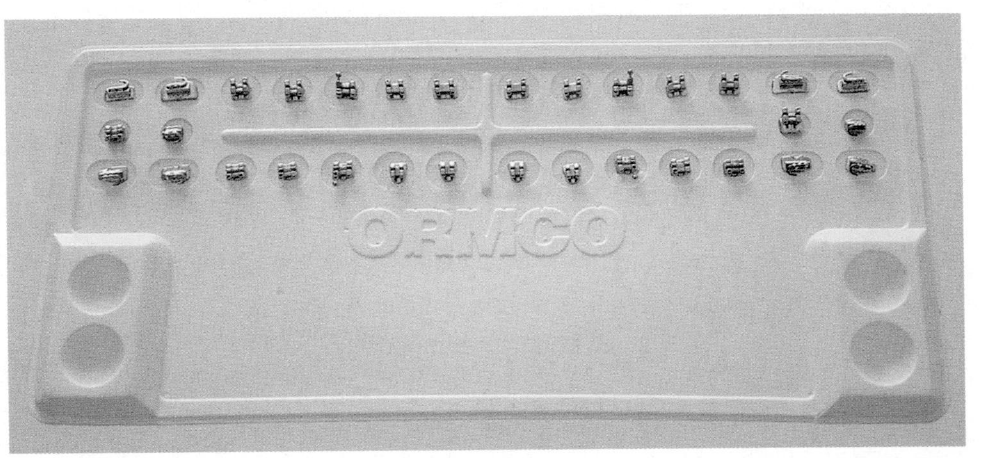
ORMCO

INSTRUMENT

Bracket Placement Card

FUNCTION To place each bracket and/or band on card according to tooth placement in mouth

CHARACTERISTIC Tape on card holds brackets in place before they are bonded to teeth.

PRACTICE NOTE Bracket Placement Card is only used on the orthodontic tray setup.

Ⓢ Bracket Placement Card should be disposed of in the garbage. Single use only.

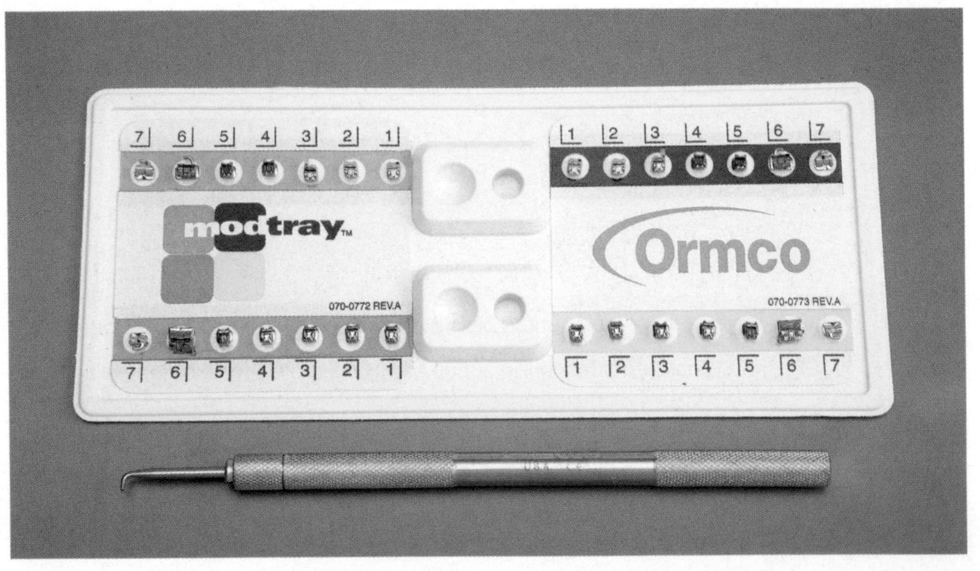
modtray™
Ormco
070-0772 REV.A
070-0773 REV.A

INSTRUMENT

Bracket Placement Card for Damon Self-Ligating Brackets with Self-Ligating Instrument

FUNCTIONS To place each bracket on card according to tooth placement in mouth
Instrument—To close bracket around arch wire; ligature tie not needed

CHARACTERISTIC Tape on card holds brackets in place before they are bonded to teeth.

PRACTICE NOTE Bracket Placement Card and Self-Ligating Instrument are used only on orthodontic bonding bracket tray setup.

S Bracket Placement Card should be disposed of in the garbage. Single use only. Self-Ligating Instrument must be cleaned, bagged individually or bagged/wrapped in a tray setup, and then sterilized. A chemical/steam indicator device should be included in the wrapping.

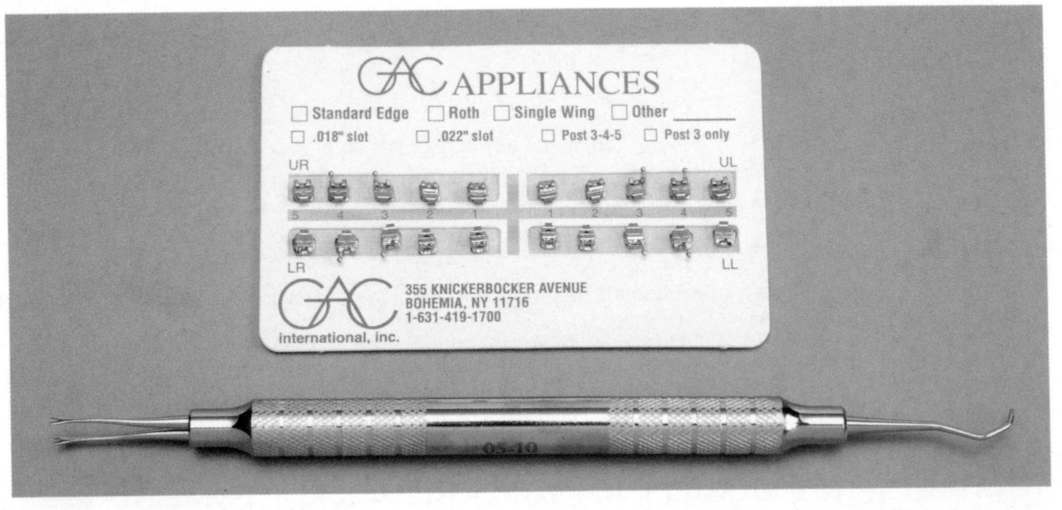

GAC APPLIANCES
Standard Edge
Roth
Single Wing
Other
.018" slot
.022" slot
Post 3-4-5
Post 3 only
UR
UL
5 4 3 2 1
1 2 3 4 5
LR
LL
355 KNICKERBOCKER AVENUE
BOHEMIA, NY 11716
1-631-419-1700
GAC international, inc.
OS-10

INSTRUMENT

Bracket Placement Card for GAC Self-Ligating Brackets with Self-Ligating Instrument

FUNCTIONS To place each bracket on card according to tooth placement in mouth
Instrument—To close bracket around arch wire; ligature tie not needed

CHARACTERISTIC Tape on card holds brackets in place before they are bonded to teeth.

PRACTICE NOTE Bracket Placement Card and Self-Ligating Instrument are used only on orthodontic bonding bracket tray setup.

Ⓢ Bracket Placement Card should be disposed of in the garbage. Single use only. Self-Ligating Instrument must be cleaned, bagged individually or bagged/wrapped in a tray setup, and then sterilized. A chemical/steam indicator device should be included in the wrapping.

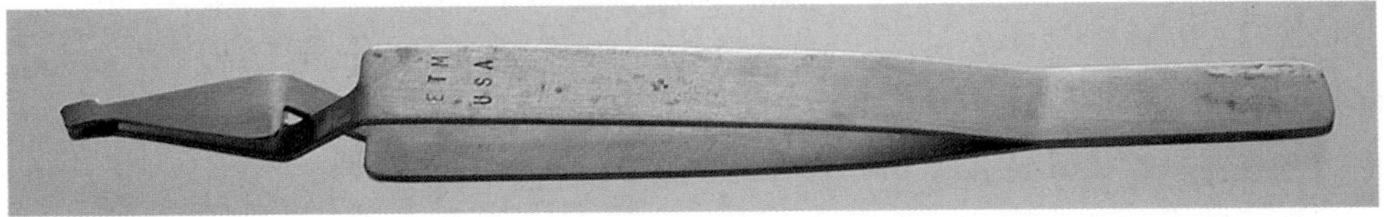
ETM
USA

INSTRUMENT

Anterior Bracket Placement Pliers

FUNCTIONS To hold and carry bracket by placing tip of pliers into slot of bracket
To place bracket on tooth for bonding

CHARACTERISTIC Range of sizes

PRACTICE NOTE Anterior Bracket Placement Pliers is only used on the orthodontic tray setup.

Ⓢ Anterior Bracket Placement Pliers must be cleaned, bagged individually or bagged/wrapped in a tray setup, and then sterilized. A chemical/steam indicator device should be included in the wrapping.

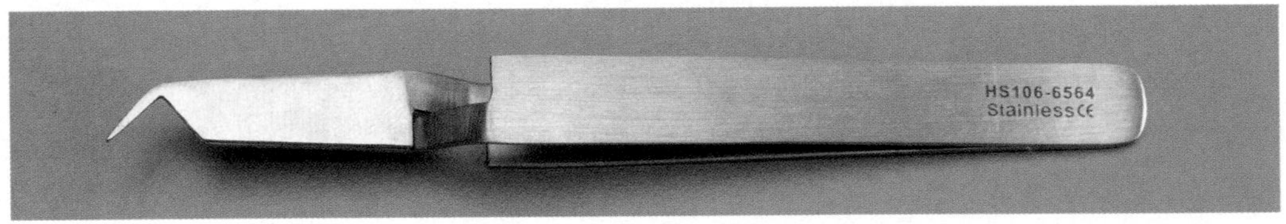
HS106-6564
Stainless CE

INSTRUMENT

Posterior Bracket Placement Pliers

FUNCTIONS To hold and carry bracket by placing tip of pliers into slot of bracket
To place bracket on tooth for bonding

CHARACTERISTIC Range of sizes

PRACTICE NOTE Posterior Bracket Placement Pliers is only used on the orthodontic tray setup.

Ⓢ Posterior Bracket Placement Pliers must be cleaned, bagged individually or bagged/wrapped in a tray setup, and then sterilized. A chemical/steam indicator device should be included in the wrapping.

392

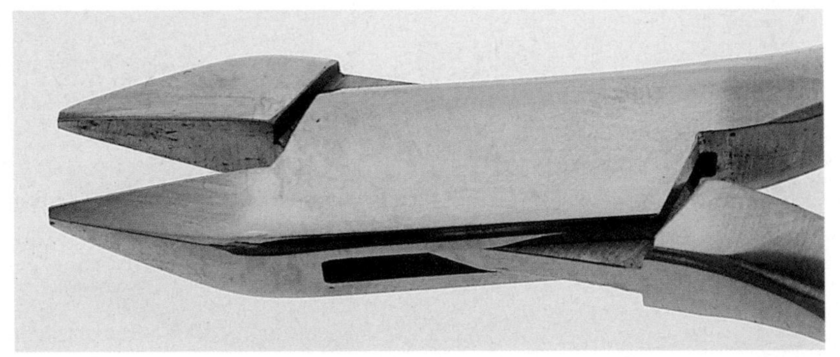

INSTRUMENT

Arch-Bending Pliers

FUNCTION To bend arch wires

CHARACTERISTIC Variety of styles, depending on type of arch wire used—Round, square, or rectangular

PRACTICE NOTE Arch-Bending Pliers is only used on the orthodontic tray setup.

S Arch-Bending Pliers must be cleaned, bagged individually or bagged/wrapped in a tray setup, and then sterilized. A chemical/steam indicator device should be included in the wrapping. Hinged instruments should be processed open and unlocked.

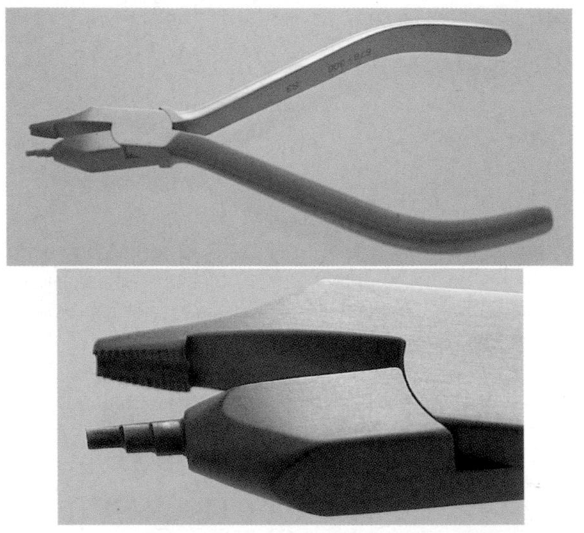

INSTRUMENT

Tweed Loop-Forming Pliers (Jarabek Pliers)

FUNCTIONS
To bend and form loops in arch wire
To bend wires for removable appliances

CHARACTERISTICS
Grooves in beak—Help to bend and form loops in wire
Variety of styles

PRACTICE NOTE
Tweed Loop-Forming Pliers is only used on the orthodontic tray setup.

S Tweed Loop-Forming Pliers must be cleaned, bagged individually or bagged/wrapped in a tray setup, and then sterilized. A chemical/steam indicator device should be included in the wrapping. Hinged instruments should be processed open and unlocked.

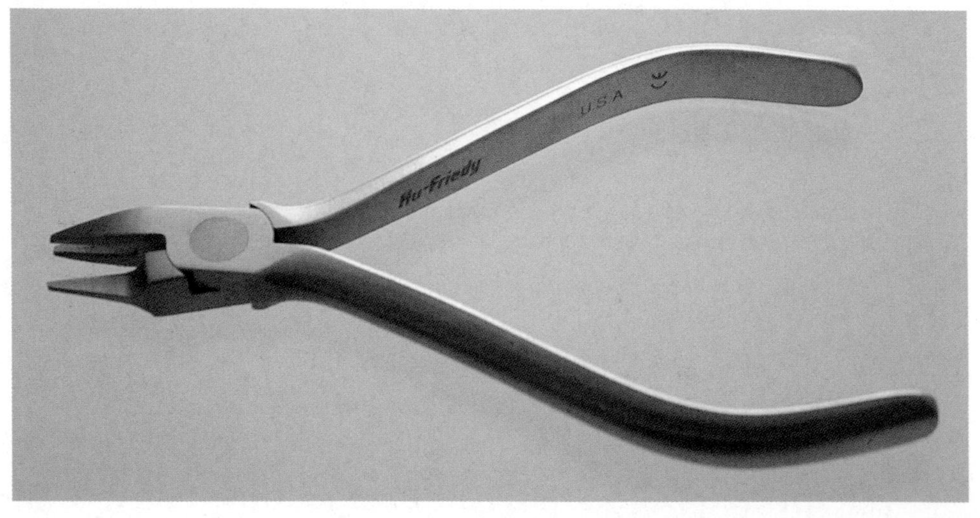
Hu-Friedy
U.S.A
CE

INSTRUMENT

Three-Prong Pliers

FUNCTION To contour and bend light wire

CHARACTERISTIC Range of sizes available

PRACTICE NOTE Three-Prong Pliers is only used on the orthodontic tray setup.

Ⓢ Three-Prong Pliers must be cleaned, bagged individually or bagged/wrapped in a tray setup, and then sterilized. A chemical/steam indicator device should be included in the wrapping. Hinged instruments should be processed open and unlocked.

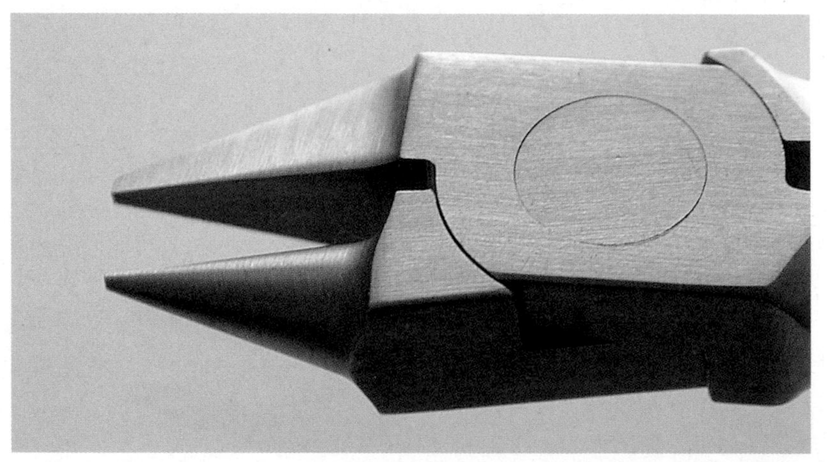

INSTRUMENT

Bird Beak Pliers evolve

FUNCTIONS To bend and form orthodontic wire
To remove bonded bracket by squeezing bracket

CHARACTERISTICS Versatile wire-bending pliers
Beaks on working end meet very precisely

PRACTICE NOTE Bird Beak Pliers is only used on the orthodontic tray setup.

Ⓢ Bird Beak Pliers must be cleaned, bagged individually or bagged/wrapped in a tray setup, and then sterilized. A chemical/steam indicator device should be included in the wrapping. Hinged instruments should be processed open and unlocked.

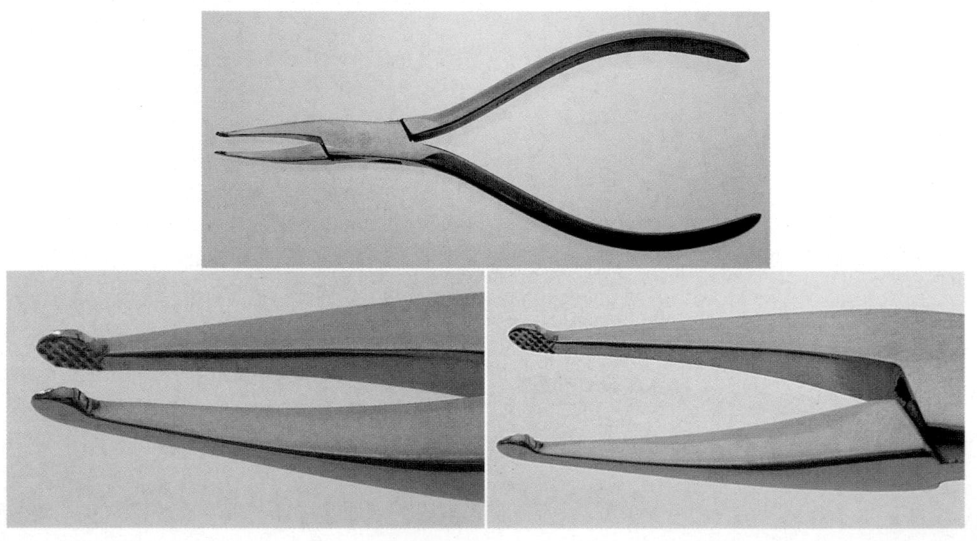

INSTRUMENT

How (or Howe) Pliers

FUNCTION

To place and remove arch wires
To check for loose bands

CHARACTERISTICS

All-purpose pliers for orthodontic procedures
Serrated tips for better grip on wire
Straight or curved beaks

PRACTICE NOTE

How Pliers is only used on the orthodontic tray setup.

S How Pliers must be cleaned, bagged individually or bagged/wrapped in a tray setup, and then sterilized. A chemical/steam indicator device should be included in the wrapping. Hinged instruments should be processed open and unlocked.

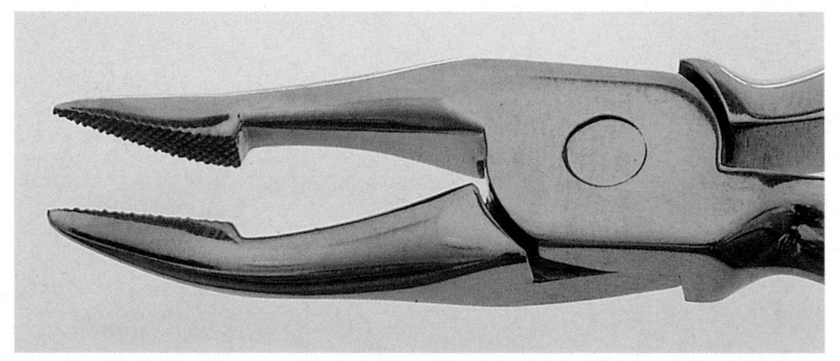

INSTRUMENT

Weingart Utility Pliers evolve

FUNCTIONS To place and remove arch wires
To aid a variety of functions for orthodontic procedures
To remove bonded brackets by squeezing bracket

CHARACTERISTIC Working ends—Tapered, slim tips to allow pliers to fit between brackets for ease of arch wire placement

PRACTICE NOTE Weingart Utility Pliers is only used on the orthodontic tray setup.

S Weingart Utility Pliers must be cleaned, bagged individually or bagged/wrapped in a tray setup, and then sterilized. A chemical/steam indicator device should be included in the wrapping. Hinged instruments should be processed open and unlocked.

404

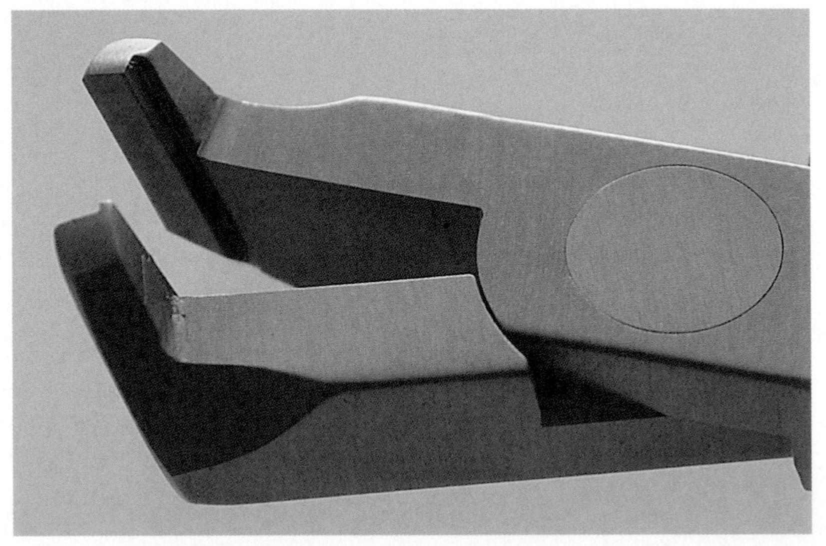

INSTRUMENT

Distal End-Cutting Pliers

FUNCTION To cut distal end of arch wire after placement in brackets and buccal tubes

CHARACTERISTIC Catch and hold excess wire after wire has been cut

PRACTICE NOTE Distal End-Cutting Pliers is only used on the orthodontic tray setup.

Ⓢ Distal End Pliers must be cleaned, bagged individually or bagged/wrapped in a tray setup, and then sterilized. A chemical/steam indicator device should be included in the wrapping. Hinged instruments should be processed open and unlocked.

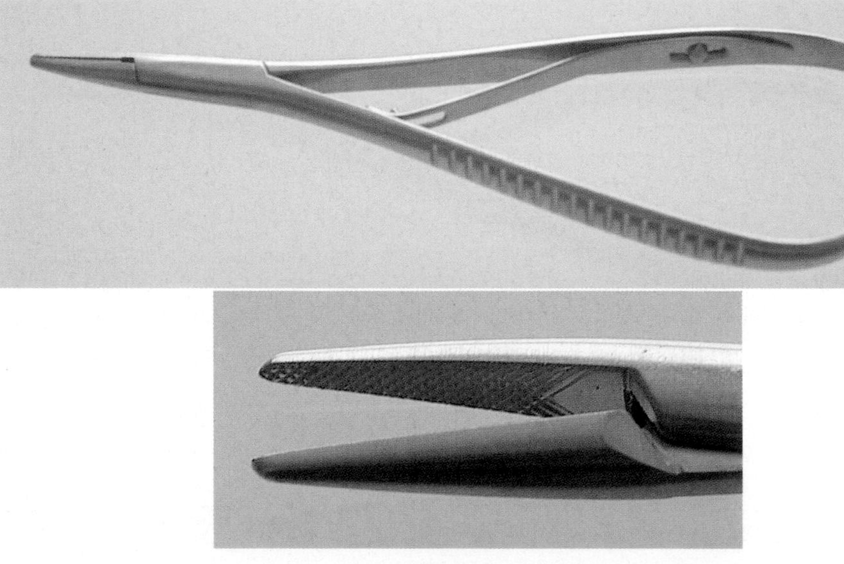

INSTRUMENT

Orthodontic Hemostat

FUNCTIONS

To hold and place separators
To hold, place, and/or tie ligatures to arch wire

CHARACTERISTIC

Multifunctional instrument for orthodontic procedures
Example: Mathieu pliers

PRACTICE NOTE

Orthodontic Hemostat is used on the orthodontic tray setup.

Ⓢ Orthodontic Hemostat must be cleaned, bagged individually or bagged/wrapped in a tray setup, and then sterilized. A chemical/steam indicator device should be included in the wrapping. Hinged instruments should be processed open and unlocked.

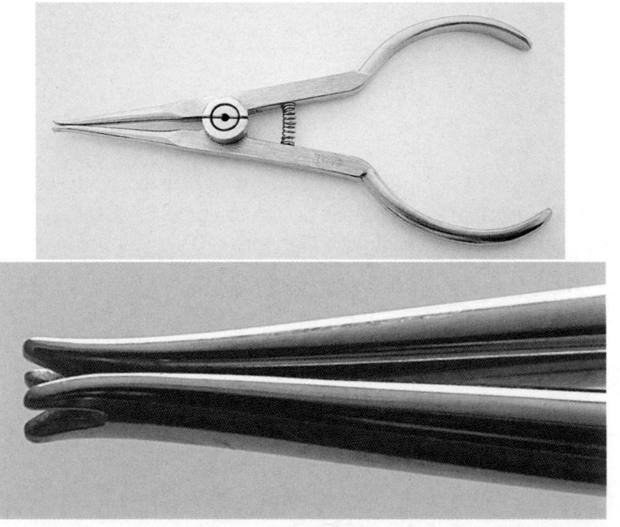

INSTRUMENT

Ligature-Tying (Coon) Pliers

FUNCTION To tie in ligature to arch wire

CHARACTERISTICS Channel on pliers—Locks wire ends in place as tips spread
Variety of styles

PRACTICE NOTE Ligature-Tying Pliers is only used on the orthodontic tray setup.

Ⓢ Ligature-Tying Pliers must be cleaned, bagged individually or bagged/wrapped in a tray setup, and then sterilized. A chemical/steam indicator device should be included in the wrapping. Hinged instruments should be processed open and unlocked.

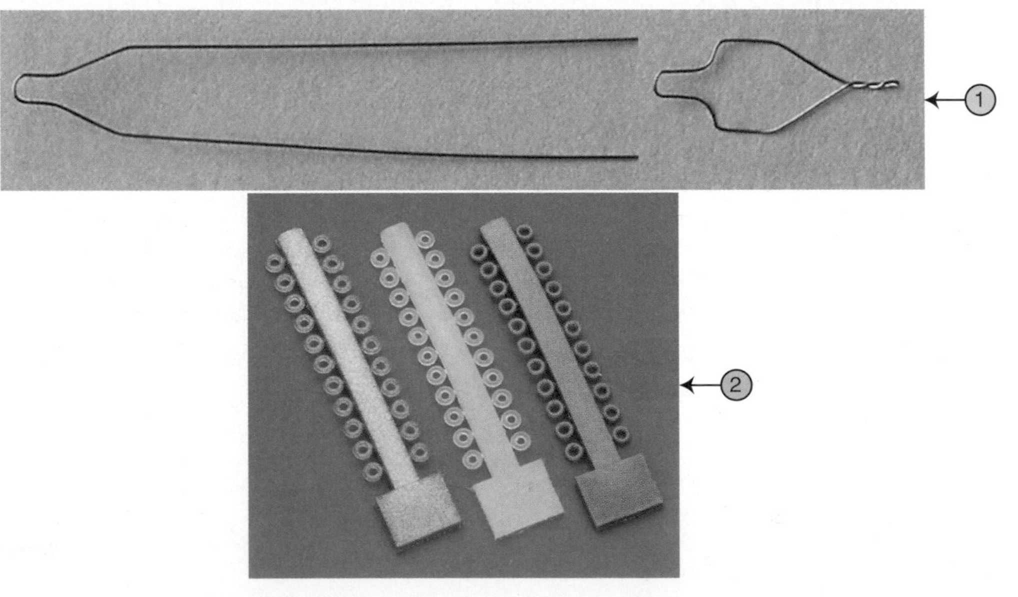
1
2

INSTRUMENT

Ligatures Ties

FUNCTION To secure the arch wire to the band or bracket

CHARACTERISTICS

① Wire Ligature Ties
Thin, flexible wire
Comes in precut length or spools

② Elastic Ligature Ties
Available in different colors
Comes on a stick (pictured), canes, and chains

PRACTICE NOTE Ligature ties are used on the orthodontic archwire placement tray setup.

Wire Ligature Ties should be disposed of in a Sharps container.
Elastic Ligature Ties should be disposed of in garbage.

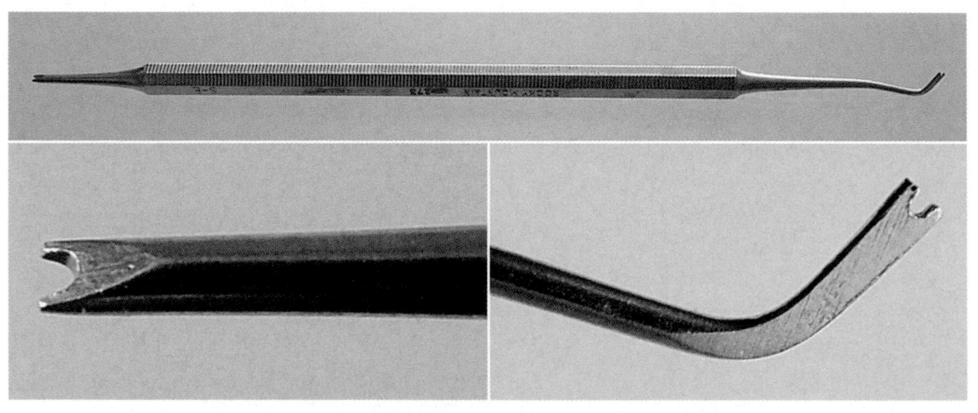
ROCKY MOUNTAIN
273

INSTRUMENT

Ligature Director

FUNCTION To place ligature wire around brackets after it has been tied to arch wire

CHARACTERISTICS Single or double ended
Ends of instrument—Have notches to assist placement of ligature tie around brackets

PRACTICE NOTE Ligature Director is used on the orthodontic archwire placement tray setup.

Ⓢ Ligature Director must be cleaned, bagged individually or bagged/wrapped in a tray setup, and then sterilized. A chemical/steam indicator device should be included in the wrapping.

414

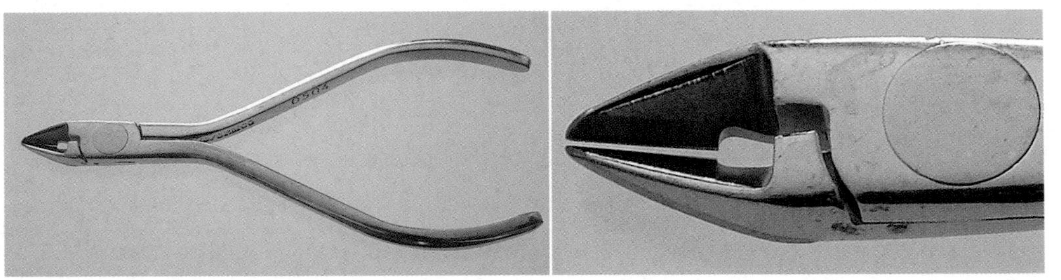

INSTRUMENT

Ligature/Wire Cutters

FUNCTIONS To cut ligature after it has been tied to arch wire
To cut ligature tie to allow removal of arch wire

CHARACTERISTIC Range of sizes available

PRACTICE NOTE Ligature/Wire Cutters is used on the orthodontic tray setup.

S Ligature/Wire Cutters must be cleaned, bagged individually or bagged/wrapped in a tray setup, and then sterilized. A chemical/steam indicator device should be included in the wrapping. Hinged instruments should be processed open and unlocked.

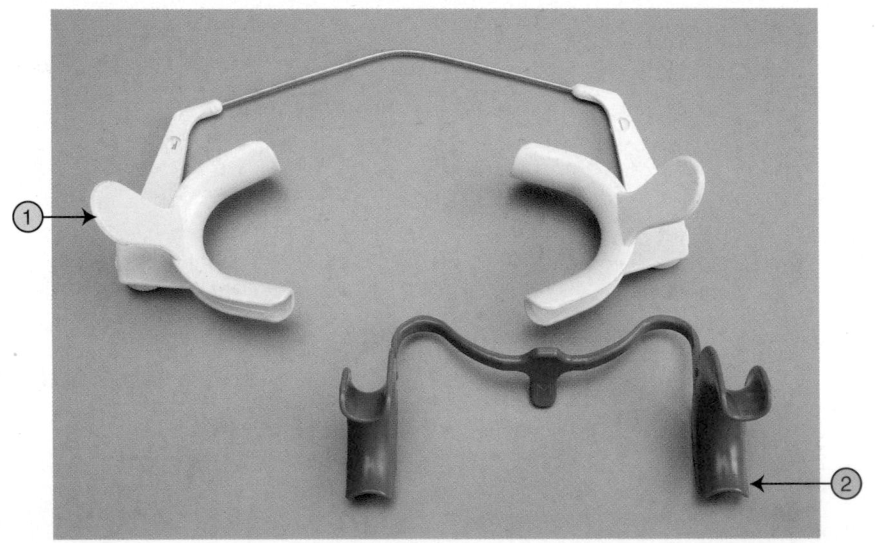
1
2

INSTRUMENT

Lip Retractors evolve

FUNCTIONS To retract lips allowing for intraoral access for bonding brackets
To retract lips for intraoral orthodontic photographs

CHARACTERISTICS
① Reusable Lip Retractors
② Disposable Lip Retractors

PRACTICE NOTE Lip Retractors are used with orthodontic procedures and other tray setups that include taking intraoral photographs.

Ⓢ Reusable Lip Retractors must be cleaned, bagged individually or bagged/wrapped in a tray setup, and then sterilized. A chemical/steam indicator device should be included in the wrapping. Disposable Lip Retractors should be disposed of in the garbage. Single use only.

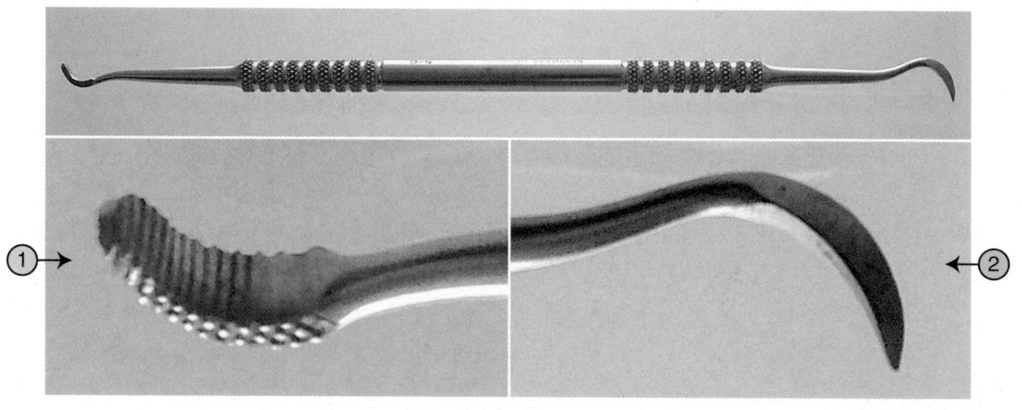
1
2

INSTRUMENT

Orthodontic (Shure) Scaler

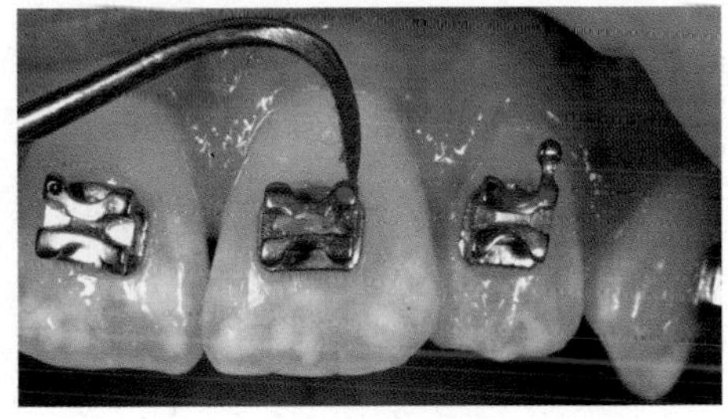

FUNCTIONS

To place brackets for bonding (both ends)
To remove separators (scaler end)
To remove elastic ligature ties (scaler end)
To remove excess cement or bonding material (scaler end)
To check for loose bands and brackets (both ends)

CHARACTERISTICS

Universal instrument used for several orthodontic functions:
- Single ended—Scaler or band pusher
- Double ended—① Band pusher
  ② Orthodontic scaler

PRACTICE NOTE

Orthodontic Scaler is used on the orthodontic tray setup.

Ⓢ Orthodontic Scaler must be cleaned, bagged individually or bagged/wrapped in a tray setup, and then sterilized. A chemical/steam indicator device should be included in the wrapping.

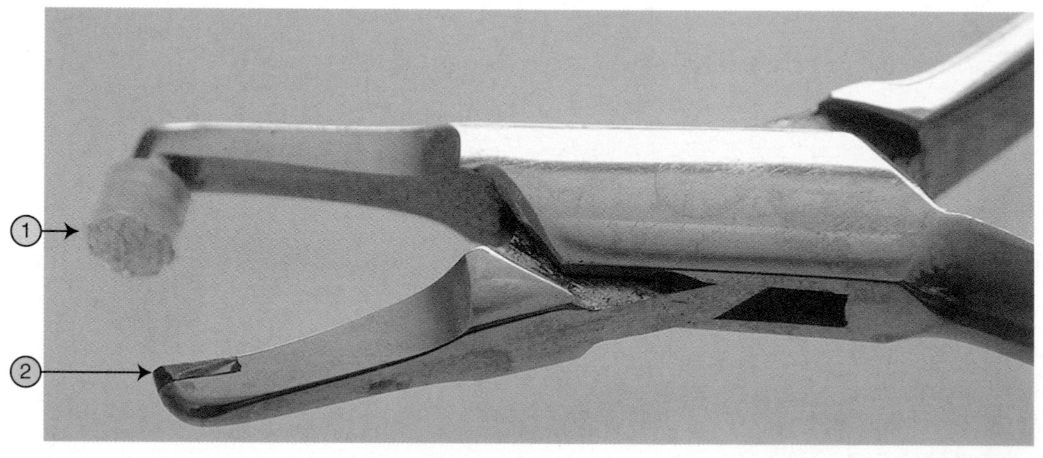
1
2

INSTRUMENT

Posterior Band Remover

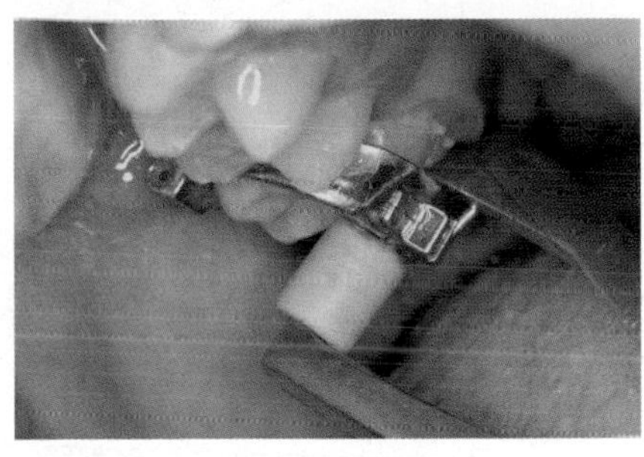

FUNCTION To remove orthodontic bands from teeth

CHARACTERISTICS Two beak types:

① One beak has round cover to place on occlusal surface of tooth to prevent damage during removal of band.

② Opposite beak is curved and is placed on gingival side of bracket to apply pressure and remove band from tooth.

PRACTICE NOTE Posterior Band Remover is used on the orthodontic tray setup.

Ⓢ Posterior Band Remover must be cleaned, bagged individually or bagged/wrapped in a tray setup, and then sterilized. A chemical/steam indicator device should be included in the wrapping. Hinged instruments should be processed open and unlocked.

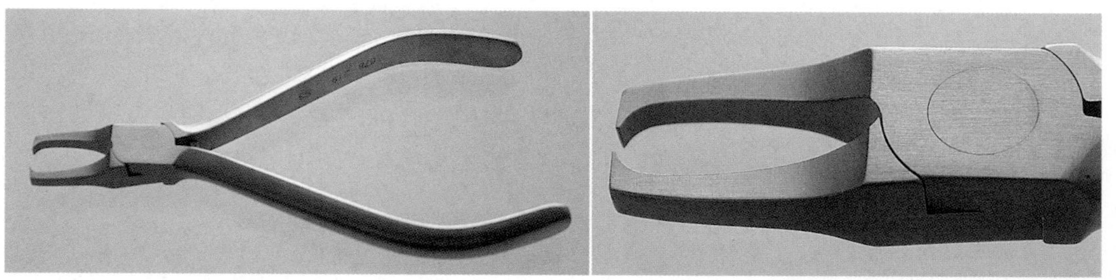

INSTRUMENT

Bracket Remover

FUNCTION To remove anterior or posterior brackets from teeth

CHARACTERISTIC Grasp bracket to remove it from tooth

PRACTICE NOTE Bracket Remover is used on the orthodontic tray setup.

Ⓢ Bracket Remover must be cleaned, bagged individually or bagged/wrapped in a tray setup, and then sterilized. A chemical/steam indicator device should be included in the wrapping. Hinged instruments should be processed open and unlocked.

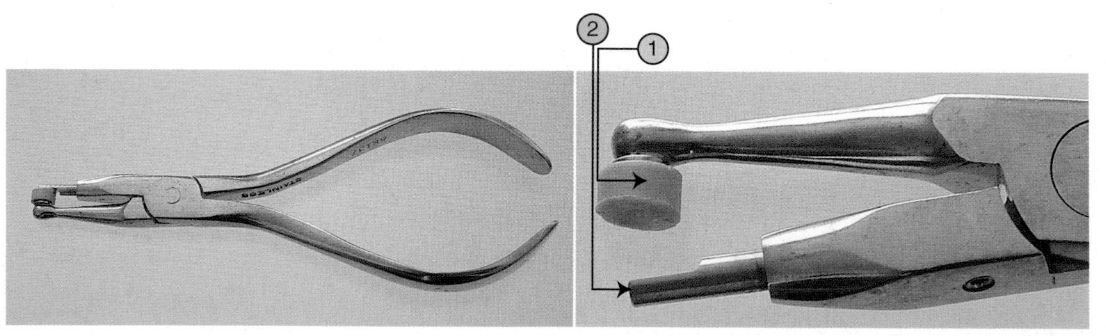

2
1

INSTRUMENT

Adhesive-Removing Pliers

FUNCTION To remove excess adhesive after debonding of brackets

CHARACTERISTICS
① Plastic pad on round end (pad can be changed)
② Carbide-inserted tip on short beak—Scrapes off the adhesive

PRACTICE NOTE Adhesive-Removing Pliers is used on the orthodontic tray setup.

Ⓢ Adhesive-Removing Pliers must be cleaned, bagged individually or bagged/wrapped in a tray setup, and then sterilized. A chemical/steam indicator device should be included in the wrapping. Hinged instruments should be processed open and unlocked.

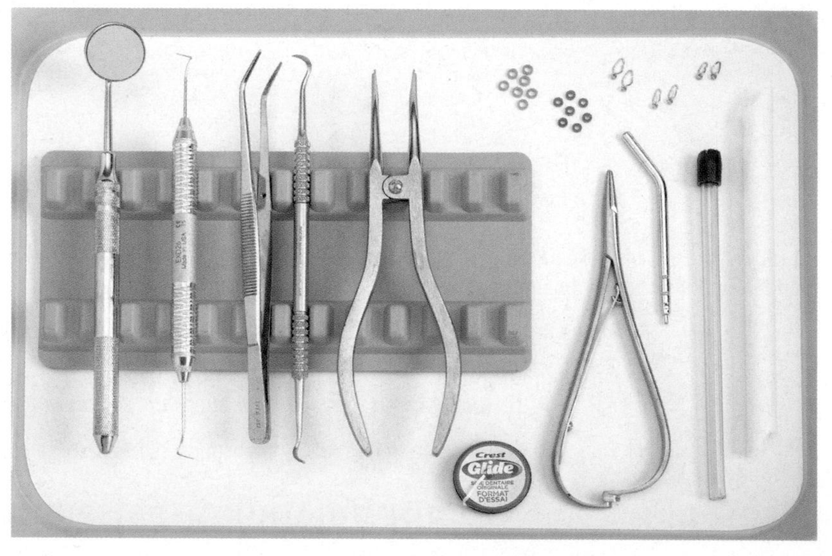
Crest
Glide
FORMAT
D'ESSAI

TRAY SETUP

Orthodontic Tooth Separating

TOP

Elastic separators, spring coil separators

BOTTOM (FROM LEFT TO RIGHT)

Mouth mirror, explorer, cotton forceps (pliers), orthodontic (Shure) scaler, elastic separating pliers, floss, orthodontic hemostat (Mathieu pliers), air/water syringe tip, low-volume saliva ejector tip, high-volume evacuation (HVE) tip

Refer to each individual picture for correct procedure for instrument sterilization or disposal of instrument or material.

Refer to other chapters for additional instruments on this tray setup that are not included in this chapter.

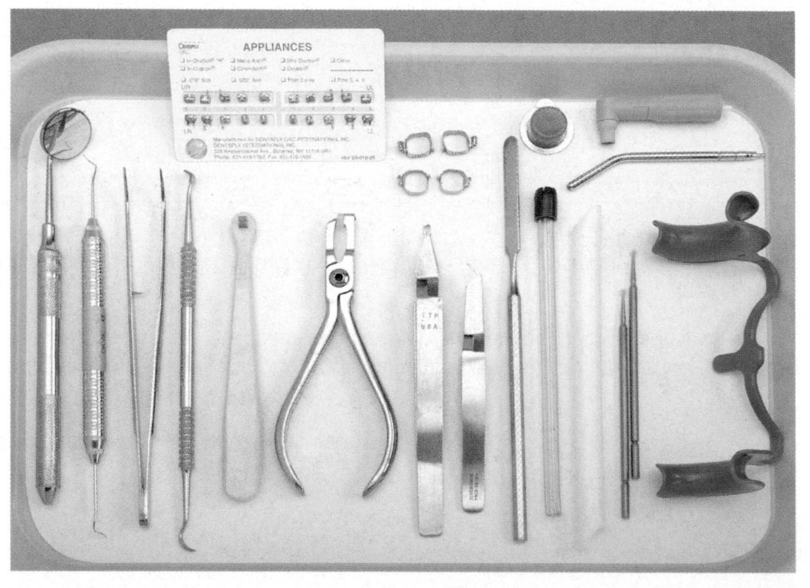
APPLIANCES

TRAY SETUP

Orthodontic Cementing and Bonding Brackets

TOP ROW (LEFT TO RIGHT)

Bracket placement card with brackets, orthodontic bands, polishing agent without fluoride, disposable prophy angle with polishing cup, air/water syringe tip

BOTTOM ROW (LEFT TO RIGHT)

Mouth mirror, explorer, cotton forceps, orthodontic scaler (Shure scaler), band seater-bite stick, posterior band remover, anterior bracket placement pliers, posterior bracket placement pliers, flexible cement spatula, low-volume saliva ejector, high-volume evacuation (HVE) tip, microbrushes, disposable cheek retractors

S Refer to each individual picture for correct procedure for instrument sterilization or disposal of instrument or material.

Refer to other chapters for additional instruments on this tray setup that are not included in this chapter.

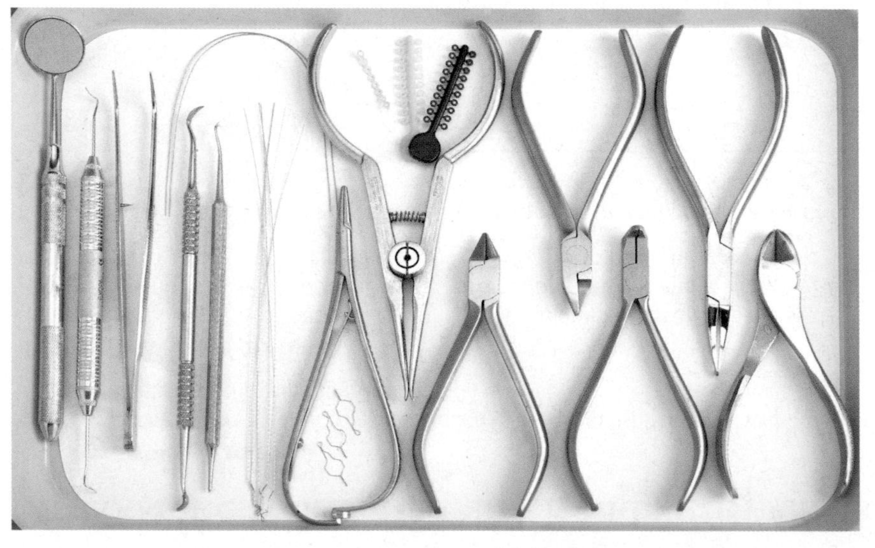

TRAY SETUP

Orthodontic Tying-in Arch Wire

TOP (FROM LEFT TO RIGHT)

Preformed archwire, elastic ligature ties

BOTTOM (FROM LEFT TO RIGHT)

Mouth mirror, explorer, cotton forceps, orthodontic (Shure) scaler, ligature director, wire ligature ties, orthodontic hemostat (Mathieu pliers), (under orthodontic hemostat, short wire ligature ties), ligature-tying (Coon) pliers, bird beak pliers, arch-bending pliers, distal-end cutting pliers, How (Howe) pliers, ligature/wire cutters

S Refer to each picture for correct procedure for instrument sterilization or disposal of instrument or material.

Refer to other chapters for additional instruments on this tray setup that are not included.

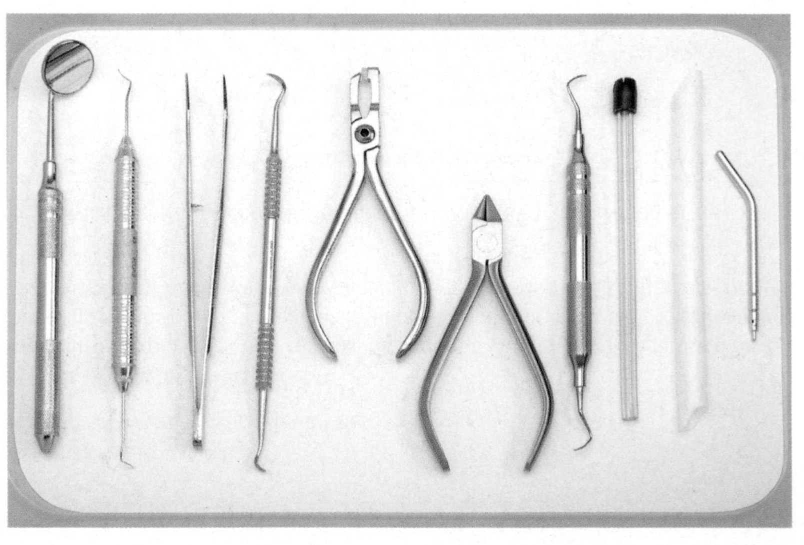

TRAY SETUP

Orthodontic Removing Bands and Brackets

LEFT TO RIGHT

Mouth mirror, explorer, cotton forceps, orthodontic (Shure) scaler, posterior band remover, bird beak pliers, universal curette, low-volume saliva ejector, high-volume evacuation (HVE) tip, air/water syringe tip

Refer to each picture for correct procedure for instrument sterilization or disposal of instrument or material.

Refer to other chapters for additional instruments on this tray setup that are not included.

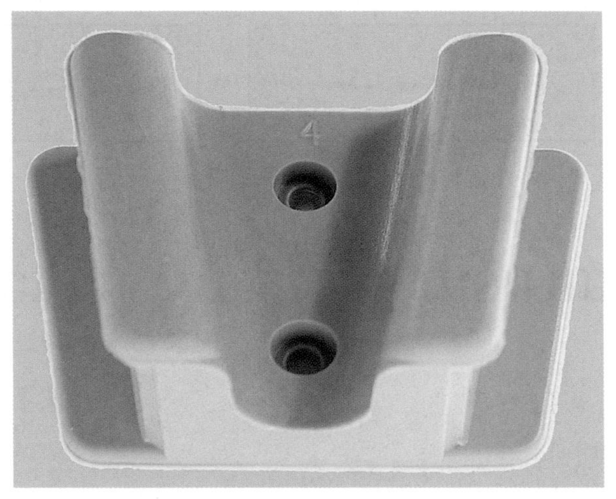
4

INSTRUMENT

Mouth Prop

FUNCTION To hold patient's mouth open during dental procedure

CHARACTERISTICS Placed in posterior part of mouth while patient bites down
Often used for sedated patients
Disposable Mouth Props available
Range of sizes—Pediatric to large adult

PRACTICE NOTE Mouth Prop could be used with any dental procedure, including, but not exclusive to, operative or surgical.

S Mouth Prop must be cleaned, bagged individually or bagged/wrapped in a tray setup, and then sterilized. A chemical/steam indicator device should be included in the wrapping. Disposable Mouth Prop should be disposed of in the garbage.

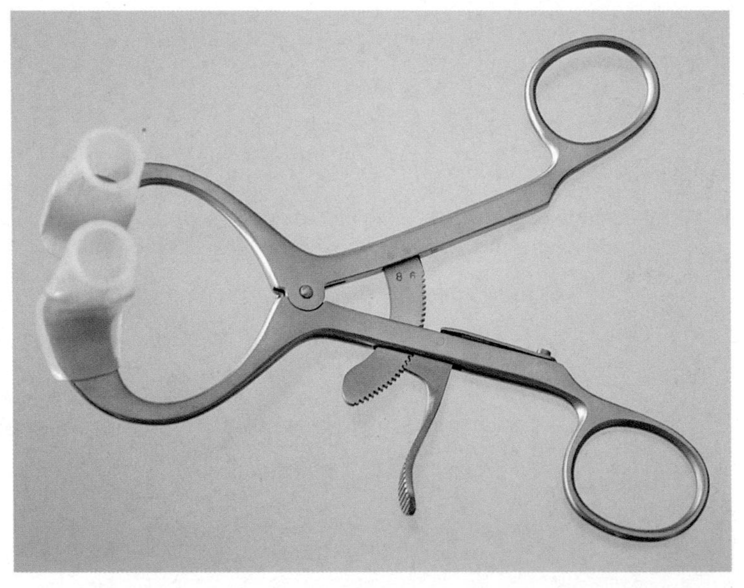

INSTRUMENT

Mouth Gag

FUNCTION To hold patient's mouth open during dental procedure

CHARACTERISTICS Often used for sedated patients
Locking device
Range of sizes available

PRACTICE NOTE Mouth Gag is mostly used on oral surgery and periodontal surgical procedures when patient is sedated.

S Mouth Gag must be cleaned, bagged individually or bagged/wrapped in a tray setup, and then sterilized. A chemical/steam indicator device should be included in the wrapping. Hinged instruments should be processed open and unlocked.

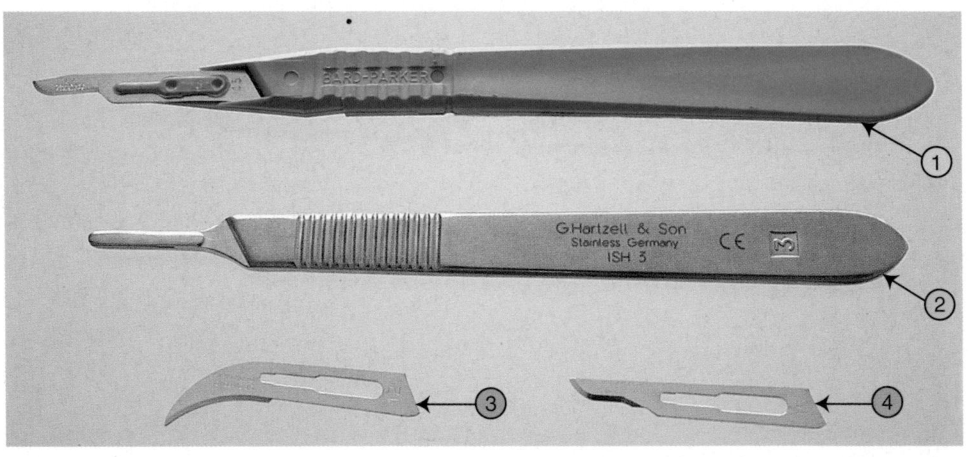
BARD-PARKER
G.Hartzell & Son
Stainless Germany
ISH 3
CE
1
2
3
4

INSTRUMENT

Scalpel Handle with Blades

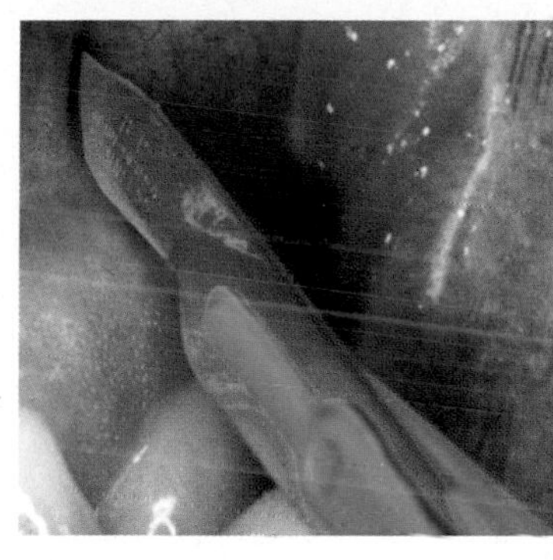

FUNCTIONS

To hold blade in place
To cut tissue with blade
To trim interproximal restorations

CHARACTERISTICS

① Disposable handle/blade in one unit
② Scalpel Handle
Commonly used blades: ③ No. 12, ④ no. 15
Blades—Disposable, variety of shapes and sizes

PRACTICE NOTE

Scalpel with Blades is mostly used on oral surgery and periodontal surgical tray setups and occasionally used with composite tray setups for removing flash material and interproximal carving.

Ⓢ Scalpel Handle must be cleaned, bagged individually or bagged/wrapped in a tray setup, and then sterilized. A chemical/steam indicator device should be included in the wrapping. Scalpel Blade must be disposed of in a Sharps container. Disposable Handle and Blade in one unit must be disposed of in a Sharps container.

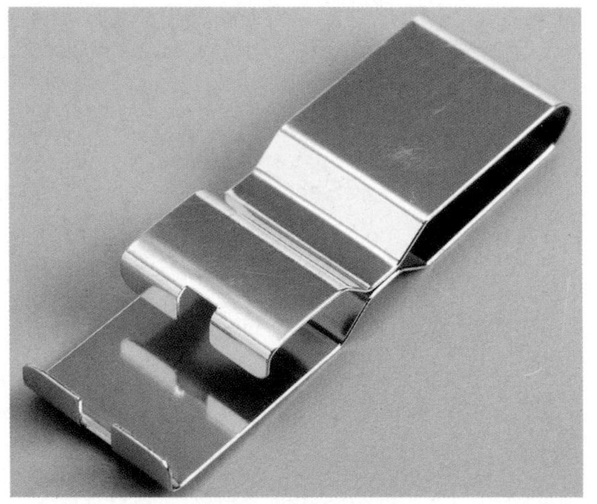

INSTRUMENT

Scalpel Blade Remover

FUNCTION To remove blade from scalpel handle safely

CHARACTERISTICS Removes all sizes of blades
Autoclavable

PRACTICE NOTES Steps for removing blade:

- Insert blade with blade side up; align to notch
- Press down on blade remover
- Pull handle away from blade

Scalpel Blade Remover is mostly used on oral surgery and periodontal surgical tray setups

S Scalpel Blade Remover must be cleaned, bagged individually or bagged/wrapped in a tray setup, and then sterilized. A chemical/steam indicator device should be included in the wrapping. Scalpel Blade must be disposed of in a Sharps container.

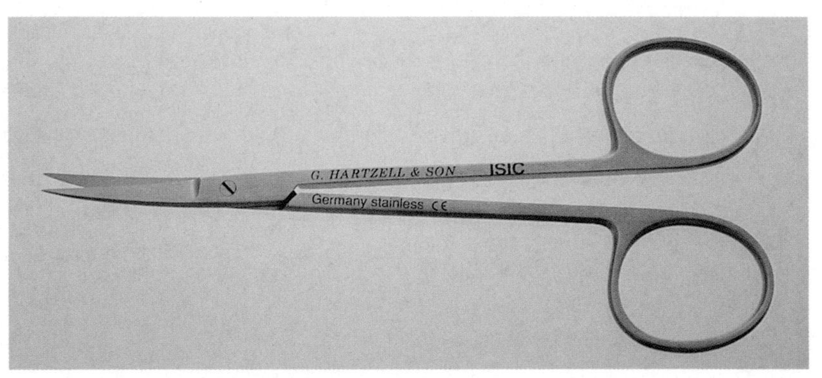
G. HARTZELL & SON
ISIC
Germany stainless CE

INSTRUMENT

Tissue Scissors

evolve

FUNCTION To cut tissue

CHARACTERISTICS Straight or curved
Variety of shapes and sizes
Variety of uses

PRACTICE NOTE Tissue Scissors is mostly used on oral surgery and periodontal surgical tray setups.

S Tissue Scissors must be cleaned, bagged individually or bagged/wrapped in a tray setup, and then sterilized. A chemical/steam indicator device should be included in the wrapping. Hinged instruments should be processed open and unlocked.

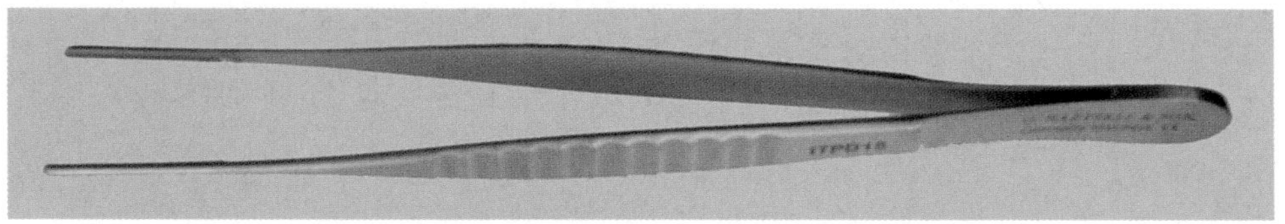

INSTRUMENT

Tissue Forceps

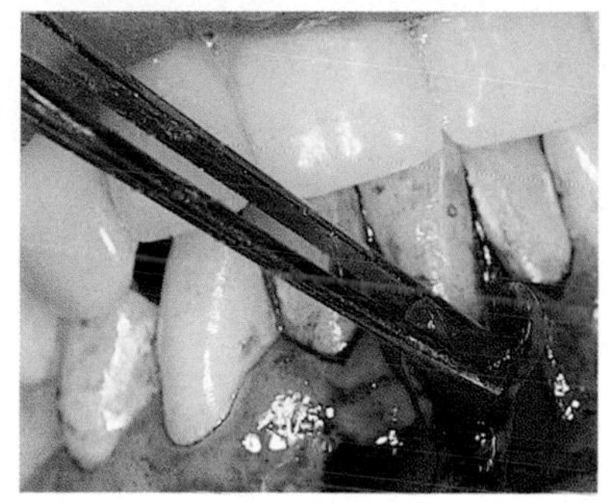

FUNCTION To hold tissue during surgical procedures

CHARACTERISTICS Serrated or rat-tooth tips
Range of sizes available

PRACTICE NOTE Tissue Forceps is mostly used on oral surgery and periodontal surgical tray setups.

S Tissue Forceps must be cleaned, bagged individually or bagged/wrapped in a tray setup, and then sterilized. A chemical/steam indicator device should be included in the wrapping.

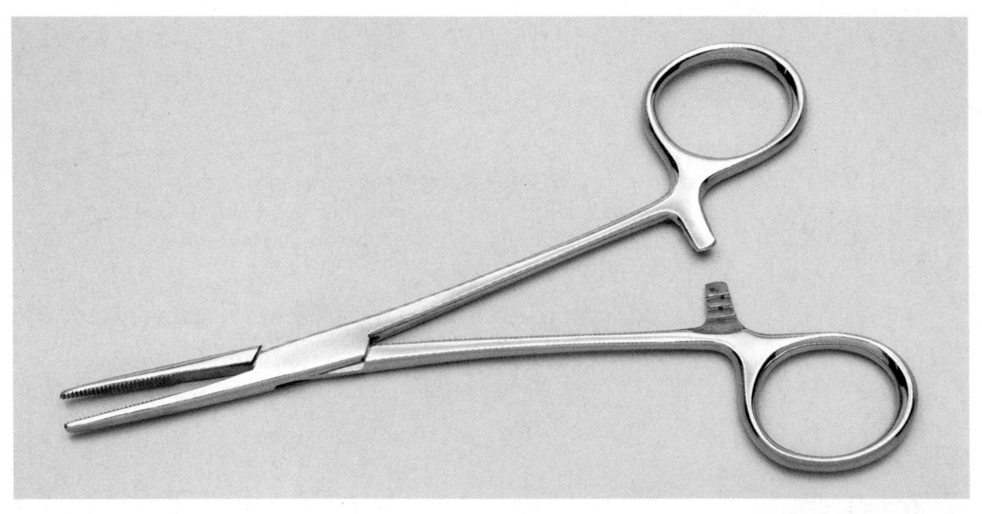

INSTRUMENT

Hemostat

FUNCTION

To grasp tissue or bone fragments
To hold and grasp material in and out of the oral cavity

CHARACTERISTICS

Straight or curved
Working end—Serrated, locking
Variety of functions in other dental procedures
Range of sizes available

PRACTICE NOTE

Hemostat is mostly used on oral surgery and periodontal surgical tray setups. Hemostat is also used on restorative and many other tray setups.

S Hemostat must be cleaned, bagged individually or bagged/wrapped in a tray setup, and then sterilized. A chemical/steam indicator device should be included in the wrapping. Hinged instruments should be processed open and unlocked.

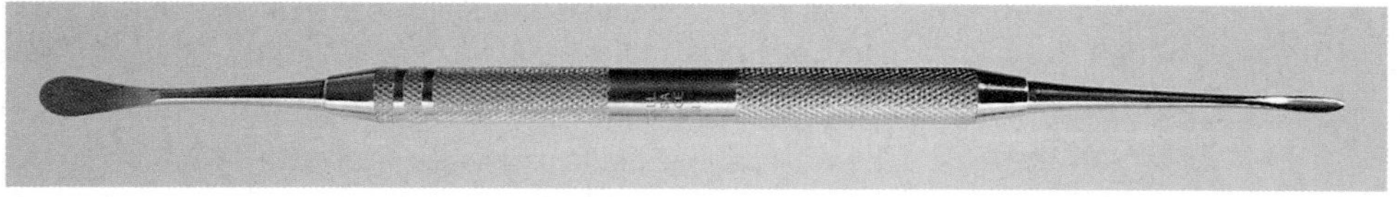

INSTRUMENT

Periosteal Elevator evolve

FUNCTIONS

To separate tissue from tooth or bone
To hold tissue away from surgical site

CHARACTERISTICS

Working end—Pointed or round
Range of sizes available

PRACTICE NOTE

Periosteal Elevator is used on oral surgery and periodontal surgical tray setups.

Periosteal Elevator must be cleaned, bagged individually or bagged/wrapped in a tray setup, and then sterilized. A chemical/steam indicator device should be included in the wrapping.

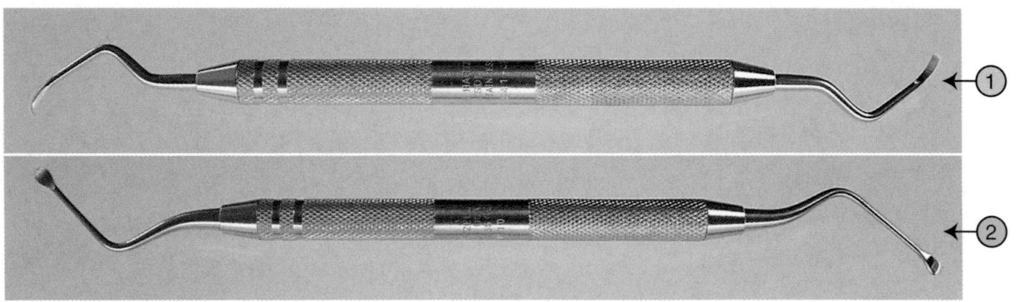
1
2

INSTRUMENT

Surgical Curette evolve

FUNCTIONS

To remove debris or granulation tissue from surgical site
To remove cyst from extraction site or surgical site
To perform gross tissue debridement

CHARACTERISTICS

Single or double ended
Variety of sizes and shapes

Examples:

1. Commonly used type: Prichard
2. Miller

PRACTICE NOTE

Surgical Curette is mostly used on oral surgery and periodontal surgical tray setups.

Surgical Curette must be cleaned, bagged individually or bagged/wrapped in a tray setup, and then sterilized. A chemical/steam indicator device should be included in the wrapping.

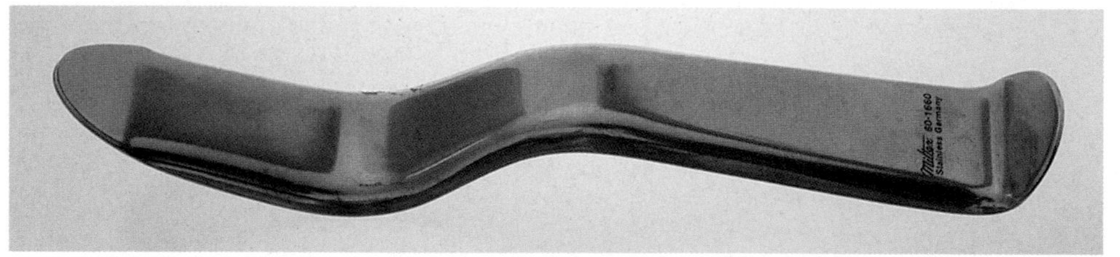
Miltex 60-1660
Stainless Germany

INSTRUMENT

Tongue and Cheek Retractor

FUNCTION To hold and retract tongue or cheek during surgery

CHARACTERISTIC Variety of styles and sizes

Example: Common type used: Minnesota

PRACTICE NOTE Tongue and Cheek Retractor is mostly used on oral surgery and periodontal surgical tray setups.

Tongue and Cheek Retractor must be cleaned, bagged individually or bagged/wrapped in a tray setup, and then sterilized. A chemical/steam indicator device should be included in the wrapping.

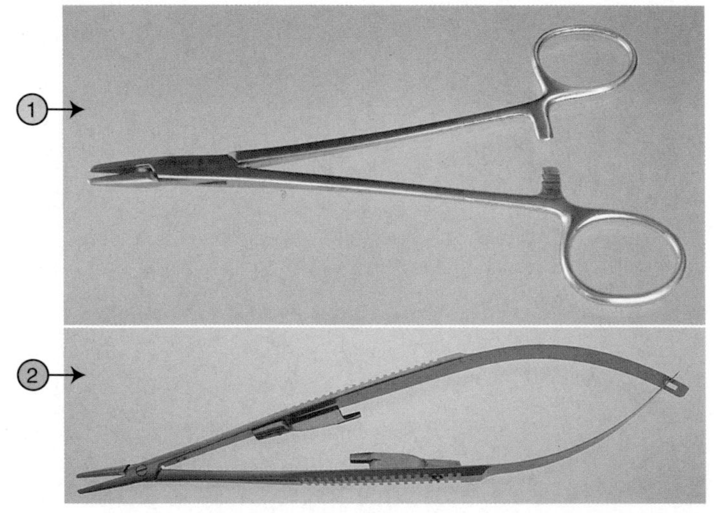
1
2

INSTRUMENT

Needle Holder

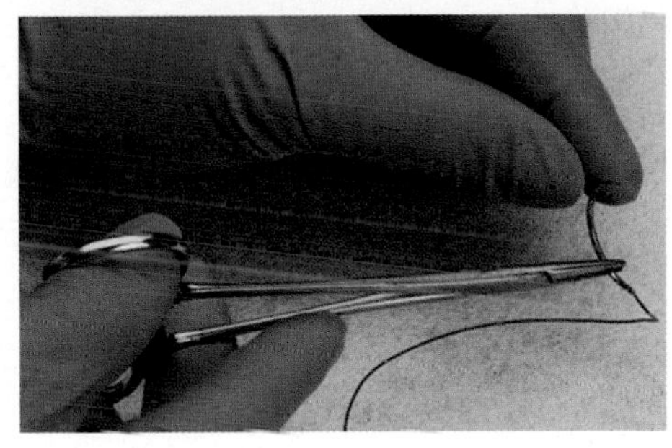

FUNCTION To grasp and manipulate suture needle during use

CHARACTERISTICS Working end—Different lengths, curved or straight
Notched ends available (to accommodate needle)
Range of sizes—Micro for microsurgery to large
Variety of styles:
- ① Universal
- ② Castroviejo

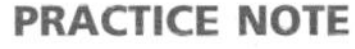

PRACTICE NOTE Needle Holder is mostly used on oral surgery and periodontal surgical tray setups.

Ⓢ Needle Holder must be cleaned, bagged individually or bagged/wrapped in a tray setup, and then sterilized. A chemical/steam indicator device should be included in the wrapping. Hinged instruments should be processed open and unlocked.

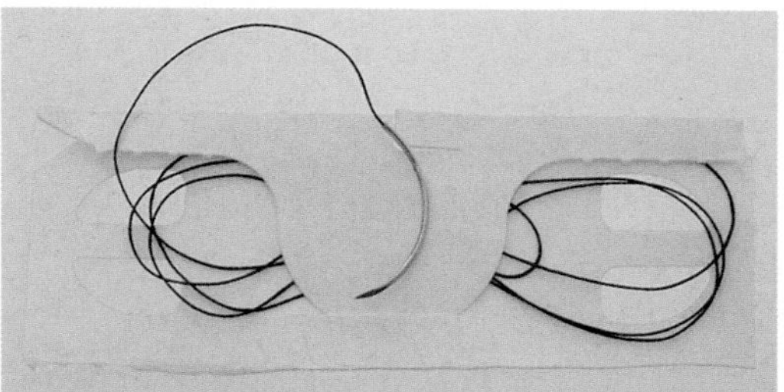

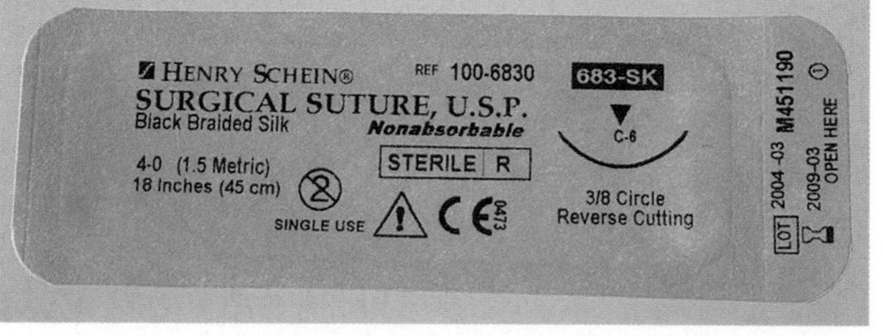
HENRY SCHEIN®
REF 100-6830
683-SK
SURGICAL SUTURE, U.S.P.
Black Braided Silk
Nonabsorbable
4-0 (1.5 Metric)
18 Inches (45 cm)
STERILE R
SINGLE USE
CE 0473
C-6
3/8 Circle
Reverse Cutting
LOT 2004 -03 M451190
2009-03
OPEN HERE

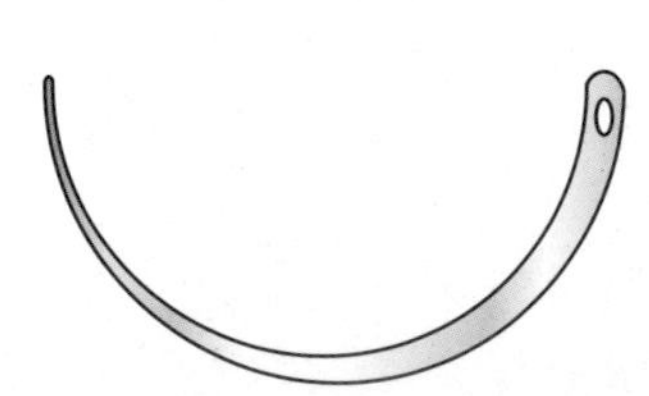

INSTRUMENT

Suture Needle and Sutures 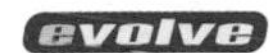

FUNCTION To suture surgical site

CHARACTERISTICS Resorbable sutures—Gut plain, chromic gut, polyglycolic (PGA)
Nonresorbable sutures—Silk, nylon, polyester, polypropylene
Available in sterile package
Variety of suture needle sizes available with different sutures

PRACTICE NOTE Suture Needle and Sutures are mostly used on oral surgery and periodontal surgical tray setups.

S Suture Needle and Sutures must be disposed of in a Sharps container.

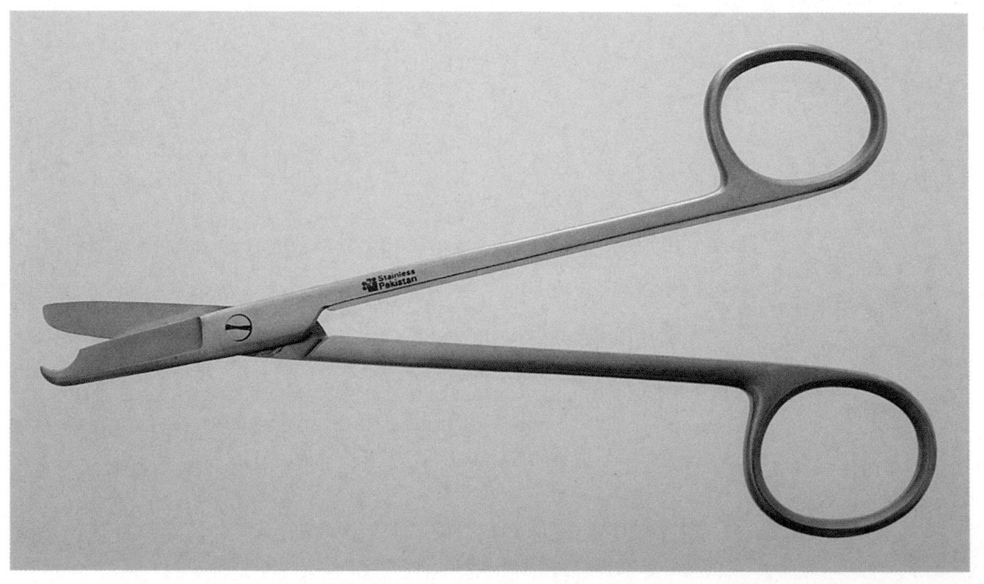
Stainless
Pakistan

INSTRUMENT

Suture Scissors

FUNCTION To cut sutures

CHARACTERISTICS Cutting edges—Straight or angled
May have notch on end of cutting edge (shown in picture)
Range of sizes

PRACTICE NOTE Suture Scissors is mostly used on oral surgery and periodontal surgical tray setups.

S Suture Scissors must be cleaned, bagged individually or bagged/wrapped in a tray setup, and then sterilized. A chemical/steam indicator device should be included in the wrapping. Hinged instruments should be processed open and unlocked.

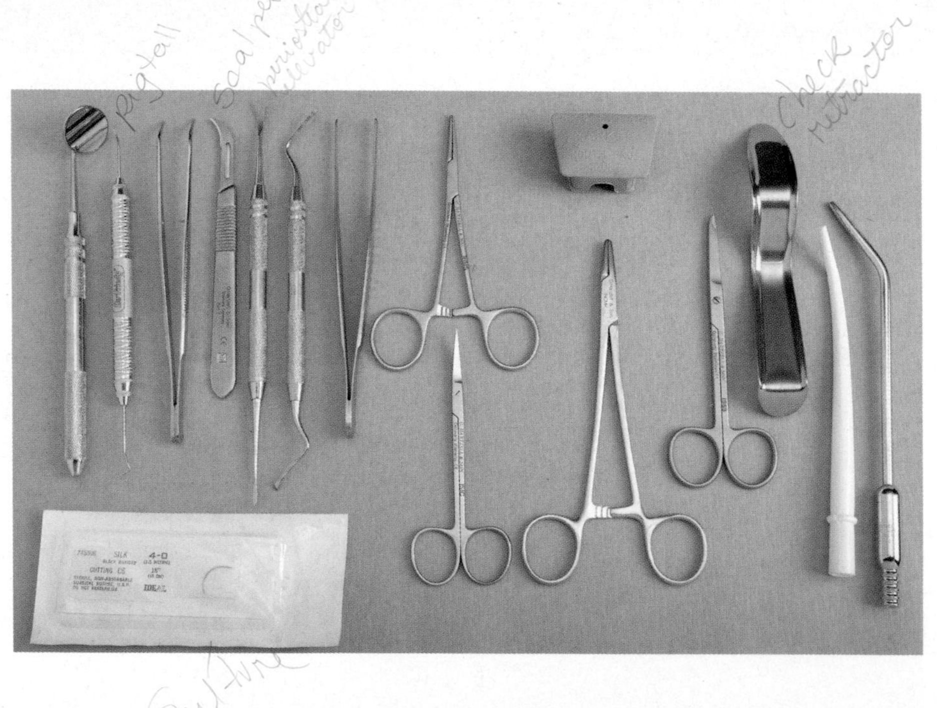
SILK
4-0
CUTTING CS
IDEAL

TRAY SETUP

Universal Surgical

TOP ROW (FROM LEFT TO RIGHT)

Mouth mirror, explorer, cotton forceps (pliers), scalpel with blade #12, periosteal elevator, surgical curette (Prichard), tissue holder, hemostat, tissue scissors, mouth prop, needle holder, suture scissors, tongue and check retractor, disposable high-volume surgical evacuation tip, high-volume surgical evacuation tip

BOTTOM ROW (FROM LEFT TO RIGHT)

Silk suture with needle in sterile package

Refer to each picture for correct procedure for instrument sterilization or disposal of instrument or material.

Refer to other chapters for additional instruments on this tray setup that are not included in this chapter.

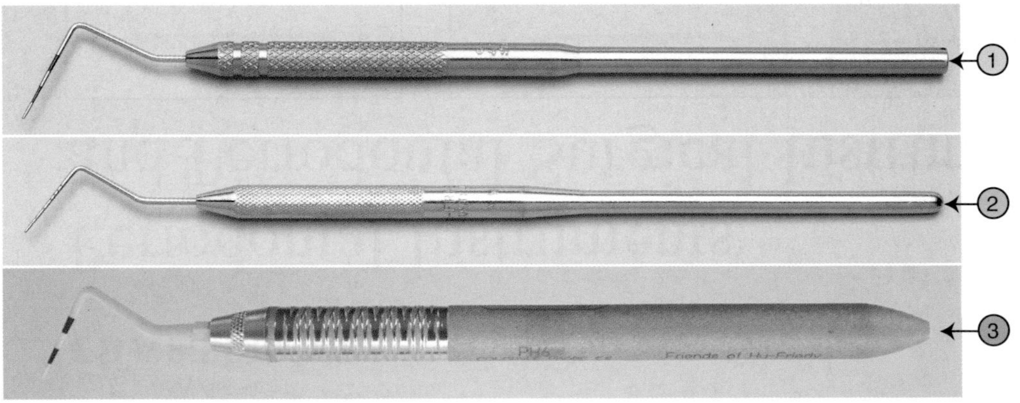
1
2
3
PH6

INSTRUMENT

Periodontal Probes evolve

FUNCTION To measure periodontal pocket depth in millimeter increments

CHARACTERISTICS Flat or rounded ends

Millimeter-increment markings vary for each style:

1. Color coded—Black markings for millimeter measurements
2. Other styles—Indentations in metal for millimeter measurement
3. Color-ended probe with black visible markings—Replaceable tip, different tip designs, plastic tip safe for implant probing

Double-ended style available with probe on one end, explorer on the other

Computerized probes available

PRACTICE NOTE Periodontal Probe is used on basic setup, dental hygiene, and periodontal tray setups.

S Periodontal Probe must be cleaned, bagged individually or bagged/wrapped in a tray setup, and then sterilized. A chemical/steam indicator device should be included in the wrapping.

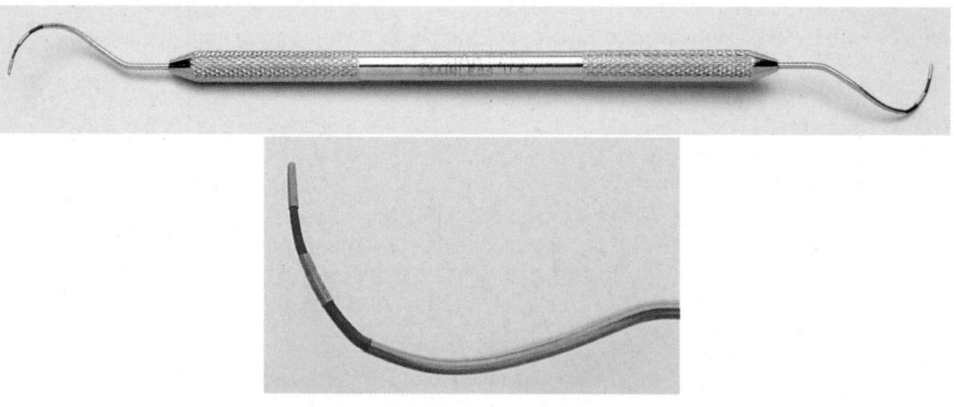

INSTRUMENT

Furcation Probe

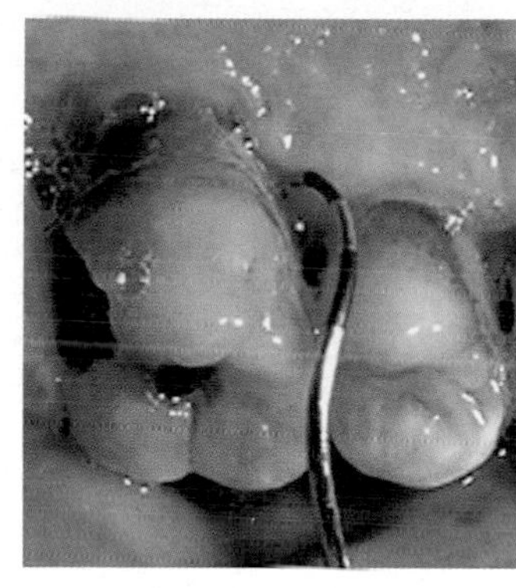

FUNCTION To measure horizontal and vertical pocket depth of multirooted teeth in furcation areas

CHARACTERISTICS Flat or rounded ends
Single or double ended
Millimeter-increment markings vary for each style:

- Color-coded—Black markings for millimeter measurements
- Other styles—Indentations in metal for millimeter measurements

Example: Nabors probe (color coded)

PRACTICE NOTE Furcation Probe is used on basic, dental hygiene, and periodontal tray setups.

Ⓢ Furcation Probe must be cleaned, bagged individually or bagged/wrapped in a tray setup, and then sterilized. A chemical/steam indicator device should be included in the wrapping.

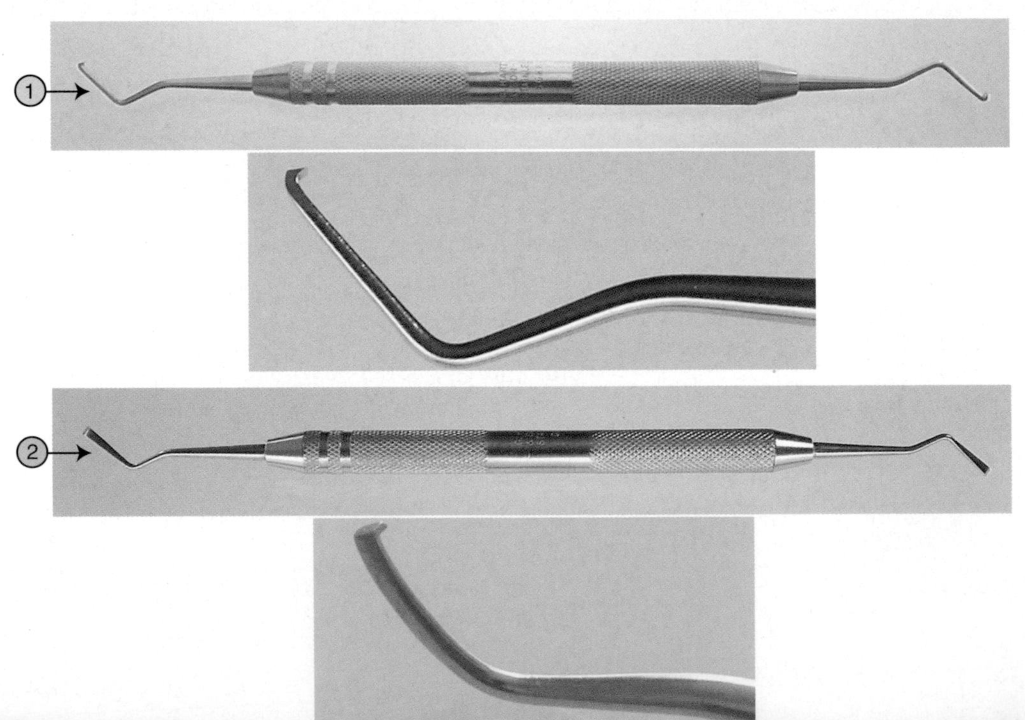
1
2

Hoe—Mesial/Distal and Buccal/Lingual

INSTRUMENT

FUNCTION To remove subgingival and supragingival calculus

CHARACTERISTICS
① Mesial/Distal Hoe
② Buccal/Lingual Hoe
Used with pulling motion
Straight cutting edge
Single or double ended
Designed to function in anterior or posterior locations
- Anterior hoe—Shorter, straighter shanks
- Posterior hoe—Longer, angled shanks

PRACTICE NOTE Mesial/Distal and Buccal/Lingual Hoes, according to procedure performed, could be used on dental hygiene and periodontal tray setups.

Ⓢ Mesial/Distal and Buccal/Lingual Hoes must be cleaned, bagged individually or bagged/wrapped in a tray setup, and then sterilized. A chemical/steam indicator device should be included in the wrapping.

472

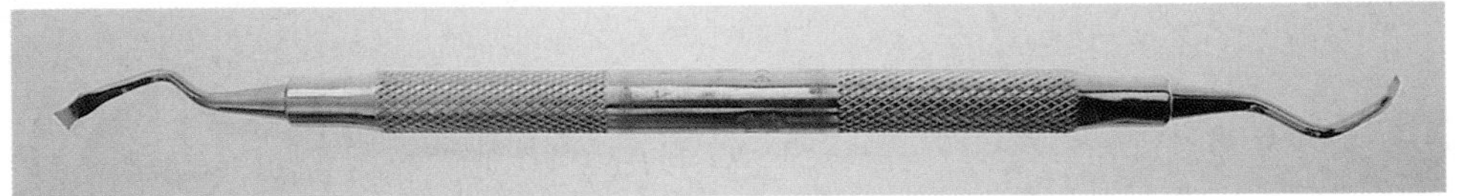

INSTRUMENT

Back-Action Hoe

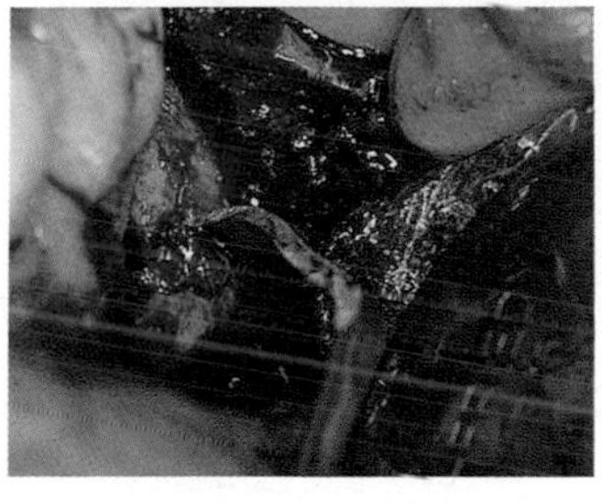

FUNCTIONS To remove bone adjacent to teeth without causing trauma

CHARACTERISTICS Double ended
Variety of sizes and shapes

PRACTICE NOTE Back-Action Hoe, according to procedure performed, could be used on dental hygiene and periodontal tray setups.

Ⓢ Back-Action Hoe must be cleaned, bagged individually or bagged/wrapped in a tray setup, and then sterilized. A chemical/steam indicator device should be included in the wrapping.

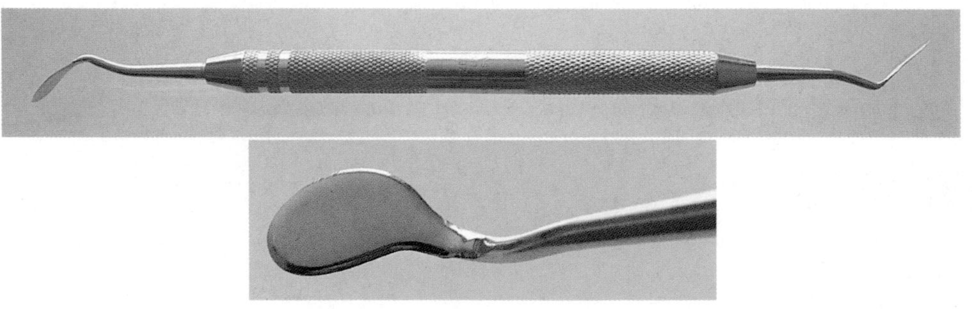

INSTRUMENT

Periodontal Knife—Kidney Shaped

FUNCTIONS

To use for bevel incision for gingivectomy
To use for gingivoplasty

CHARACTERISTICS

Variety of sizes and shapes
Name by designer: Kirkland, Goldman-Fox, Buck, Solt

PRACTICE NOTE

Periodontal Knife—Kidney Shaped is used on periodontal surgical tray setups.

Ⓢ Periodontal Knife—Kidney Shaped must be cleaned, bagged individually or bagged/wrapped in a tray setup, and then sterilized. A chemical/steam indicator device should be included in the wrapping.

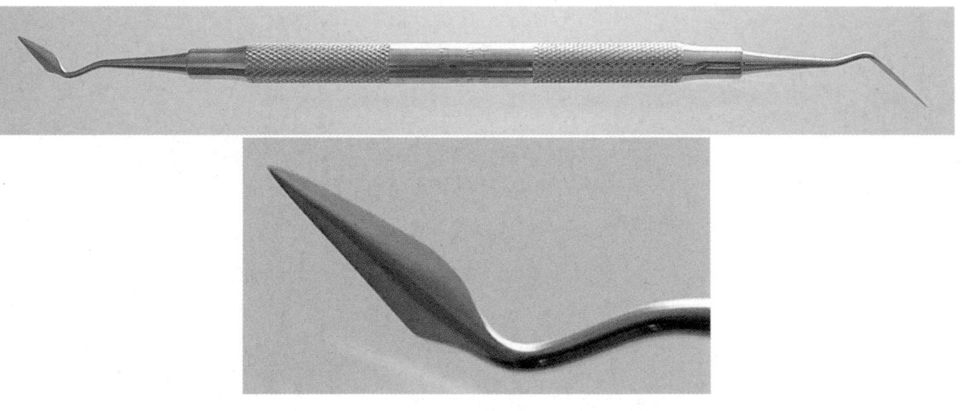

INSTRUMENT

Interdental Knife—Spear Point

FUNCTIONS

To use for interdental cutting of gingiva
To remove tissue

CHARACTERISTICS

Blade angulated for easier use
Name by designer: Orban, Goldman-Fox, Buck, Sanders
Single or double ended
Range of sizes
Example: Buck 5/6

PRACTICE NOTE

Interdental Knife—Spear Point is used on periodontal surgical tray setup.

S Interdental Knife—Spear Point must be cleaned, bagged individually or bagged/wrapped in a tray setup, and then sterilized. A chemical/steam indicator device should be included in the wrapping.

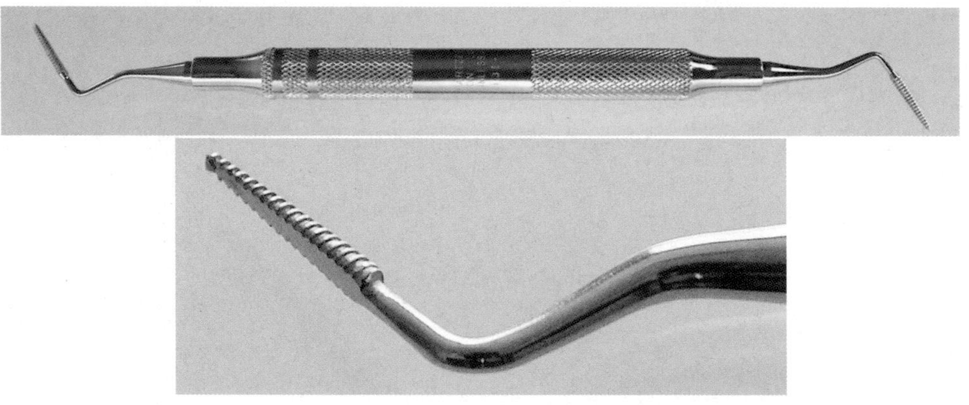

INSTRUMENT

Interdental File

FUNCTION To crush and remove heavy deposits from subgingival and supragingival interproximal areas

CHARACTERISTICS Used with push or pull motion

Various angles—Curved, straight, mesial/distal, and buccal/lingual

Examples: Sugarman, Schluger, Buck

Range of sizes available

PRACTICE NOTE Interdental File is used on periodontal surgical tray setups.

Interdental File must be cleaned, bagged individually or bagged/wrapped in a tray setup, and then sterilized. A chemical/steam indicator device should be included in the wrapping.

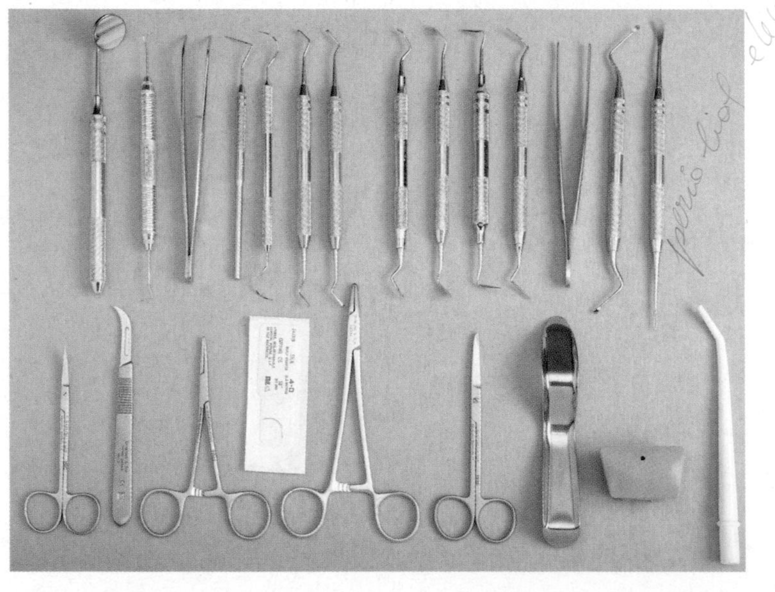

TRAY SETUP

Periodontal Surgical

TOP ROW—FROM LEFT TO RIGHT

Mouth mirror, explorer, cotton forceps (pliers), periodontal probe, furcation probe, mesial/distal hoe, buccal/lingual hoe, back-action hoe, kidney-shape periodontal knife, interproximal knife, bone file, tissue forceps, surgical curette, periosteal elevator

BOTTOM ROW—FROM LEFT TO RIGHT

Tissue scissors, scalpel with #12 blade, hemostat, silk sutures with needle, needle holder, suture scissors, check and tongue retractor (Minnesota), mouth prop, disposable high-volume surgical evacuation tip

S Refer to each picture for correct procedure for instrument sterilization or disposal of instrument or material.

Refer to Chapter 15: Universal Surgical Instruments for complete instruments used in periodontal surgery.

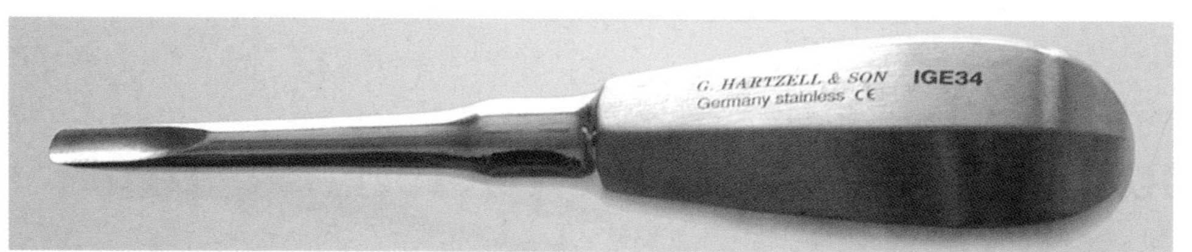
G. HARTZELL & SON
Germany stainless CE
IGE34

INSTRUMENT

Straight Elevator evolve

FUNCTIONS To loosen tooth from periodontal ligaments before extraction
To separate and lift tooth from socket

CHARACTERISTICS Single ended
Range of sizes available

PRACTICE NOTE Straight Elevator is used on surgical extraction tray setups.

S Straight Elevator must be cleaned, bagged individually or bagged/wrapped in a tray setup, and then sterilized. A chemical/steam indicator device should be included in the wrapping.

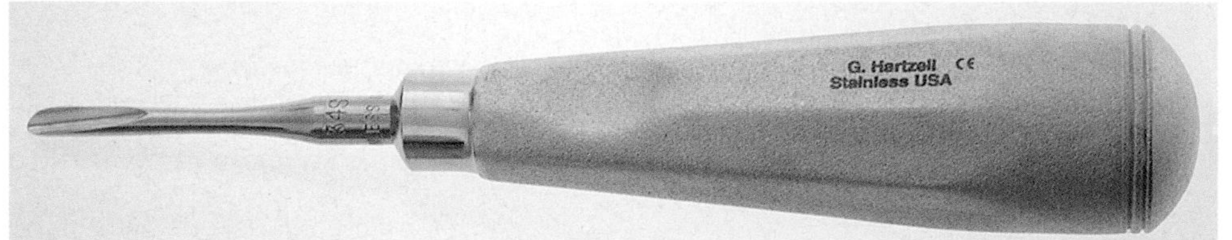
G. Hartzell CE
Stainless USA

INSTRUMENT

Luxating Elevator

FUNCTIONS
To cut periodontal ligaments before extraction
To rock tooth back and forth before extraction

CHARACTERISTICS
Single ended
Sharp blade on working end
Range of sizes available

PRACTICE NOTE
Luxating Elevator is used on surgical extraction tray setups.

S Luxating Elevator must be cleaned, bagged individually or bagged/wrapped in a tray setup, and then sterilized. A chemical/steam indicator device should be included in the wrapping.

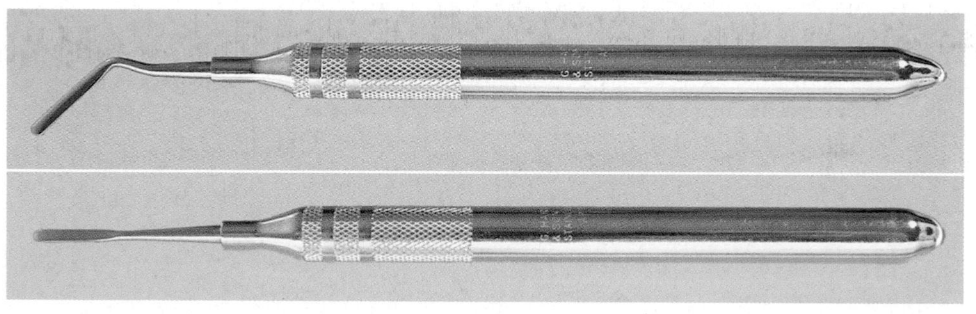

INSTRUMENT

Periotomes

FUNCTIONS

To cut periodontal ligaments for atraumatic tooth extraction
To use when dental implant placement is indicated

CHARACTERISTICS

Thin, sharp blades—Cause minimal damage to periodontal ligaments and surrounding alveolar bone
Straight or angled blades
Single or double ended
Range of sizes available
Some manufacturers make replaceable tip

PRACTICE NOTE

Periotomes are used on surgical extraction tray setups.

Ⓢ Periotomes must be cleaned, bagged individually or bagged/wrapped in a tray setup, and then sterilized. A chemical/steam indicator device should be included in the wrapping.

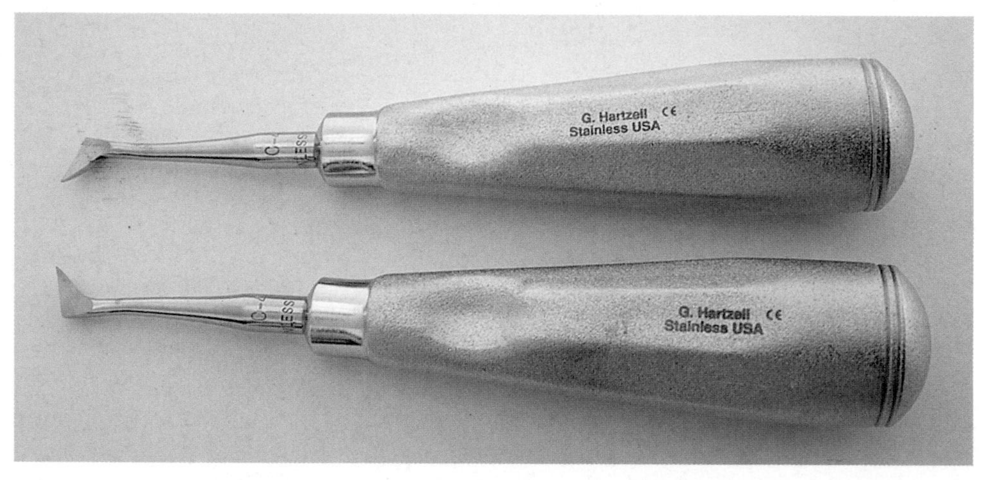
G. Hartzell CE
Stainless USA
G. Hartzell CE
Stainless USA

INSTRUMENT

Root Elevators

FUNCTIONS

To loosen root
To separate and lift root from socket
To use on posterior teeth

CHARACTERISTICS

Single ended
Right and left pairs
Range of sizes available
Example: Cryer (commonly type used)

PRACTICE NOTE

Root Elevators are used on surgical extraction tray setups.

Root Elevators must be cleaned, bagged individually or bagged/wrapped in a tray setup, and then sterilized. A chemical/steam indicator device should be included in the wrapping.

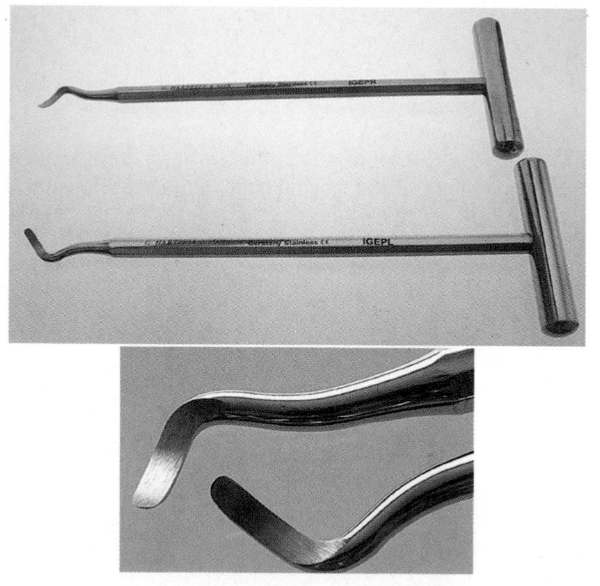
IGEPR
Germany Stainless CE
IGEPL

INSTRUMENT

T-Bar Elevators

Usely use for 3rd molar

FUNCTIONS

To loosen tooth from periodontal ligaments before extraction
To separate tooth from alveolus
To use on posterior teeth

CHARACTERISTICS

Single ended
Rounded or pointed
Right or left pairs
Range of sizes available

PRACTICE NOTE

T-Bar Elevators are used on surgical extraction tray setups.

S T-Bar Elevators must be cleaned, bagged individually or bagged/wrapped in a tray setup, and then sterilized. A chemical/steam indicator device should be included in the wrapping.

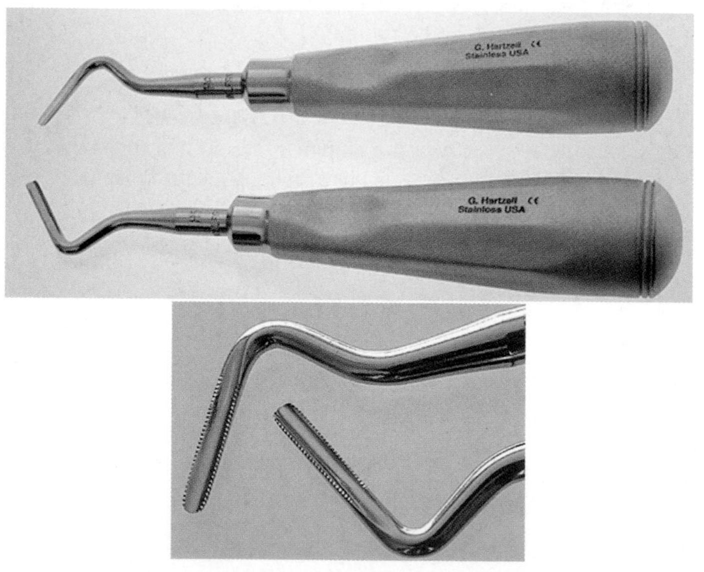
G. Hartzell CE
Stainless USA
G. Hartzell CE
Stainless USA

INSTRUMENT

Root-Tip Elevators

FUNCTION To lift and remove fragments of root

CHARACTERISTICS Single ended
Rounded or pointed
Straight or right and left pairs

PRACTICE NOTE Root-Tip Elevators are used on surgical extraction tray setups.

(S) Root-Tip Elevators must be cleaned, bagged individually or bagged/wrapped in a tray setup, and then sterilized. A chemical/steam indicator device should be included in the wrapping.

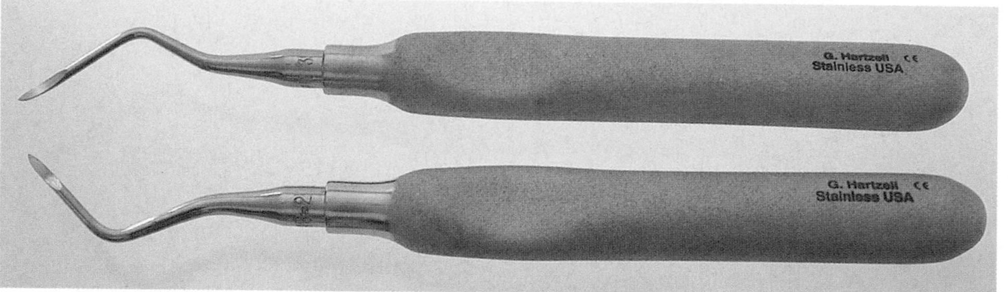
G. Hartzell
Stainless USA
G. Hartzell
Stainless USA

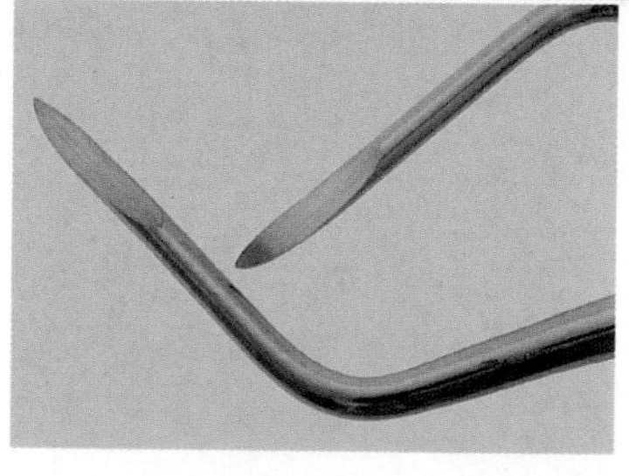

INSTRUMENT

Root-Tip Picks

FUNCTION To lift and remove small root tips in difficult areas

CHARACTERISTICS Pointed at working end
Straight or right and left pairs

PRACTICE NOTE Root-Tip Picks are used on surgical extraction tray setups.

S Root-Tip Picks must be cleaned, bagged individually or bagged/wrapped in a tray setup, and then sterilized. A chemical/steam indicator device should be included in the wrapping.

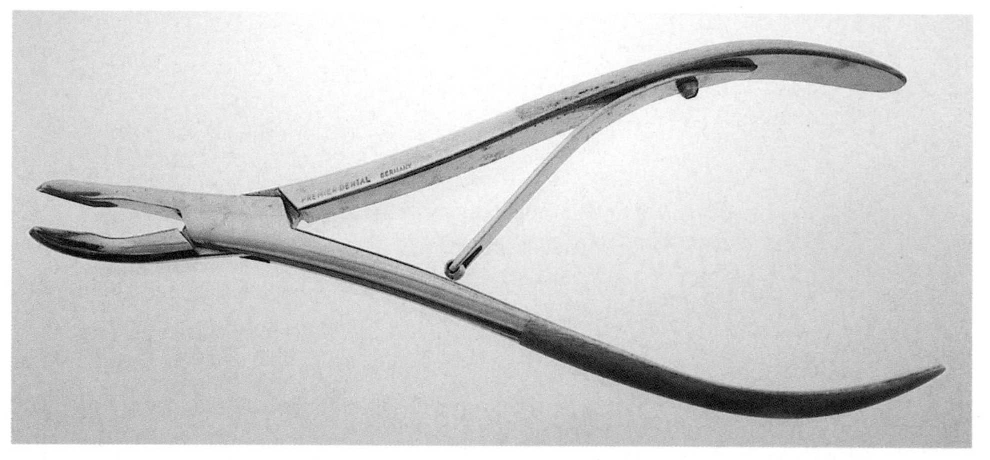
PREMIER DENTAL GERMANY

INSTRUMENT

Rongeurs

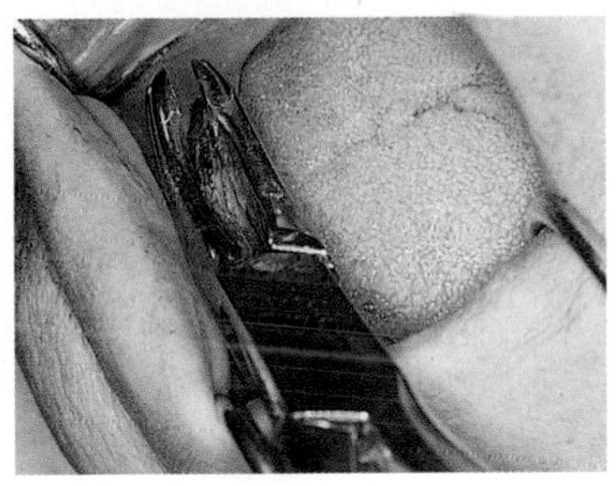

FUNCTIONS To trim and remove excess alveolar bone after extraction of teeth
To contour alveolar bone after single or multiple extractions

CHARACTERISTICS Variety of sizes and angles

PRACTICE NOTE Rongeurs is used on surgical extraction tray setups.

S Rongeurs must be cleaned, bagged individually or bagged/wrapped in a tray setup, and then sterilized. A chemical/steam indicator device should be included in the wrapping. Hinged instruments should be processed open and unlocked

500

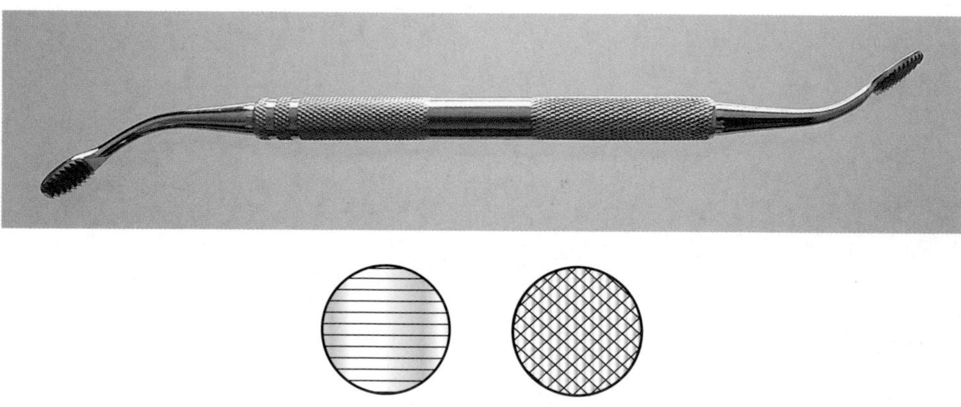

INSTRUMENT

Bone File

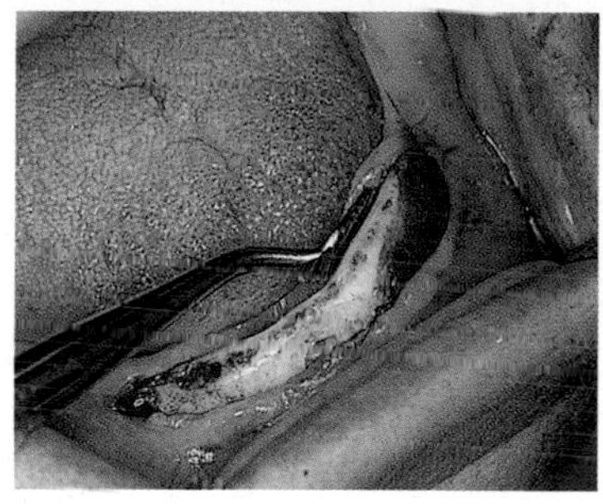

FUNCTION To remove or smooth rough edges of alveolar bone

CHARACTERISTICS Used with push-pull motion
Straight-cut or crosscut cutting end
Variety of sizes, angles, and shapes

PRACTICE NOTE Bone File is used on surgical extraction tray setups.

S Bone File must be cleaned, bagged individually or bagged/wrapped in a tray setup, and then sterilized. A chemical/steam indicator device should be included in the wrapping.

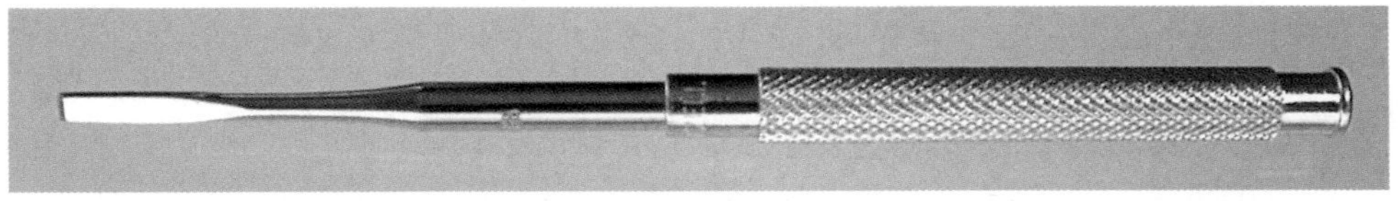

INSTRUMENT

Surgical Chisel

FUNCTIONS

To split or section a tooth for easier removal by tapping on chisel with mallet
To reshape or contour alveolar bone

CHARACTERISTICS

Single-bevel chisel—For contouring or removing alveolar bone
Bi-bevel chisel—For splitting teeth
Styles—Surgical chisels, bone splitter
Range of sizes available

PRACTICE NOTE

Surgical Chisel is used on surgical extraction and other types of surgical procedure tray setups.

S Surgical Chisel must be cleaned, bagged individually or bagged/wrapped in a tray setup, and then sterilized. A chemical/steam indicator device should be included in the wrapping.

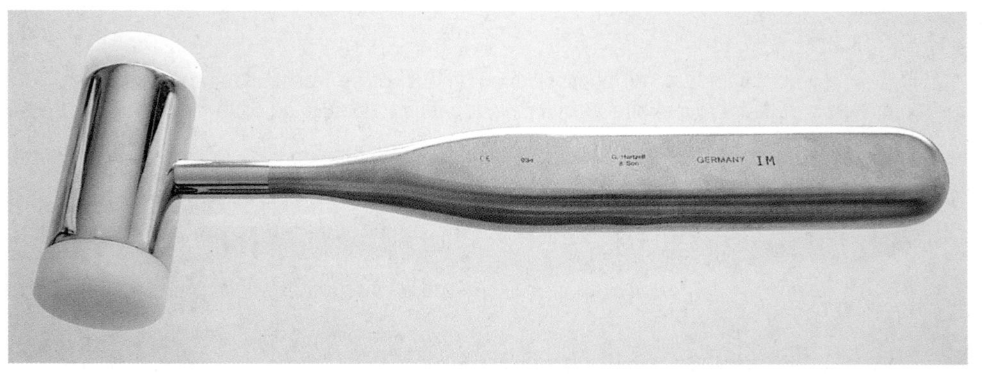
G. Hartzell
& Son
GERMANY IM

INSTRUMENT

Surgical Mallet evolve

FUNCTIONS To use with bone chisel to section tooth for easier removal by tapping on chisel with surgical mallet
To use with bone chisel to reshape or contour alveolar bone

CHARACTERISTIC Range of sizes available

PRACTICE NOTE Surgical Mallet is used on surgical extraction and other types of surgical procedure tray setups.

Ⓢ Surgical Mallet must be cleaned, bagged individually or bagged/wrapped in a tray setup, and then sterilized. A chemical/steam indicator device should be included in the wrapping.

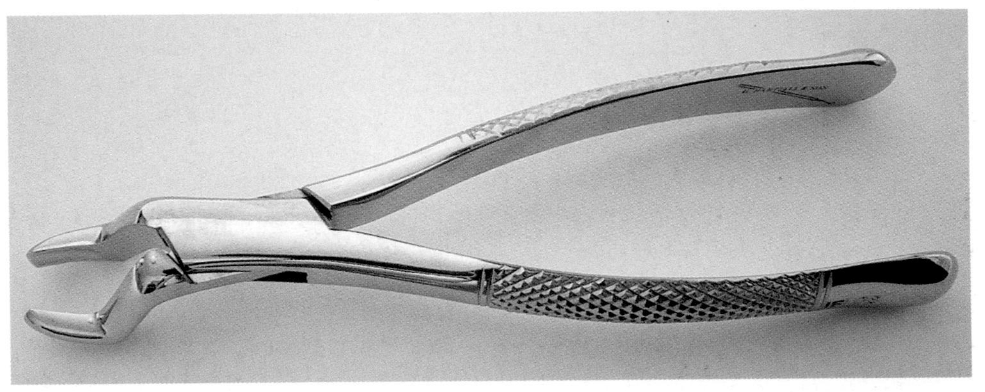

INSTRUMENT

Universal Maxillary Forceps No. 10S

FUNCTION To extract maxillary molars

CHARACTERISTIC Straight handle

PRACTICE NOTE Universal Maxillary Forceps No. 10S is used on surgical extraction tray setups.

Universal Maxillary Forceps No. 10S must be cleaned, bagged individually or bagged/wrapped in a tray setup, and then sterilized. A chemical/steam indicator device should be included in the wrapping. Hinged instruments should be processed open and unlocked.

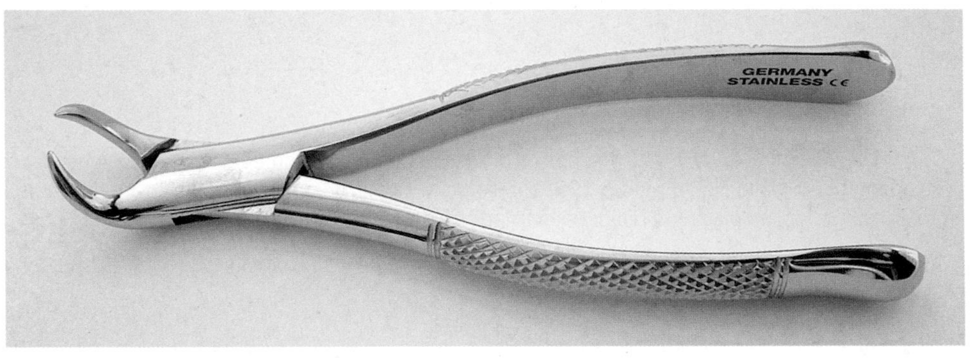
GERMANY
STAINLESS CE

INSTRUMENT

Universal Mandibular Forceps No. 16

FUNCTION To extract mandibular first and second molars

CHARACTERISTICS Straight handles or one curved handie
Referred to as *cowhorn forceps*

PRACTICE NOTE Universal Mandibular Forceps No. 16 (cowhorn) is used on surgical extraction tray setups.

Ⓢ Universal Mandibular Forceps No. 16 must be cleaned, bagged individually or bagged/wrapped in a tray setup, and then sterilized. A chemical/steam indicator device should be included in the wrapping. Hinged instruments should be processed open and unlocked.

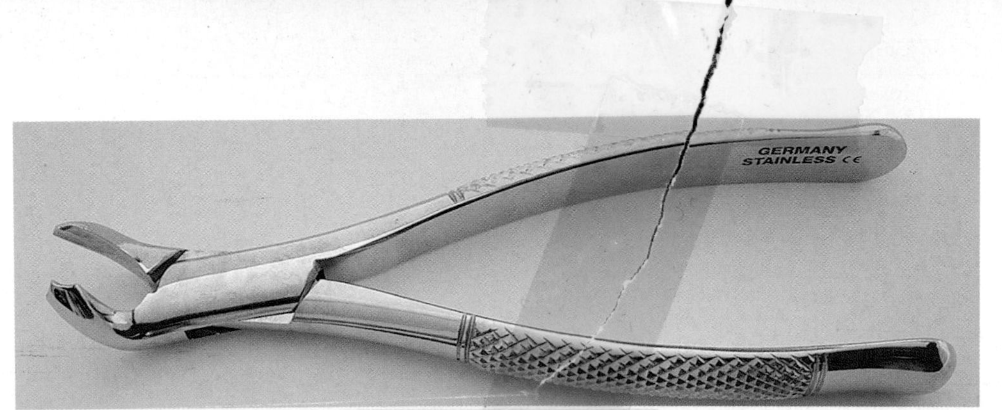
GERMANY
STAINLESS CE

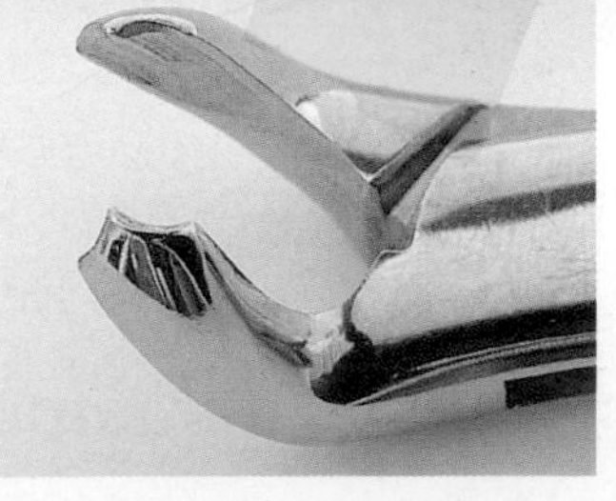

INSTRUMENT

Mandibular Forceps No. 17

FUNCTION To extract bifurcated mandibular right first or second molars

CHARACTERISTIC Straight handles

PRACTICE NOTE Mandibular Forceps No. 17 is used on surgical extraction tray setups.

Ⓢ Mandibular Forceps No. 17 must be cleaned, bagged individually or bagged/wrapped in a tray setup, and then sterilized. A chemical/steam indicator device should be included in the wrapping. Hinged instruments should be processed open and unlocked.

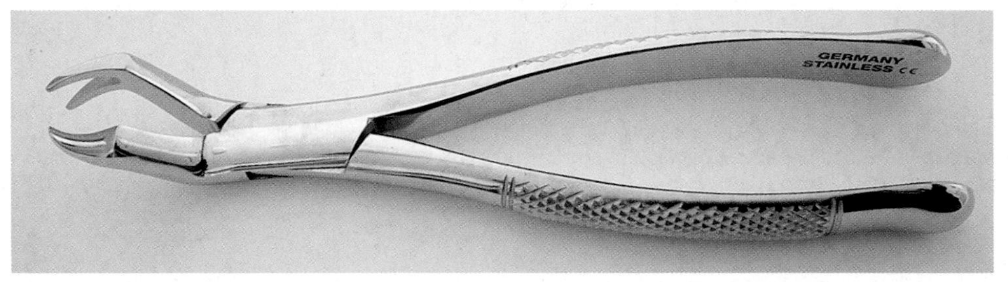
GERMANY
STAINLESS CE

INSTRUMENT

Maxillary Right Forceps No. 88R

FUNCTION To extract trifurcated maxillary right first or second molars

CHARACTERISTIC Right-split beak—For engaging lingual root

PRACTICE NOTE Maxillary Right Forceps No. 88R is used on surgical extraction tray setups.

Ⓢ Maxillary Right Forceps No. 88R must be cleaned, bagged individually or bagged/wrapped in a tray setup, and then sterilized. A chemical/steam indicator device should be included in the wrapping. Hinged instruments should be processed open and unlocked.

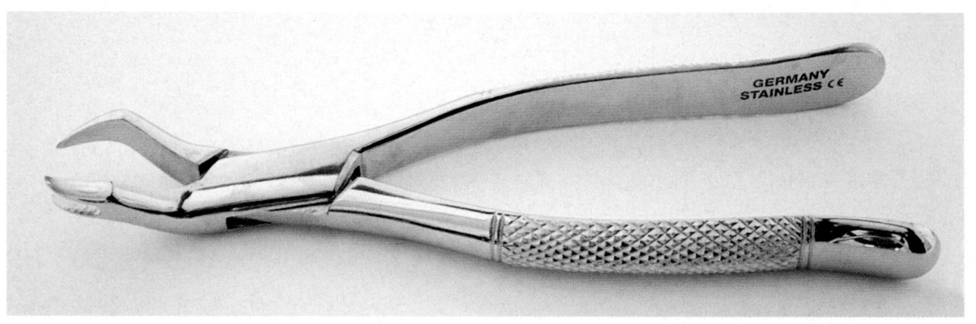
GERMANY
STAINLESS CE

INSTRUMENT

Maxillary Left Forceps No. 88L

FUNCTION To extract trifurcated maxillary left first or second molars

CHARACTERISTIC Left-split beak—For engaging lingual root

PRACTICE NOTE Maxillary Left Forceps No. 88L is used on surgical extraction tray setups.

S Maxillary Left Forceps No. 88L must be cleaned, bagged individually or bagged/wrapped in a tray setup, and then sterilized. A chemical/steam indicator device should be included in the wrapping. Hinged instruments should be processed open and unlocked.

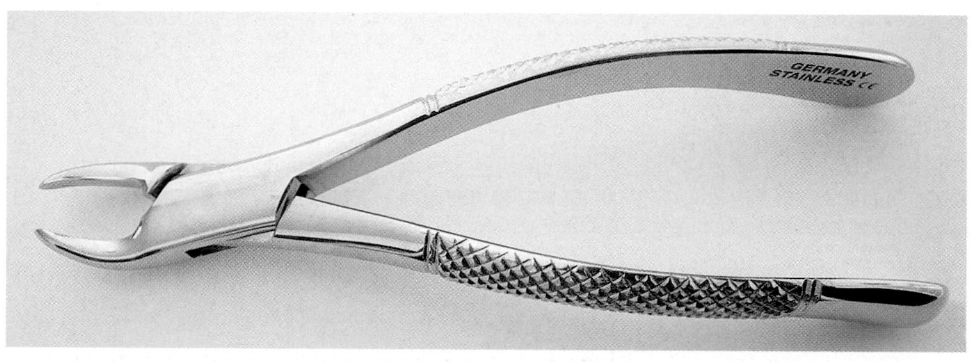
GERMANY
STAINLESS CE

INSTRUMENT

Maxillary Universal Forceps—Cryer 150 evolve

FUNCTION To extract maxillary centrals, laterals, cuspids, premolars, and roots

CHARACTERISTICS Straight handles or one curved handle

PRACTICE NOTE Maxillary Universal Forceps—Cryer 150 is used on surgical extraction tray setups.

S Maxillary Universal Forceps—Cryer 150 must be cleaned, bagged individually or bagged/wrapped in a tray setup, and then sterilized. A chemical/steam indicator device should be included in the wrapping. Hinged instruments should be processed open and unlocked.

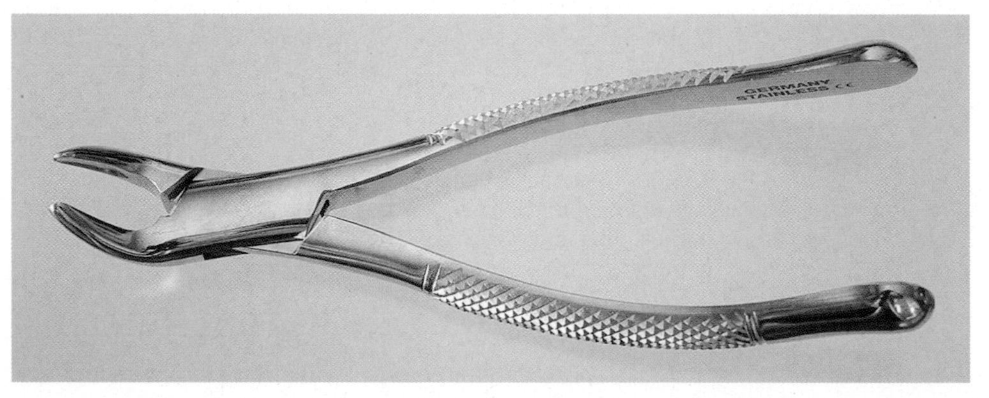
GERMANY
STAINLESS

INSTRUMENT

Mandibular Universal Forceps—Cryer 151 evolve

FUNCTION To extract mandibular centrals, laterals, cuspids, premolars, and roots

CHARACTERISTICS Straight handles or one curved handle

PRACTICE NOTE Mandibular Universal Forceps—Cryer 151 is used on surgical extraction tray setups.

S Mandibular Universal Forceps—Cryer 151 must be cleaned, bagged individually or bagged/wrapped in a tray setup, and then sterilized. A chemical/steam indicator device should be included in the wrapping. Hinged instruments should be processed open and unlocked.

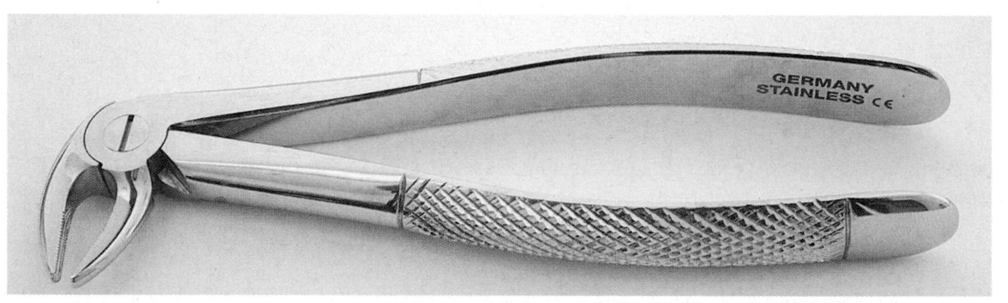
GERMANY
STAINLESS CE

INSTRUMENT

Mandibular Anterior Forceps

FUNCTION To extract mandibular anterior teeth

CHARACTERISTIC Serrated beaks

PRACTICE NOTE Mandibular Anterior Forceps is used on surgical extraction tray setups.

Ⓢ Mandibular Anterior Forceps must be cleaned, bagged individually or bagged/wrapped in a tray setup, and then sterilized. A chemical/steam indicator device should be included in the wrapping. Hinged instruments should be processed open and unlocked.

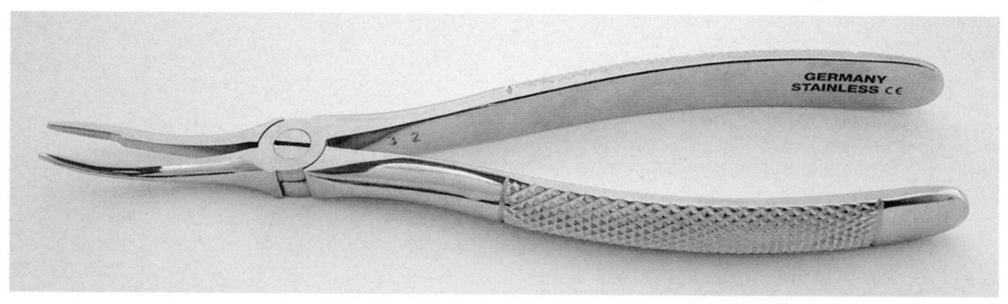
GERMANY
STAINLESS CE
3 2

INSTRUMENT

Maxillary Root Forceps

FUNCTION To extract maxillary roots

CHARACTERISTICS Narrow, serrated beaks
Straight handles

PRACTICE NOTE Maxillary Root Forceps is used on surgical extraction tray setups.

S Maxillary Root Forceps must be cleaned, bagged individually or bagged/wrapped in a tray setup, and then sterilized. A chemical/steam indicator device should be included in the wrapping. Hinged instruments should be processed open and unlocked.

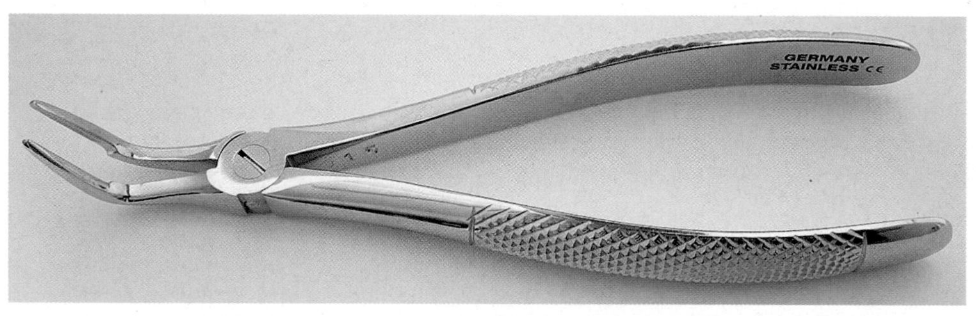
GERMANY
STAINLESS

INSTRUMENT

Mandibular Root Forceps

FUNCTION To extract mandibular roots

CHARACTERISTICS Narrow, serrated beaks
Straight handles

PRACTICE NOTE Mandibular Root Forceps is used on surgical extraction tray setups.

Ⓢ Mandibular Root Forceps must be cleaned, bagged individually or bagged/wrapped in a tray setup, and then sterilized. A chemical/steam indicator device should be included in the wrapping. Hinged instruments should be processed open and unlocked.

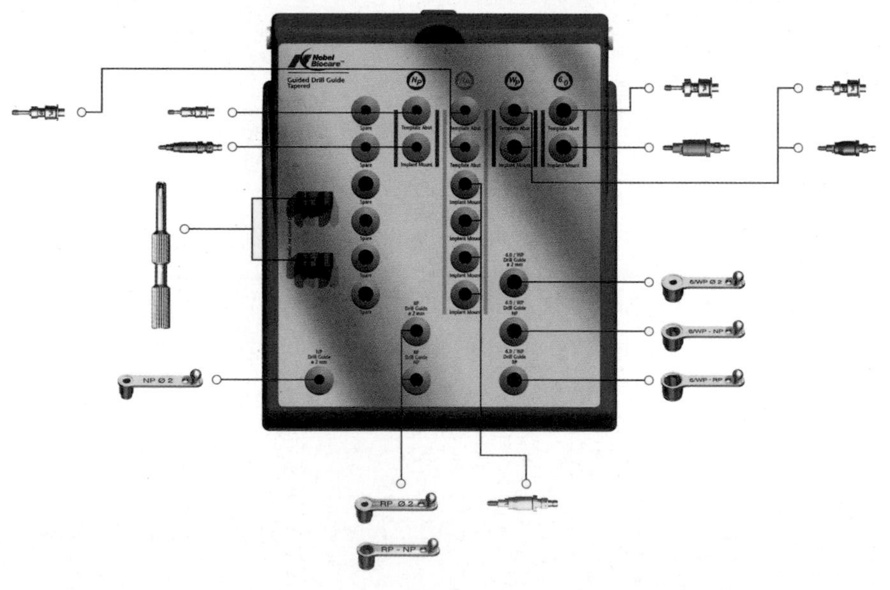
Nobel Biocare™
Guided Drill Guide
Tapered
Template Abut
Implant Mount
Spare
NP Ø 2
RP Ø 2
RP - NP
6/WP Ø 2
6/WP - NP
6/WP - RP

INSTRUMENT

Implant System

FUNCTION To use for implant surgery

CHARACTERISTICS Components—Depth drills, thread formers, hand wrench, ratchet, ratchet adapter, hex driver

PRACTICE NOTES Implant System is used on a surgical tray setup. Sterile technique must be kept during procedure.

S Implant System must be cleaned, bagged individually or bagged/wrapped in a tray setup, and then sterilized. A chemical/steam indicator device should be included in the wrapping.

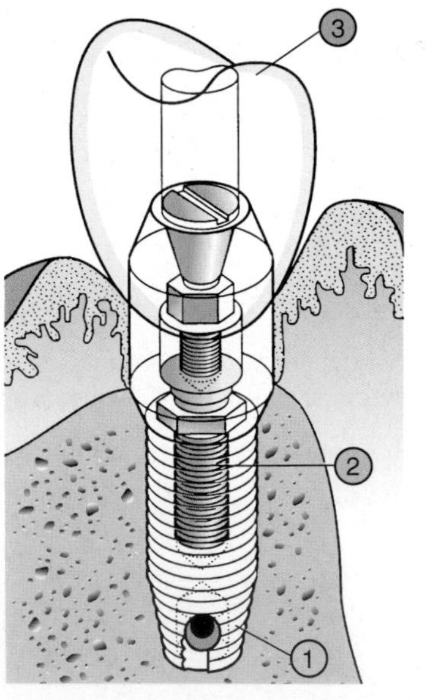
3
2
1

INSTRUMENT

Implant

FUNCTION To use for implant surgery

CHARACTERISTICS Endosteal Implant—An implant surgically embedded into the bone

Osseointegration—The attachment of healthy bone to a dental implant also referred to as stably integrated.

Two other types of implants—Subperiosteal and transosteal

Components—

1. Implant fixture (titanium) embedded into bone
2. Center screw
3. Crown

PRACTICE NOTES Implant is used on a surgical tray setup. Sterile technique must be kept during procedure.

S Implant must be bagged individually and then sterilized. A chemical/steam indicator device should be included in the wrapping. Use a biological indicator for every sterilizer load that contains an implantable device. Verify results before using the implantable device, whenever possible according to the MMWR Guidelines for Infection Control in Dental Health-Care Settings—2003, Recommendations, Category IB. Strongly recommended for implementation and supported by experimental, clinical, or epidemiologic studies and a strong theoretical rationale.

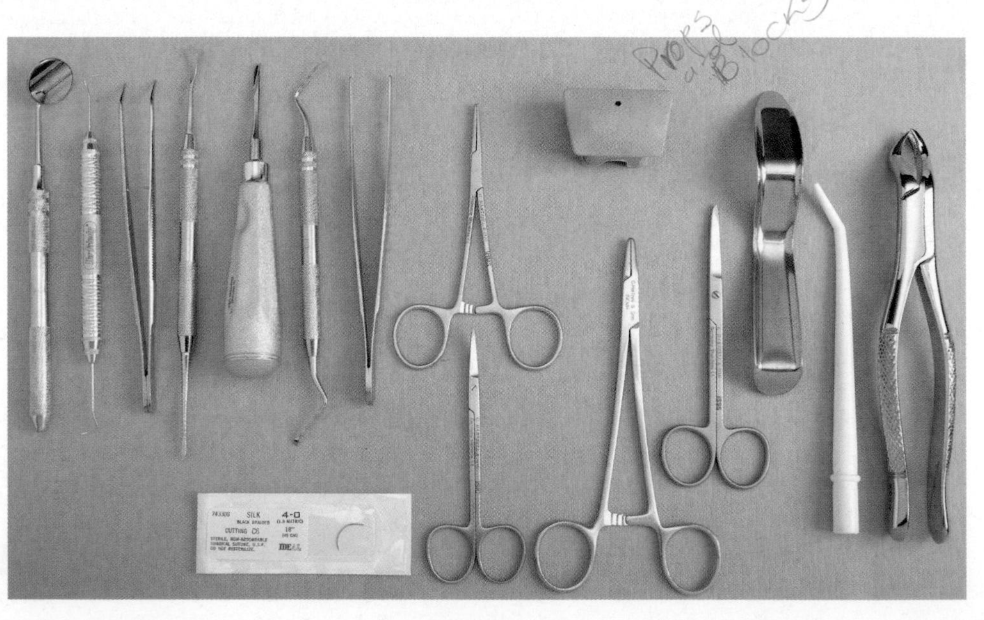
SILK
4-0
CUTTING C6
18"

TRAY SETUP

Extraction of Maxillary Right First Molar

TOP ROW (FROM LEFT TO RIGHT)

Mouth mirror, explorer, cotton forceps periosteal elevator, straight elevator, surgical curette, tissue forceps, hemostat, tissue scissors, mouth prop, needle holder, suture scissors, tongue and cheek retractor (Minnesota), disposable high-volume surgical evacuation tip, and maxillary right forceps No. 88R

BOTTOM ROW

Silk suture with needle in sterile package

Ⓢ Refer to each picture for correct procedure for instrument sterilization or disposal of instrument or material.

Refer to Chapter 15: Universal Surgical Instruments to see additional instruments used in Oral Surgery Extractions.

For mandibular first or second molar extraction, the tray setup is identical to the tray setup for the extraction of a maxillary right first molar except that a mandibular right forceps no. 17 is used in place of a maxillary right forceps no. 88R.

532

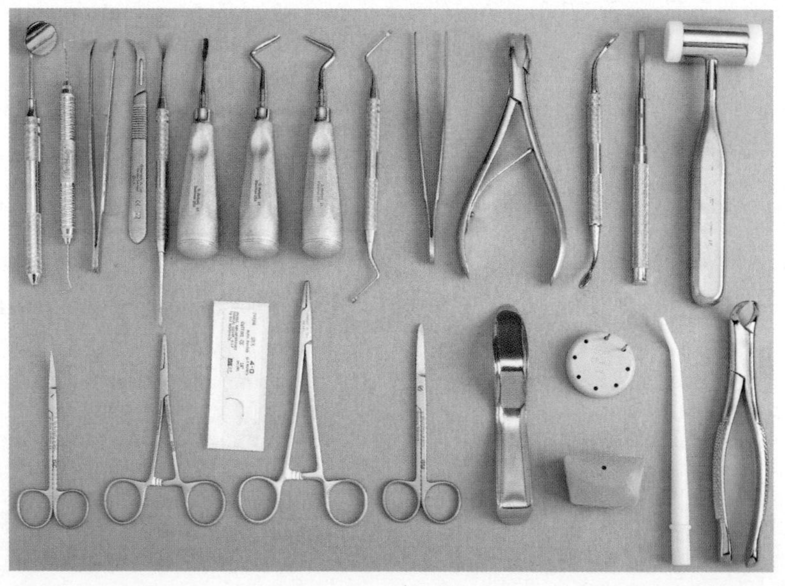

TRAY SETUP

Extraction of Impacted Mandibular Molar

TOP ROW (FROM LEFT TO RIGHT)

Mouth mirror, explorer, cotton forceps (pliers), scalpel with No. 12 blade, periosteal elevator, straight elevator, right and left root tip elevators, surgical curette, tissue forceps, Rongeurs, bone file, surgical chisel, surgical mallet

BOTTOM ROW (FROM LEFT TO RIGHT)

Tissue scissors, hemostats, silk suture with needle in sterile package, needle holder, suture scissors, tongue and cheek retractor (Minnesota), surgical long shank burs in bur holder, mouth prop, disposable high-volume surgical evacuation tip, universal mandibular forceps No. 16

Ⓢ Refer to each picture for correct procedure for instrument sterilization or disposal of instrument or material.

Refer to Chapter 15: Universal Surgical Instruments to see additional instruments used in Oral Surgery Extractions. Also, refer to other chapters for additional instruments on this tray setup.

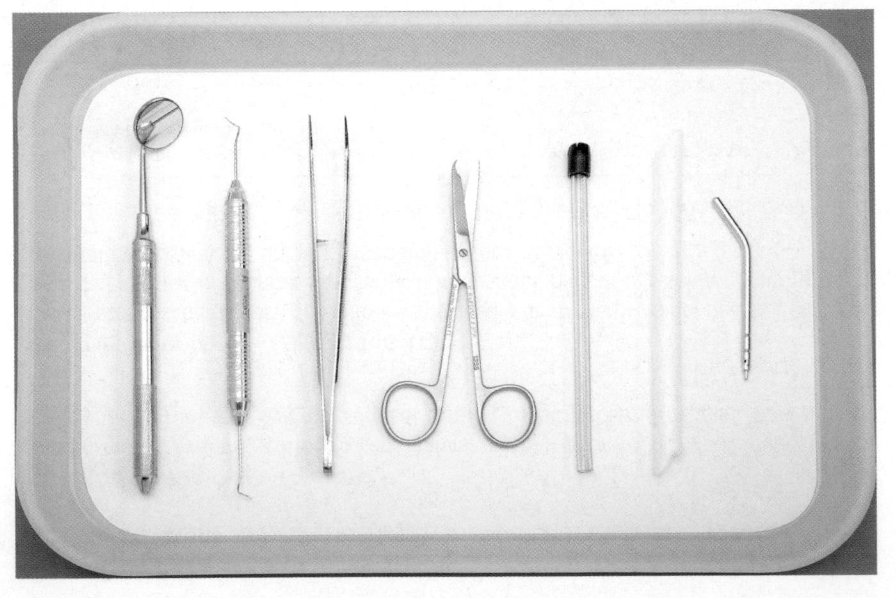

TRAY SETUP

Suture Removal

LEFT TO RIGHT

Mouth mirror, pigtail explorer, cotton forceps (pliers), suture scissors, saliva ejector, high-volume evacuator (HVE) tip, air/water syringe tip

Refer to each picture for correct procedure for instrument sterilization or disposal of instrument or material.

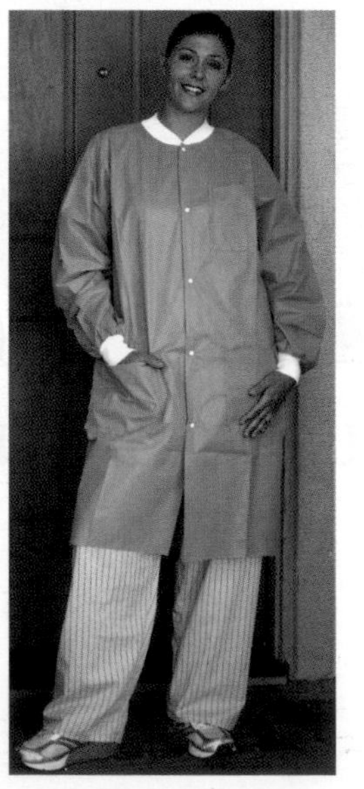

INSTRUMENT

Laboratory Coat

FUNCTION To protect clothing, surgical scrubs, and skin during patient care and sterilization process to prevent contamination from blood and body substances

CHARACTERISTICS Disposable or cloth (cloth gown must be made of polyester and cotton in accordance with state and federal regulations)
Cuffed long sleeves
Closure at neckline
Moisture resistant (against contamination by liquids)

PRACTICE NOTES All protective clothing should be removed before leaving the work place.
Follow regulations within the state for standard precautions.

S Dispose of lab coat in garbage at the end of the day.
If lab coat becomes visibly soiled during the work day, change to a new lab coat.

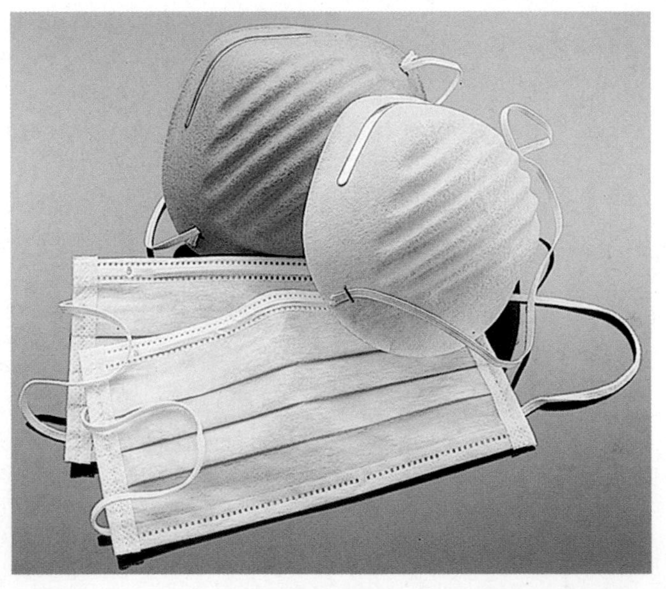

INSTRUMENT

Protective Mask

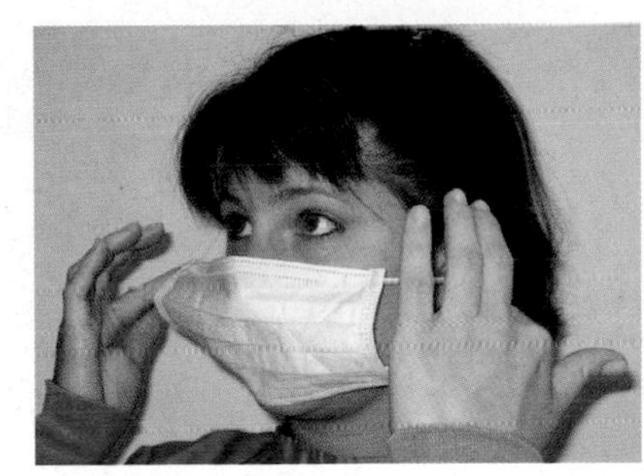

FUNCTIONS

To protect against chemicals, airborne pathogens, bacteria, and viruses during processing of instruments for sterilization

To protect against airborne pathogens, bacteria, and viruses and against scrap filling material during all phases of patient treatment

CHARACTERISTIC

Dome shaped or flat

PRACTICE NOTES

Protective Mask must cover nose and mouth.

Protective Mask must be worn during dental procedures with a patient and during any exposure to dental material that is airborne.

S Protective Mask should be disposed of in the garbage.

A new mask must be used with each patient.

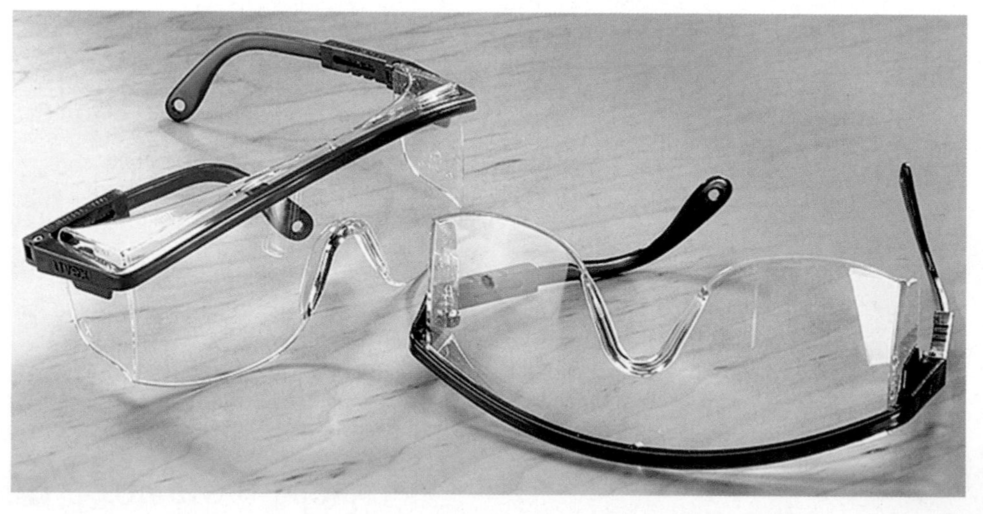

INSTRUMENT

Protective Glasses/Eye Wear

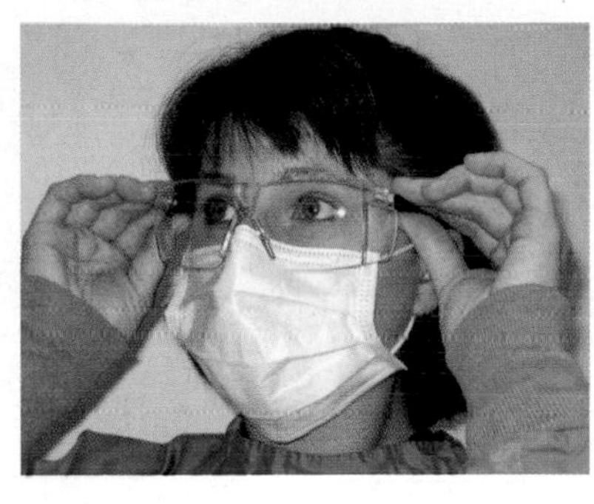

FUNCTIONS

To protect against chemicals, airborne pathogens, bacteria, and viruses during processing of instruments for sterilization

To protect against airborne pathogens, bacteria, and viruses during patient care and against scrap-filling material during restorative and rinsing phases of patient treatment

CHARACTERISTICS

Extend to sides, top, and bottom of eyes for complete protection

Variety of styles available—some styles are larger to fit over prescription glasses

PRACTICE NOTES

Facial shields available for eye protection (mask must be worn)

Protective Glasses must be worn during dental procedures with a patient and during any exposure to dental material that is airborne.

S Glasses are disinfected between patients according to the manufacturer's recommendation.

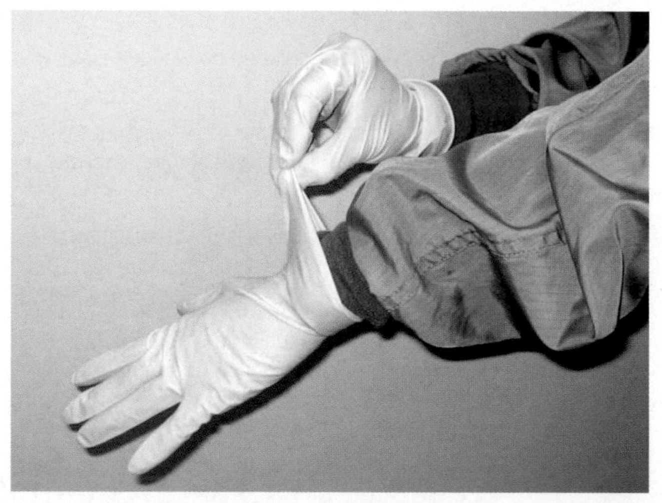

INSTRUMENT

Examination Gloves

FUNCTIONS

To wear during patient care
To wear as a protective barrier
To wear during treatment room disinfection

CHARACTERISTICS

Latex or vinyl
Nonsterile gloves worn for most dental procedures; sterile gloves may be worn for surgical procedures
Various sizes available

PRACTICE NOTE

Examination Gloves are single use only. Wash hands prior to putting on gloves and after removing gloves. Must change if leaving patient care or use overgloves (refer to page 547). Replace worn or torn gloves immediately. If procedure is long, change gloves every hour. Gloves must go over cuff of lab coat.

S Examination Gloves must be disposed of in the garbage.

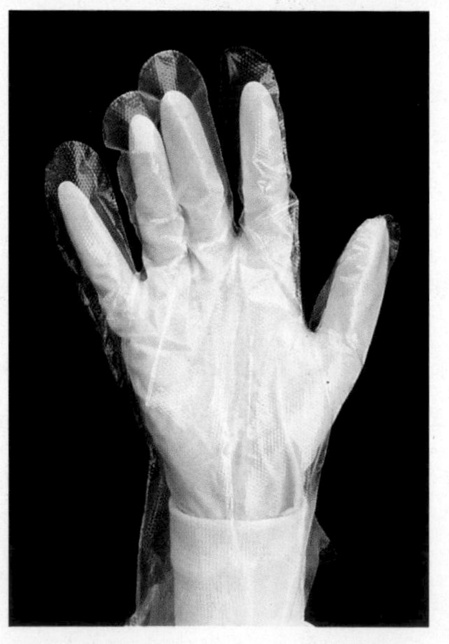

INSTRUMENT

Overgloves

FUNCTIONS To wear over examination gloves when leaving the patient
To wear as a protective barrier over the examination gloves so as not to cross contaminate

CHARACTERISTICS Lightweight clear gloves
Not to be worn for dental procedures
Various sizes available

PRACTICE NOTES New overgloves for each patient. Keep overgloves in an uncontaminated area of the treatment room. Must be careful not to contaminate outside of overgloves when putting on over examination gloves.

S Overgloves must be disposed of in the garbage.

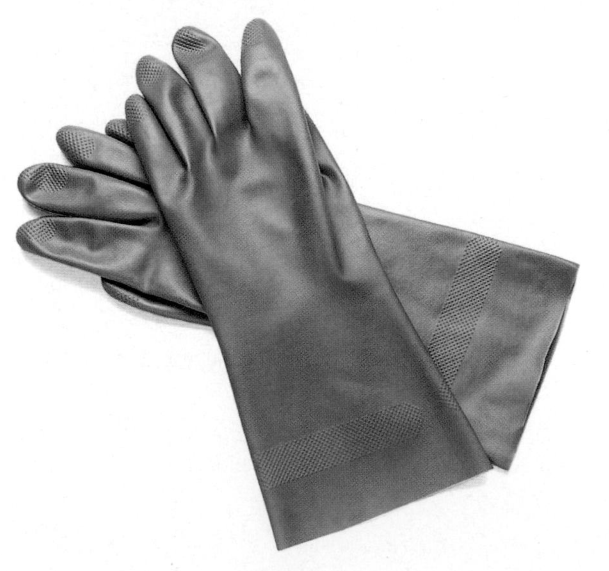

INSTRUMENT

Nitrile Utility Gloves evolve

FUNCTIONS
To protect hands during processing of instruments for sterilization procedures
To wear for preparation and handling of chemicals

CHARACTERISTICS
Chemical resistant
Puncture resistant
Ribbed for nonslip grip
Range of sizes and colors

PRACTICE NOTE
Nitrile Utility Gloves should be kept in sterilization area of office.

S
Nitrile Utility Gloves are disinfected after each use.
Sterilize according to the manufacturer's recommendation and refer to local and state regulations.

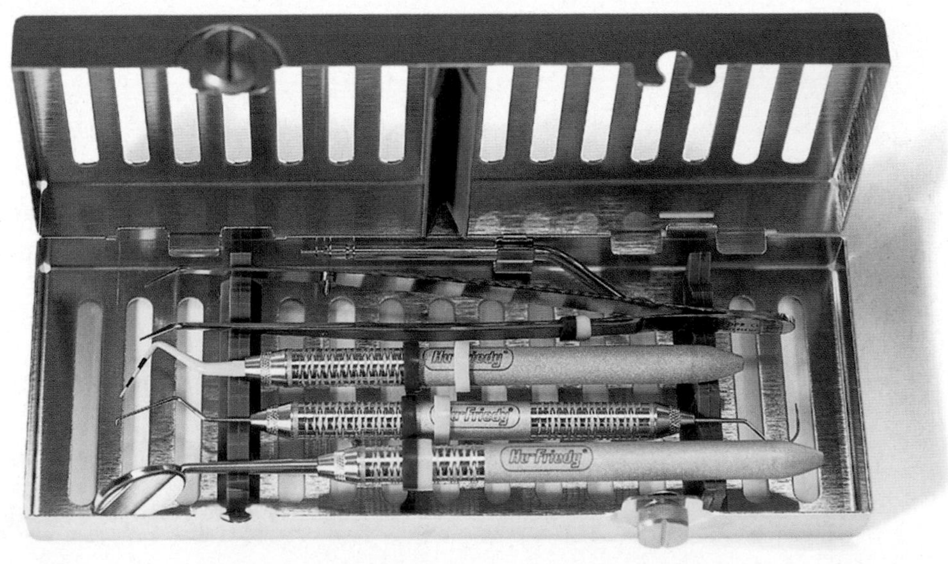
Hu-Friedy
Hu-Friedy
Hu-Friedy

INSTRUMENT

Cassette

FUNCTIONS

To use for instruments as tray setup
To use for instrument sterilization

CHARACTERISTICS

Available in metal or resin
Color coded
Range of sizes

PRACTICE NOTES

Instruments in the cassette may be cleaned in an ultrasonic cleaner and then wrapped and sterilized.
Color-coding aids in the identification of tray setups and which instrument belongs with which case.

S Cassette with instruments should be bagged/wrapped and then sterilized. A chemical/steam indicator device should be included in the wrapping.

Cassette above shows color-coded mouth mirror, explorer, periodontal probe, cotton forceps, and air/water syringe tip.

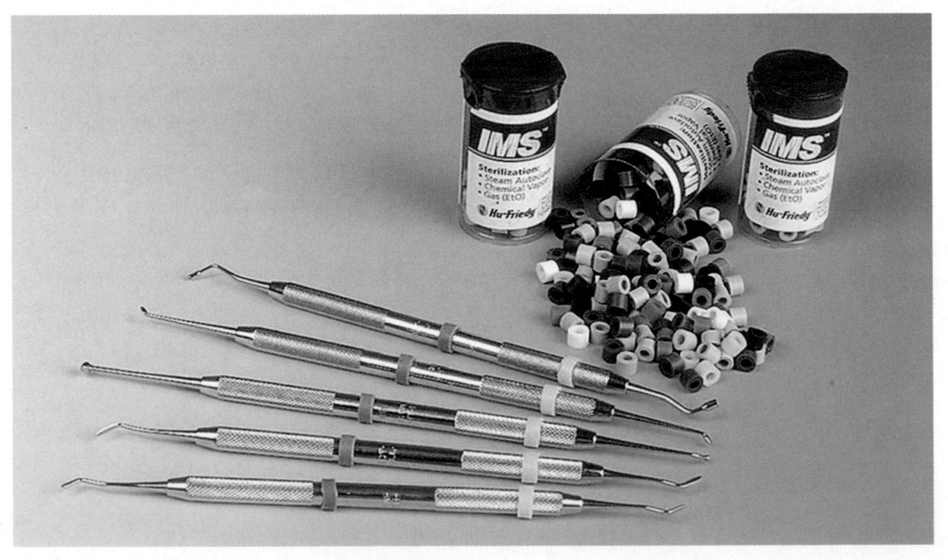
IMS
Sterilization:
• Steam Autoclave
• Chemical Vapor
• Gas (EtO)
Hu-Friedy
IMS
Sterilization:
• Steam Autoclave
• Chemical Vapor
• Gas (EtO)
Hu-Friedy

INSTRUMENT

Color Coding System for Instruments evolve

FUNCTION To color code instruments for organization and identification of tray setups

CHARACTERISTIC Variety of colors—Color coding coordinates with color cassettes

PRACTICE NOTE The color coding system makes it easier to identify tray setups and instruments within the tray setup.

S Color coding can withstand all heat sterilization methods

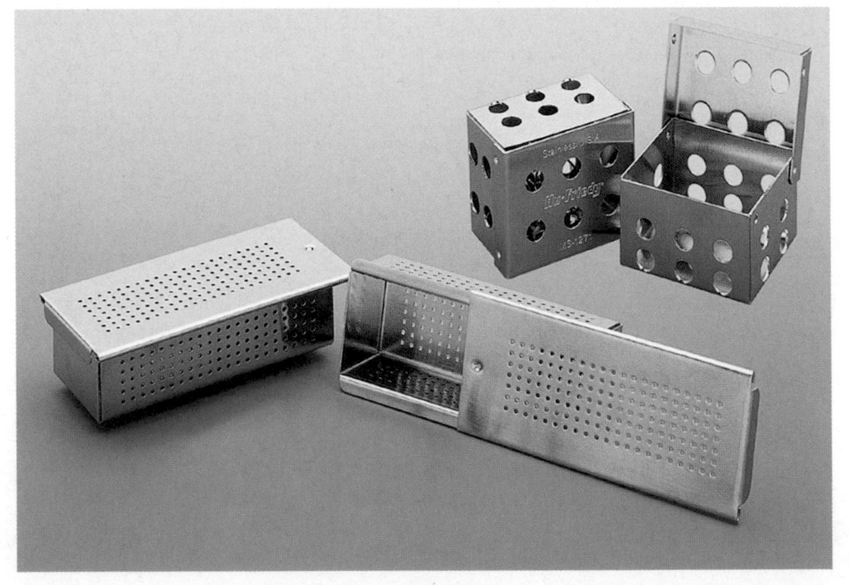

INSTRUMENT

Parts Box for Sterilization

FUNCTION To use for sterilization of small items

Example: burs, dental dam clamps

CHARACTERISTIC Range of sizes to accommodate sterilization needs

PRACTICE NOTE Parts Boxes helps hold and organize small items for tray setups.

S Parts Box or Boxes must be cleaned, bagged individually or bagged/wrapped in a tray setup, and then sterilized. A chemical/steam indicator device should be included in the wrapping.

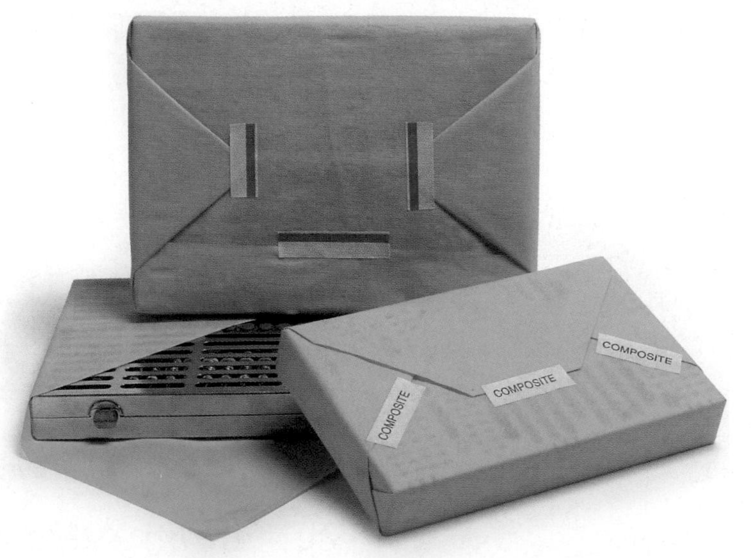
COMPOSITE
COMPOSITE
COMPOSITE

INSTRUMENT

Cassette Wrap

FUNCTIONS
To use to wrap cassette during sterilization
To store cassette in wrapping after sterilization
To use for tray cover during dental procedure

CHARACTERISTIC
Range of sizes—To accommodate cassettes

PRACTICE NOTE
Cassettes should be kept in sterile wrap until the patient is seated. Refer to local and state regulations.

S A chemical indicator device should be included in the inside of the wrapping. When the indicator device cannot be seen from the outside, a chemical indicator tape should be placed on the outside of the wrapping, as shown in picture.

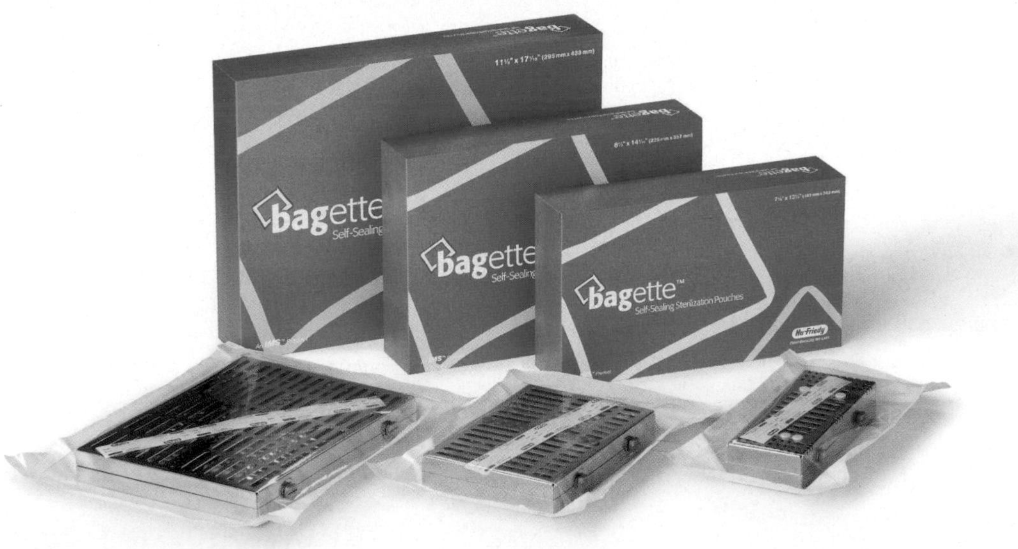
bagette
Self-Sealing
bagette
Self-Sealing
bagette™
Self-Sealing Sterilization Pouches
Hu-Friedy

INSTRUMENT

Sterilization Pouches

evolve

FUNCTION To be used for sterilization of instruments and cassettes

CHARACTERISTIC Pouches have range of sizes to accommodate all sizes of instruments and cassettes.

PRACTICE NOTE Instruments should be kept in the pouches until the patient is seated. Refer to state regulations.

S Indicator strips may be placed on the inside of pouch if it can be seen, OR indicator tape may be placed on outside of pouch. Indicator strips turn colors to verify time and temperature of the sterilization process; they do not determine the actual sterilization. Refer to sterilization monitoring.

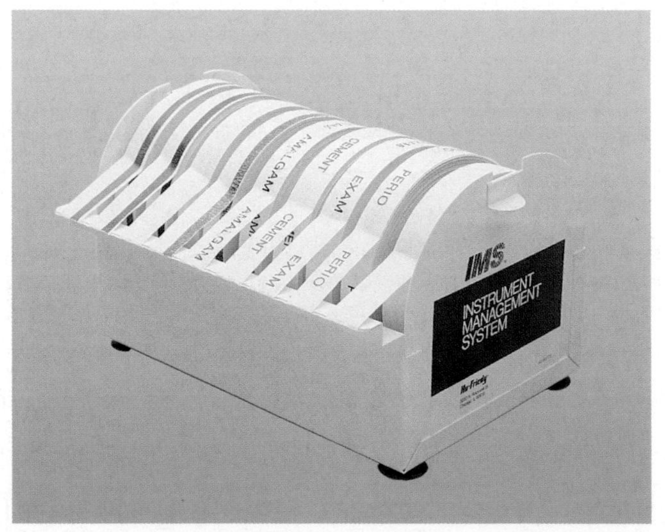
PERIO
EXAM
CEMENT
AMALGAM
PERIO
EXAM
CEMENT
AMALGAM
IMS
INSTRUMENT
MANAGEMENT
SYSTEM
Hu-Friedy

INSTRUMENT

Indicator Tape and Dispensing Unit

FUNCTIONS

To secure wrap on outside of cassette

To use outside cassettes or sterilization pouches to indicate exposure of instruments to a certain temperature—color will change on the tape

CHARACTERISTICS

Available in preprinted tray setup procedures

Available with color coding

Available blank for labeling tape with procedure and/or instrument content

PRACTICE NOTE

Instruments should be kept in the pouches until the patient is seated. Refer to state regulations.

S When indicator tape is placed outside a cassette, the strips change color with exposure to temperature of the sterilization process; they do not determine the actual sterilization. Refer to sterilization monitoring.

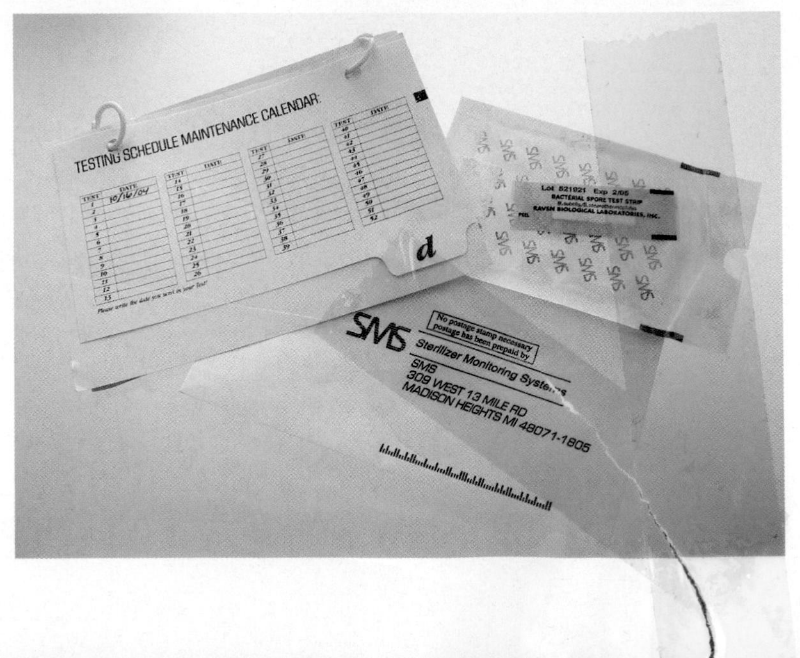
TESTING SCHEDULE MAINTENANCE CALENDAR:
TEST
DATE
10/16/04
d
Please write the date you sent in your Test
Lot 521921 Exp 2/05
BACTERIAL SPORE TEST STRIP
RAVEN BIOLOGICAL LABORATORIES, INC.
SMS
No postage stamp necessary
postage has been prepaid by
Sterilizer Monitoring Systems
SMS
309 WEST 13 MILE RD
MADISON HEIGHTS MI 48071-1805

INSTRUMENT

Biological Monitors for Sterilizers

FUNCTION To confirm efficacy of sterilization, documentation of results is recorded in office sterilization log

CHARACTERISTICS Many systems available

PRACTICE NOTES Biological Monitor testing device is placed in the sterilizer for one cycle of instruments. It is then mailed to the manufacturer, which mails back the findings. The results are logged in the office sterilization records.

S The Centers for Disease Control and Prevention (CDC), the American Dental Association (ADA), and the Office Safety and Asepsis Procedures Research Foundation (OSAP) recommend at least weekly testing of sterilizers. Local and state requirements may be different.

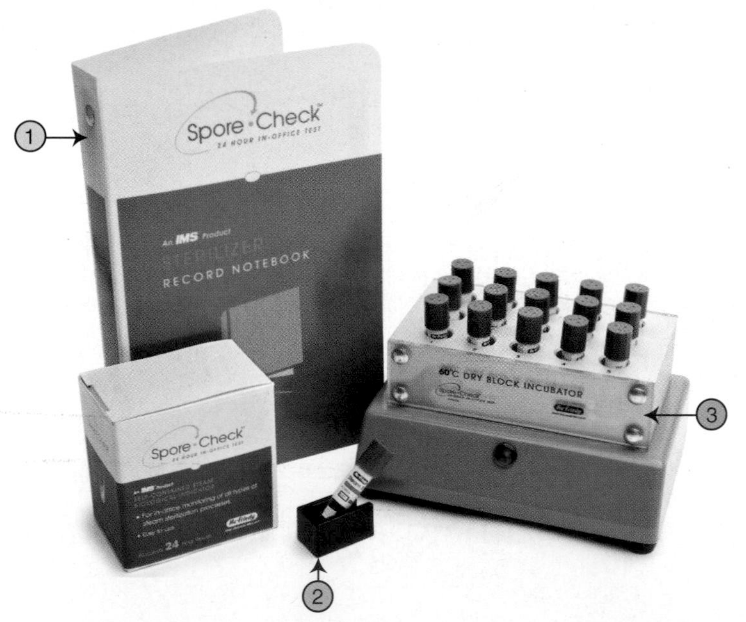

1
2
3
Spore Check
24 HOUR IN-OFFICE TEST
An IMS Product
STERILIZER
RECORD NOTEBOOK
60°C DRY BLOCK INCUBATOR

INSTRUMENT

Sterilization Spore Check—In Office

FUNCTION To monitor and confirm the effectiveness of steam sterilizers

CHARACTERISTICS

① Record book
② Self contained biological indicator
③ Dry block incubator

A vial with the solution is marked and placed in a sterilization pouch, and the sterilization cycle is processed. After the cycle is complete, follow the directions, then place vial in incubator. Results will occur in 24 hours. Record results.

Ⓢ Steam sterilizers should be checked for effectiveness every week. Every load of implants should be monitored for effectiveness when possible.

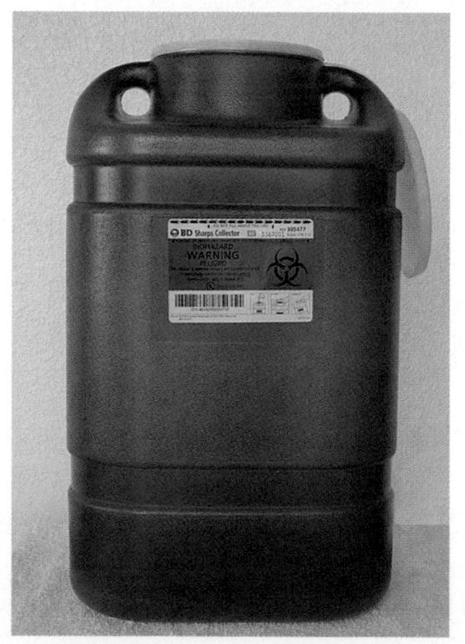
BD Sharps Collector
BIOHAZARD
WARNING
PELIGRO

INSTRUMENT

Sharps Container

FUNCTION To serve as storage receptacle for used needles, old burs, scalpel blades, orthodontic wires, endodontic files, and all other disposable sharp items used intraorally

CHARACTERISTICS Must be puncture resistant
Must be labeled "Biohazard"
Must have a reclosable top

PRACTICE NOTE Sharps containers must be disposed of according to local, state, and federal regulations.

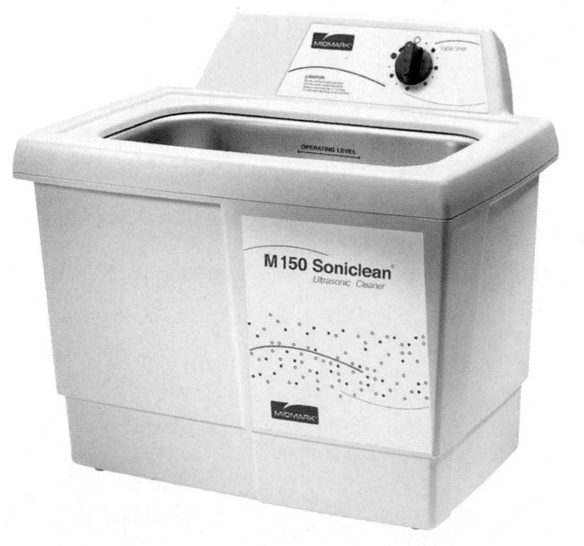
MIDMARK
Cycle timer
CAUTION
OPERATING LEVEL
M150 Soniclean
Ultrasonic Cleaner
MIDMARK

INSTRUMENT

Ultrasonic Cleaning Unit

FUNCTION To remove debris and bioburden from instruments

CHARACTERISTIC Reduces risk of exposure to pathogens during the cleaning stage of the sterilization process

PRACTICE NOTES Tank is filled with antimicrobial or general all-purpose solution especially designed for the ultrasonic unit.

Debris is removed by mechanical means; sound waves create tiny bubbles that cause inward collapse (implosion) and removal of material.

S After cleaning, the instruments must be placed in a sterilizer for processing.

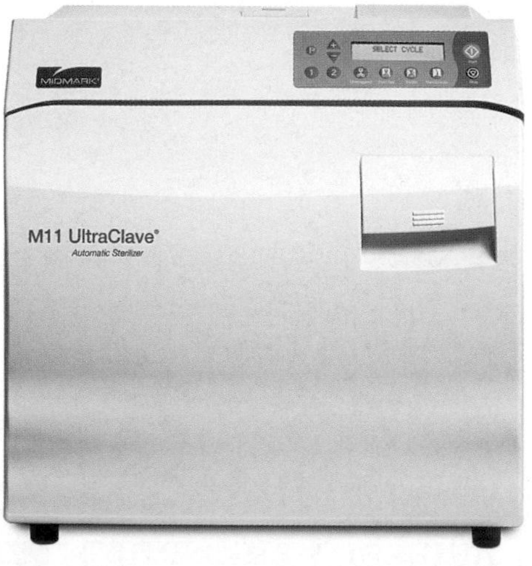
MIDMARK
SELECT CYCLE
M11 UltraClave®
Automatic Sterilizer

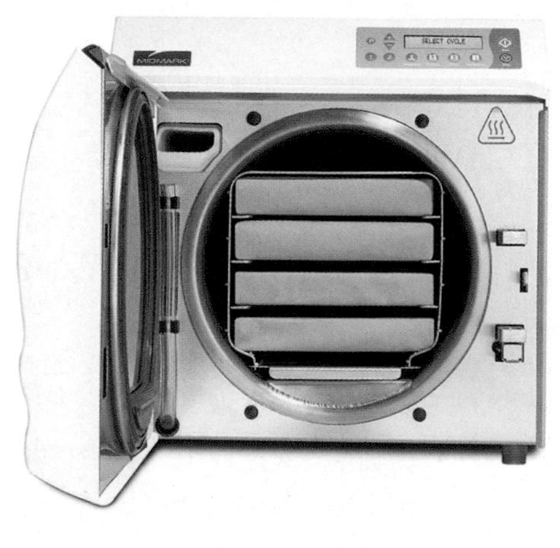
MIDMARK
SELECT CYCLE

INSTRUMENT

Sterilizer—Autoclave (Saturated Steam)

FUNCTION To kill all microbes, viruses, bacteria, and fungi, thereby sterilizing instruments

CHARACTERISTICS Uses steam under pressure—15 pounds per square inch (psi) at 250° F for 20 minutes
Shelves available for cassettes
Various styles and manufacturers
Range of sizes

S The Centers for Disease Control and Prevention (CDC), the American Dental Association (ADA), and the Office Safety and Asepsis Procedures Research Foundation (OSAP) recommend at least weekly testing of sterilizers. Local and state requirements may be different.

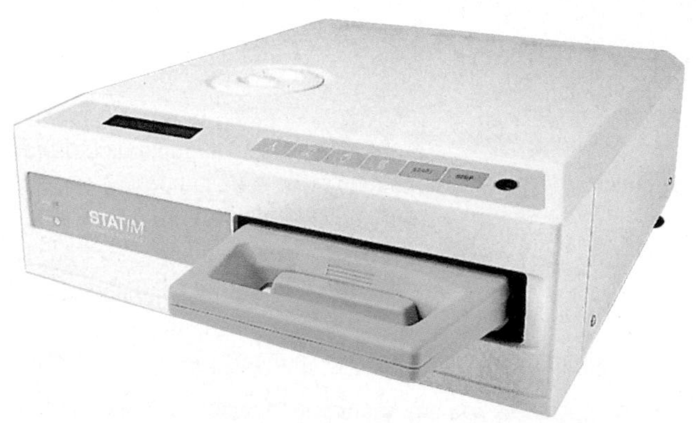
STATIM

INSTRUMENT

Sterilizer—Autoclave ("Flash")

FUNCTIONS

To kill all microbes, viruses, bacteria, and fungi, thereby sterilizing instruments
To use for quick sterilization of instruments and handpieces

CHARACTERISTICS

Unwrapped instruments:
Steam under pressure—15 psi at 270° F for 3 minutes
Wrapped instruments:
Steam under pressure—15 psi at 250° F for 15 minutes or 15 psi at 270° F for 11 minutes
Shelves available for cassettes
Various styles and manufacturers
Range of sizes

This method is not recommended for use as a routine sterilization procedure.
The Centers for Disease Control and Prevention (CDC), the American Dental Association (ADA), and the Office Safety and Asepsis Procedures Research Foundation (OSAP) recommend at least weekly testing of sterilizers. Local and state requirements may be different.

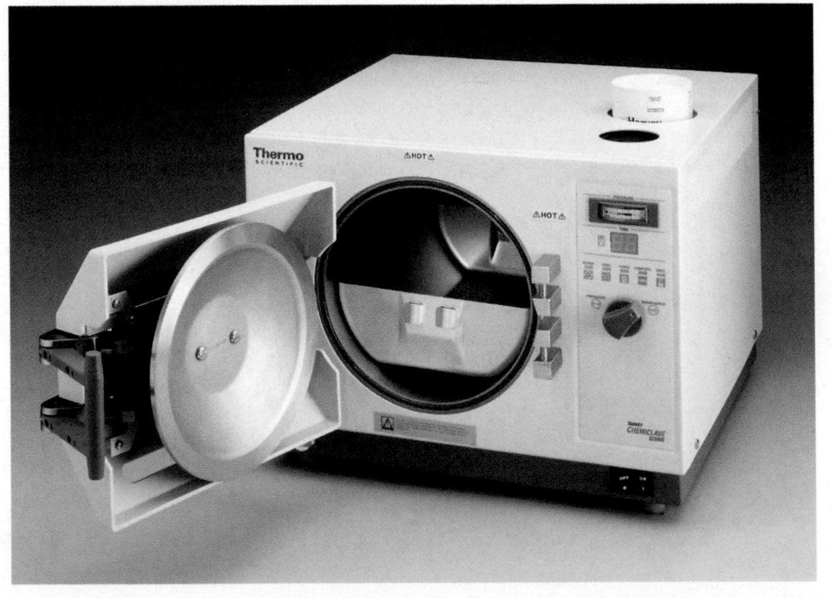
Thermo
SCIENTIFIC
HOT
HOT
CHEMICLAVE

INSTRUMENT

Sterilizer—Chemiclave (Unsaturated Chemical Vapor)

FUNCTION To kill all microbes, viruses, bacteria, and fungi, thereby sterilizing instruments

CHARACTERISTICS Uses chemical solution (alcohol, 0.23% formaldehyde, ketone, acetone, water) in a pressurized chamber—20 to 40 psi at 270° F for 20 minutes

Shelves available for cassette

Various styles and manufacturers

Range of sizes

PRACTICE NOTE State and local agencies require proper hazardous waste disposal. A Material Safety Data Sheet (MSDS) is required for the solution.

Ⓢ The Centers for Disease Control and Prevention (CDC), the American Dental Association (ADA), and the Office Safety and Asepsis Procedures Research Foundation (OSAP) recommend at least weekly testing of sterilizers. Local and state requirements may be different.

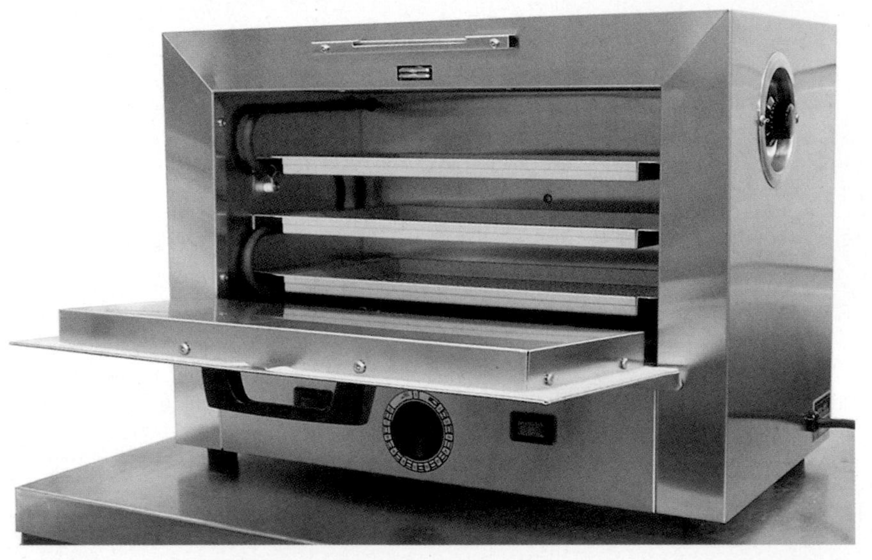

INSTRUMENT

Sterilizer—Dry Heat (Static Air)

FUNCTION To kill all microbes, viruses, bacteria, and fungi, thereby sterilizing instruments

CHARACTERISTICS
Oven-type sterilizer
320° F for 60 to 120 minutes
Shelves available for cassettes
Various styles and manufacturers
Range of sizes

PRACTICE NOTES
Packaging/wrapped material must be able to withstand high temperatures.
Door cannot be opened during sterilization cycle.
Items cannot be layered or stacked but should be placed on their edges.

The Centers for Disease Control and Prevention (CDC), the American Dental Association (ADA), and the Office Safety and Asepsis Procedures Research Foundation (OSAP) recommend at least weekly testing of sterilizers. Local and state requirements may be different.

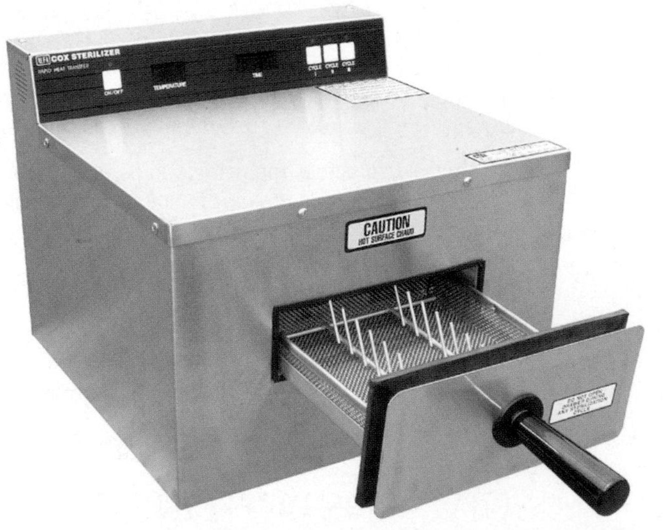
COX STERILIZER
ON/OFF
TEMPERATURE
CYCLE 1
CYCLE 2
CYCLE 3
CAUTION
HOT SURFACE
DO NOT OPEN
DRAWER DURING
ANY STERILIZATION
CYCLE

INSTRUMENT

Sterilizer—Dry Heat (Rapid Heat Transfer)

FUNCTION To kill all microbes, viruses, bacteria, and fungi, thereby sterilizing instruments

CHARACTERISTICS Forced air type sterilizer
375° F for 12 minutes (wrapped)
375° F for 6 minutes (unwrapped)
Instruments placed in preheated chamber
Various styles and manufacturers
Range of sizes

PRACTICE NOTES Packaging/wrapped material must be able to withstand high temperatures.
Door cannot be opened during sterilization cycle.

S The Centers for Disease Control and Prevention (CDC), the American Dental Association (ADA), and the Office Safety and Asepsis Procedures Research Foundation (OSAP) recommend at least weekly testing of sterilizers. Local and state requirements may be different.

CHAPTER 19

Dental Materials Equipment

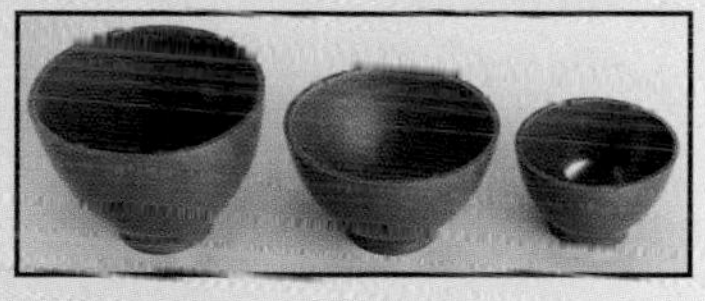

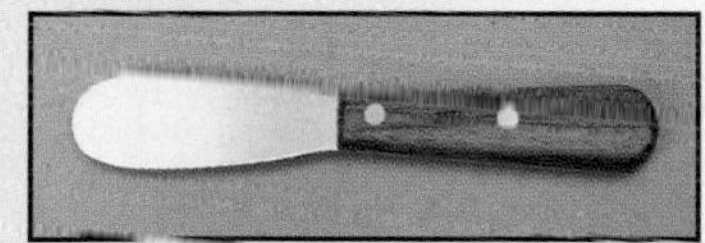

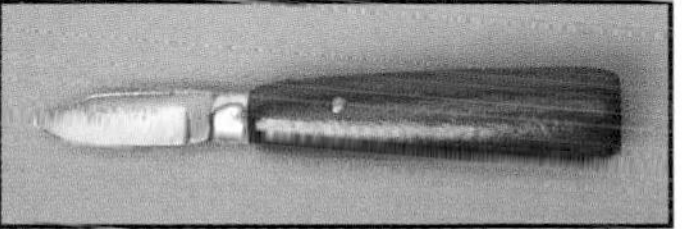

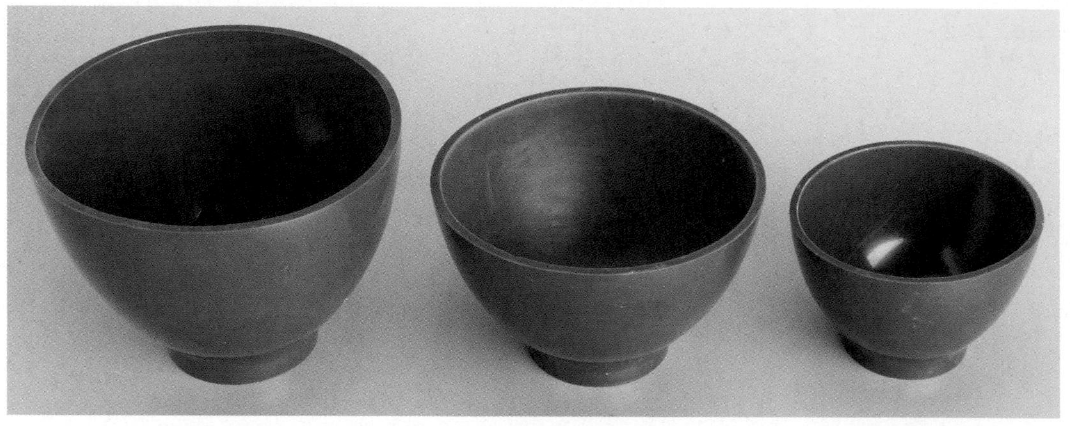

INSTRUMENT

Flexible Rubber Bowl evolve

FUNCTIONS To mix material, usually a powder and a liquid

To mix impression material and Irreversible hydrocolloid for study models, opposing models, bleaching trays, night guards, mouth guards, orthodontic appliances, custom trays for removable appliances

To mix laboratory plaster, stone, and die stone for models

CHARACTERISTICS Bowl is flexible to manipulate material.

PRACTICE NOTE Flexible Rubber Bowl is used with the flexible spatula.

S Disinfect bowls according to the manufacturer's recommendation.

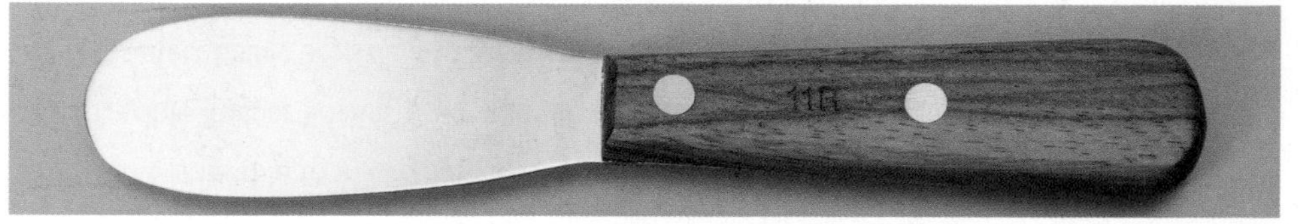

INSTRUMENT

Flexible Alginate (Irreversible Hydrocolloid) Spatula

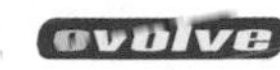

FUNCTIONS

To mix powder and a liquid in a flexible bowl
To mix impression material such as irreversible hydrocolloid (alginate)
To mix laboratory plaster, stone, and die stone for models

CHARACTERISTIC

Spatula is flexible to manipulate material.

PRACTICE NOTES

Flexible Alginate Spatula is used with the flexible rubber bowl (see page 583)

S Disinfect Flexible Alginate Spatula according to the manufacturer's recommendation. Spatula may cleaned, bagged individually, and then sterilized. A chemical/steam indicator device should be included in the wrapping.

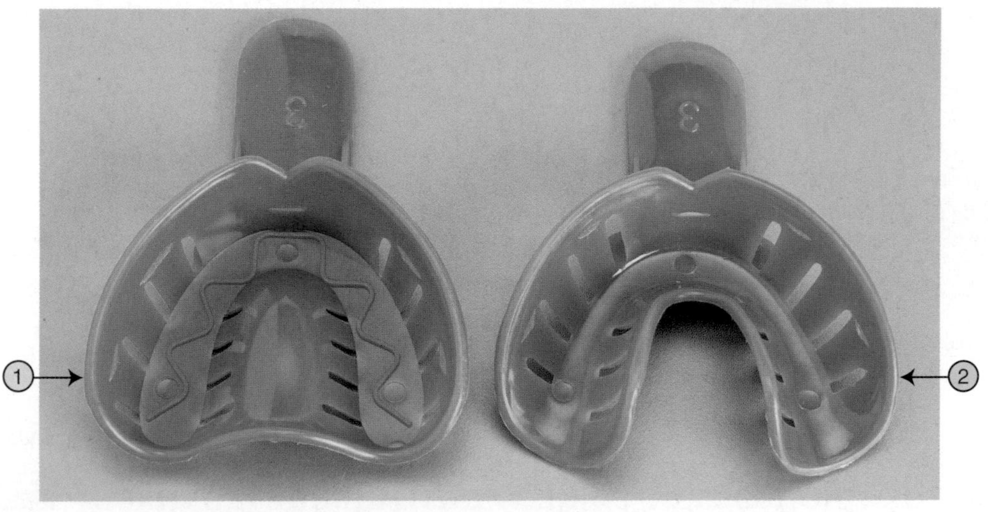
1
2

INSTRUMENT

Disposable Plastic-Perforated Full Arch Impression Trays

FUNCTION

To use for taking impressions with many types of impression material

Example: Irreversible hydrocolloid (alginate), crown, and bridge impression material

CHARACTERISTICS

① Maxillary perforated tray

② Mandibular perforated tray

Perforated trays allow material to push through the tray, creating a mechanical lock keeping the material in place.

Use only once; trays disposable

Range of sizes

PRACTICE NOTES

Plastic-Perforated Trays are used for many types of dental procedures involving taking impressions.

Impressions must be disinfected before pouring up impressions.

Ⓢ Disposable Plastic-Perforated Full Arch Impression Trays should be disposed of in the garbage.

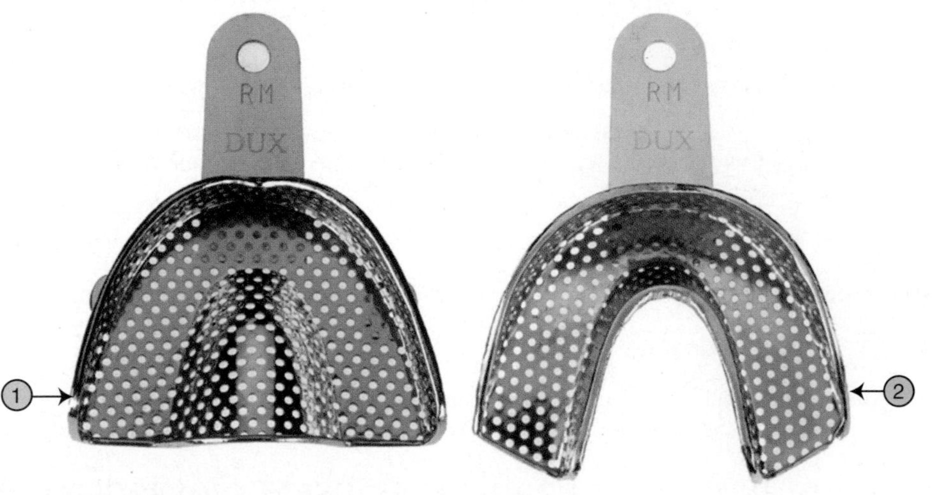
RM
DUX
RM
DUX
1
2

INSTRUMENT

Metal-Perforated Full Arch Impression Trays 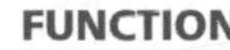

FUNCTION

To use for taking impressions with many types of impression material.

Example: Irreversible hydrocolloid (alginate), crown, and bridge impression material

CHARACTERISTICS

① Maxillary perforated tray

② Mandibular perforated tray

Perforated trays allow material to push through the tray, creating a mechanical lock keeping the material in place.

Range of sizes

PRACTICE NOTES

Metal-Perforated Full Arch Impression Trays are used for many types of dental procedures involving taking impressions.

Impressions must be disinfected before pouring up impressions.

Ⓢ Metal-Perforated Full Arch Impression Trays must be cleaned, bagged individually, then sterilized. A chemical/steam indicator device should be included in the wrapping.

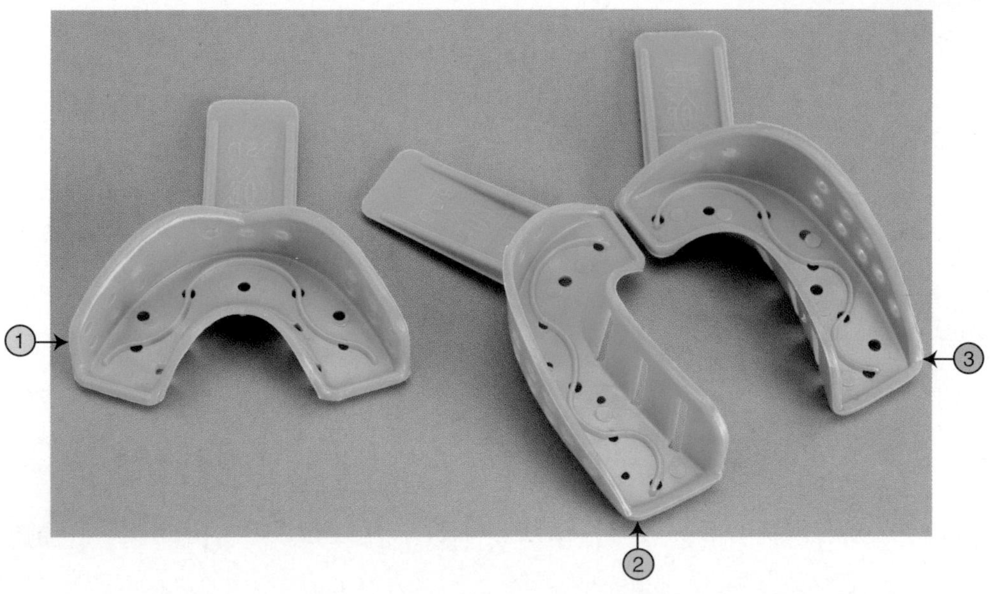
1
2
3

INSTRUMENT

Disposable Plastic-Perforated Quadrant and Anterior Impression Trays

FUNCTIONS

To use for taking impressions with many types of impression material

Example: Irreversible hydrocolloid (alginate), crown, and bridge impression material

To use for taking a quadrant or anterior portion of the mouth

CHARACTERISTICS

① Section tray for anterior maxillary or mandibular perforated tray

② Maxillary left or mandibular right perforated tray ③ Maxillary right or mandibular left perforated tray

Perforated trays allow material to push through the tray, creating a mechanical lock keeping the material in place.

Range of sizes

Use only once; trays disposable

Metal quadrant and anterior trays also available—Must be sterilized

PRACTICE NOTES

Disposable Plastic-Perforated Quadrant and Anterior Impression Trays are used for many types of dental procedures involving taking impressions.

Impressions must be disinfected before pouring out impressions.

Ⓢ Disposable Plastic-Perforated Quadrant and Anterior Impression Trays should be disposed of in the garbage. Single use only. Metal quadrant and anterior trays must be cleaned, bagged individually, and then sterilized. A chemical/steam indicator device should be included in the wrapping.

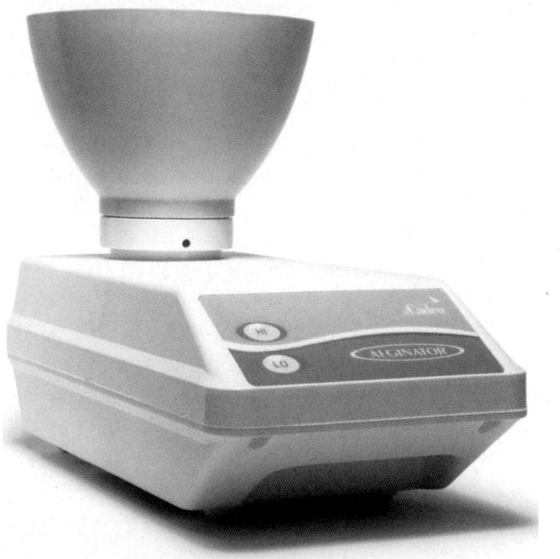
HI
LO
ALGINATOR

INSTRUMENT

Alginator

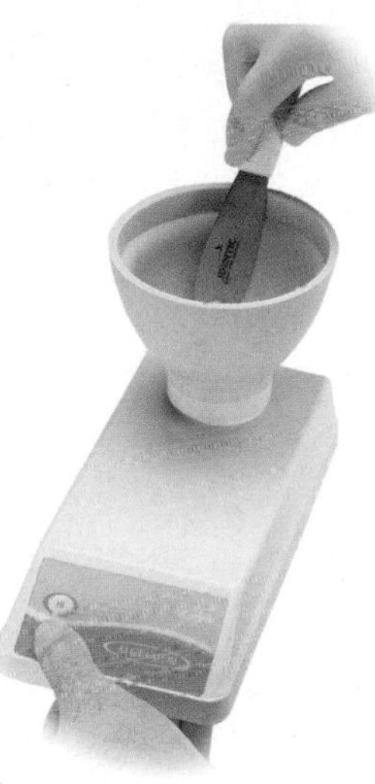

FUNCTION To mix alginate, irreversible hydrocolloid automatically

CHARACTERISTICS Flexible bowl attaches to Alginator

Low and high buttons allow bowl to rotate, mixing the alginate and water together.

Spatula pressing the material against the bowl along with the rotation of the bowl results in the material being a smooth consistency.

PRACTICE NOTES Alginator is used for many dental procedures involving taking an alginate impression.

Impressions must be disinfected before pouring up impressions.

Ⓢ Alginator and bowl should be disinfected according to the manufacturer's recommendation. Alginator spatula must be cleaned, bagged individually, and then sterilized. A chemical/steam indicator device should be included in the wrapping.

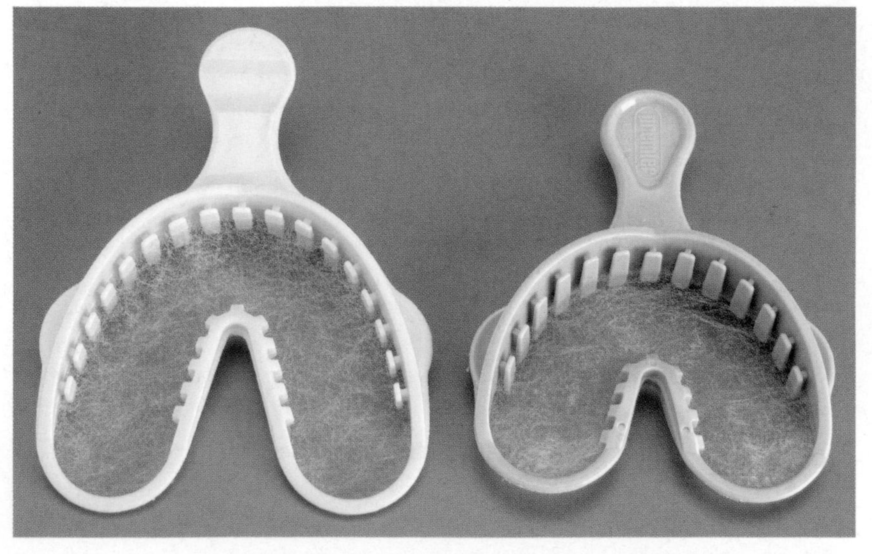

INSTRUMENT

Triple Tray (Disposable)

FUNCTIONS

To use for taking final impressions for crown and bridge restorations, opposing teeth and bite registration with one impression

To use in the mouth, taking maxillary and mandibular simultaneously

To use with many types of impression material

CHARACTERISTICS

Trays have a ledge on the side to hold sufficient amount of material for the impression.

Trays have mesh-type material in the middle of the tray to hold material in place.

Trays available:

- Quadrant used for maxillary right/left or mandibular right/left
- Maxillary left or mandibular right perforated tray
- Anterior maxillary or mandibular perforated tray

Use only once; trays disposable

PRACTICE NOTE

Triple Trays are used for many types of dental procedures.

Ⓢ Triple Trays should be disposed of in the garbage.

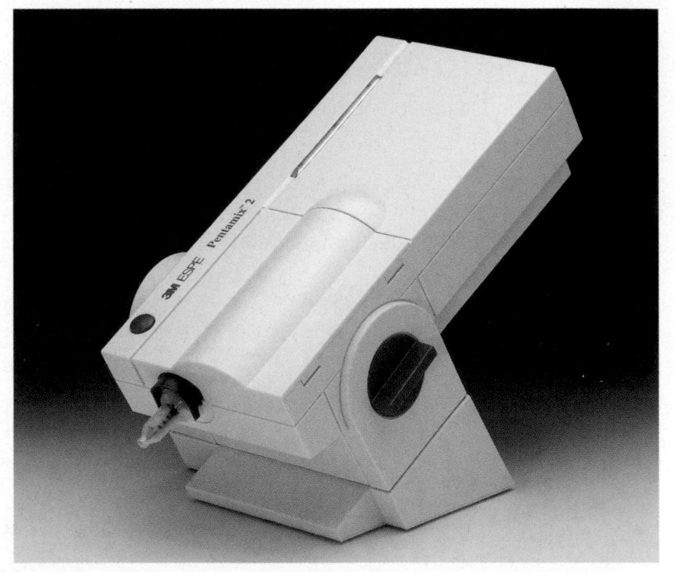
3M ESPE
Pentamix™ 2

INSTRUMENT

Automixer

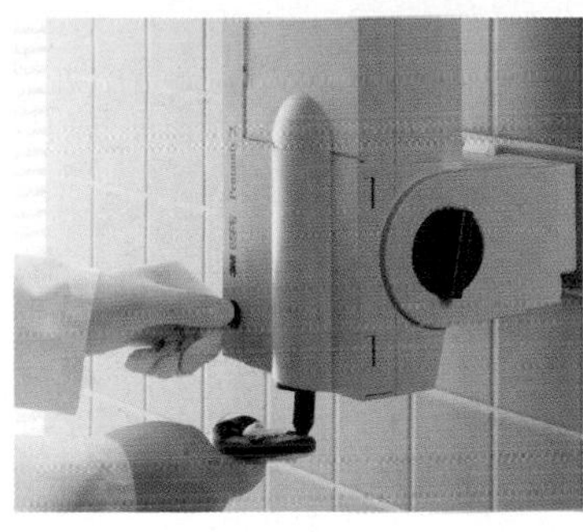

FUNCTIONS
To automatically mix final impression material
To mix base and catalyst for polyvinylsiloxane material
To place material after dispensing from Automixer in impression trays for final impressions

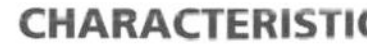

CHARACTERISTIC
Different styles of Automixers available

PRACTICE NOTES
A wash material (placed in a syringe) is placed on the prepared tooth by the operator before the tray with the impression material is placed in the patient's mouth.
Polyvinylsiloxane can also be mixed manually.

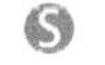

Use overgloves to handle Automixer, or disinfect according to the manufacturer's recommendation.

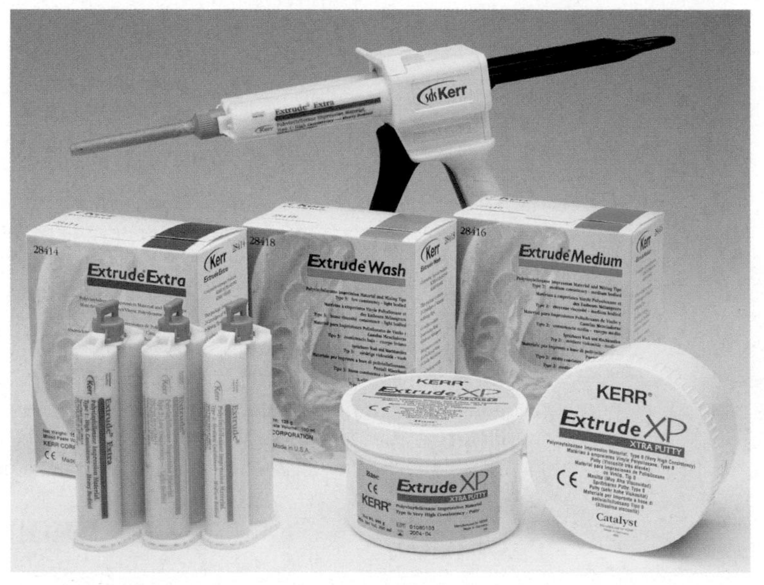
sds Kerr
Extrude Extra
28414
Extrude Extra
28418
Extrude Wash
28416
Extrude Medium
KERR
Extrude XP
XTRA PUTTY
Catalyst
Base
Made in U.S.A.

INSTRUMENT

Mixing Gun for Final Impression Material

evolve

FUNCTIONS

To mix polyvinylsiloxane material for final impression
To mix base and catalyst for impression tray
To mix wash material for the syringe
To mix material for bite registration

CHARACTERISTICS

Manufacturers have different style guns to accommodate their material.
Different technique for the tray material is to mix a putty material that is a base and a catalyst.

PRACTICE NOTES

A tube with the base and catalyst is inserted into the mixing gun with a mixing rod attached. Pressure is placed on the trigger of the gun, and the material extrudes from the tubes into the mixing rod and onto the impression tray or into the tube of the syringe.
Tray material and wash (syringe) material are different.

S Use overgloves to handle Mixing Gun or disinfect according to the manufacturer's recommendation. Mixing rod tips should be disposed of in the garbage. Single use only.

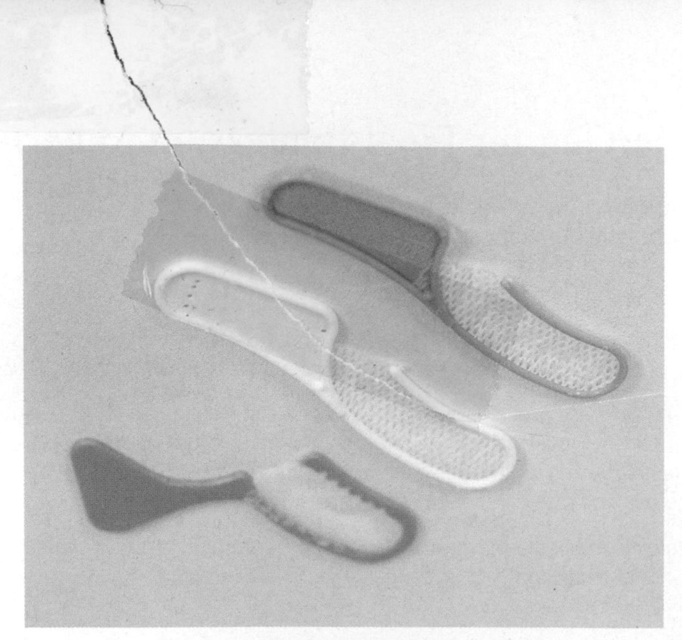

INSTRUMENT

Bite Registration Tray

FUNCTIONS

To use for taking bite registration for crown and bridge procedures
To use in the mouth taking maxillary and mandibular simultaneously
To use with many types of bite registration material

CHARACTERISTICS

Trays have mesh type material in the middle of the tray to hold material in place.
Range of sizes
Trays can be used in right or left quadrant.
Anterior section bite registration tray is also available.
Use only once; trays disposable

PRACTICE NOTES

Bite Registration Tray is used with crown and bridge tray setup.
Mixing guns may be used to mix material (see page 599).
Bite Registration Tray should be disinfected before sending to laboratory.

S Bite Registration Trays should be disposed of in the garbage.

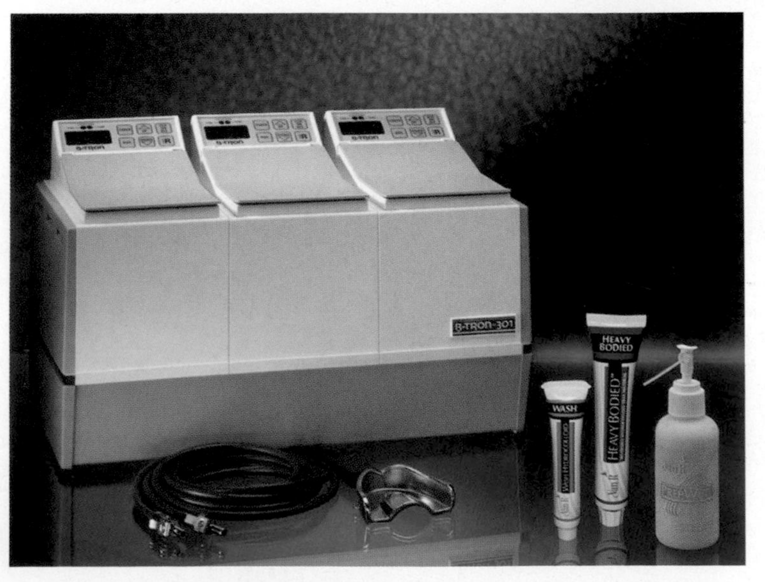

B-TRON-301
HEAVY BODIED
WASH

INSTRUMENT

Reversible Hydrocolloid Unit

FUNCTION To boil reversible hydrocolloid, store, and temper material for final impressions

CHARACTERISTICS Hydrocolloid unit has three baths:

- Liquefying the semisolid material at 212° F (100° C)
- Storage bath that cools the material and keeps it ready for impressions at 150° F (65.5° C)
- Tempering bath holds the filled impression tray for 5 minutes before it is placed in the patient's mouth at 110° F (44° C)

Tubes of the material are for the impression tray.

Small cylinders are for the wash material and are used in syringes for operator to place around tooth before impression is taken.

PRACTICE NOTE Reversible Hydrocolloid water–cooled impression trays need to be used for this type of impression material (see page 604)

Ⓢ Impression trays and syringes must be cleaned, bagged individually, and then sterilized. A chemical/steam indicator device should be included in the wrapping. Hydrocolloid Unit must be handled with overgloves.

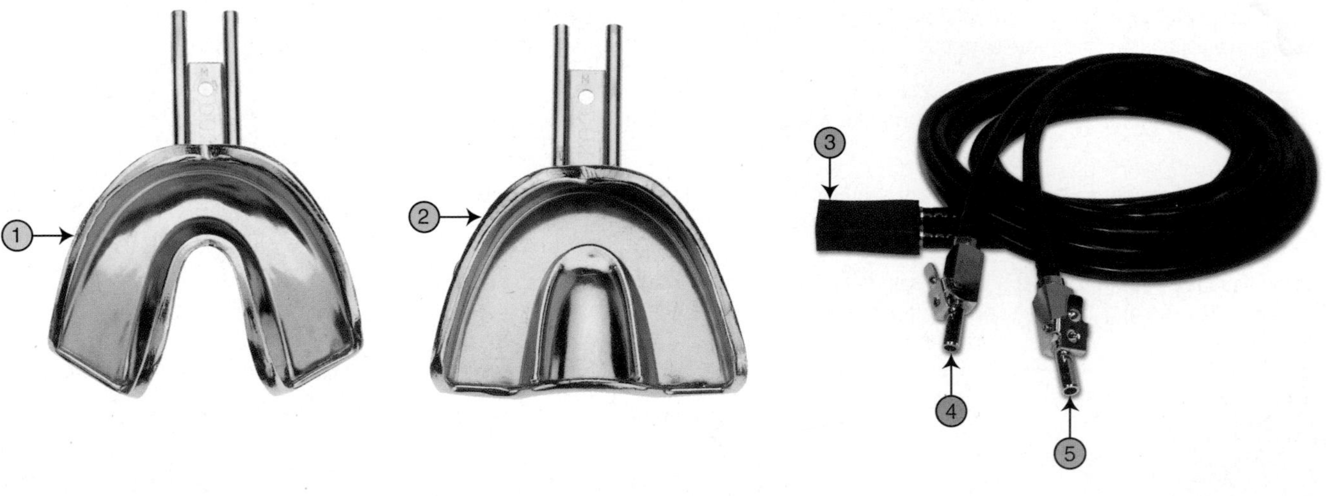
1
2
3
4
5

Irreversible Hydrocolloid Water–Cooled Impression Trays and Hose evolve

INSTRUMENT

FUNCTION To take impression with reversible hydrocolloid

CHARACTERISTICS

① Mandibular water-cooled tray
② Maxillary water-cooled tray
③ Attaches to tray
④ Attaches to water source on dental unit
⑤ Attaches to vacuum system of dental unit

A hose attaches to the tray on one end; the other end attaches to a water source and a vacuum for the water. The water runs inside the tray, which cools and sets the material once in the patient's mouth.

PRACTICE NOTE Important to connect all parts of the hose before turning on the water source

S Irreversible Hydrocolloid Water–Cooled Impression Trays and syringes must be cleaned, bagged individually, and then sterilized. A chemical/steam indicator device should be included in the wrapping. Hose should be disinfected according to the manufacturer's recommendation.

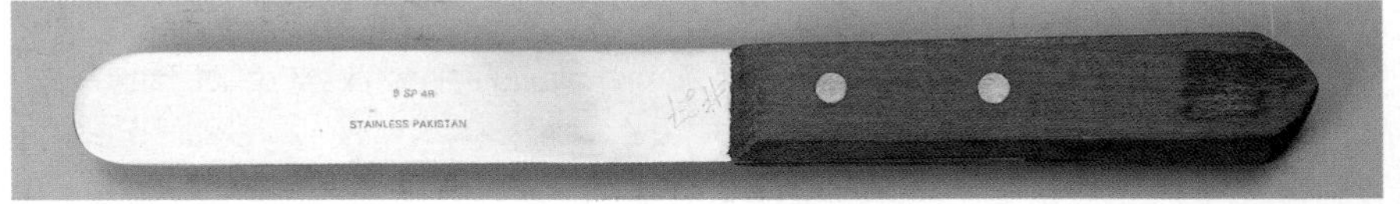
9 SP 4R
STAINLESS PAKISTAN

INSTRUMENT

Laboratory Spatula

FUNCTIONS
To mix powder and a liquid in a flexible bowl
To mix laboratory plaster, stone, and die stone for models

CHARACTERISTICS
Spatula straight to help manipulate material
Range of sizes

PRACTICE NOTE
Laboratory Spatula is used with vibrator (see page 608).

Ⓢ Disinfect Laboratory Spatula according to the manufacturer's recommendation. Laboratory Spatula may be cleaned, bagged individually, and then sterilized. A chemical/steam indicator device should be included in the wrapping.

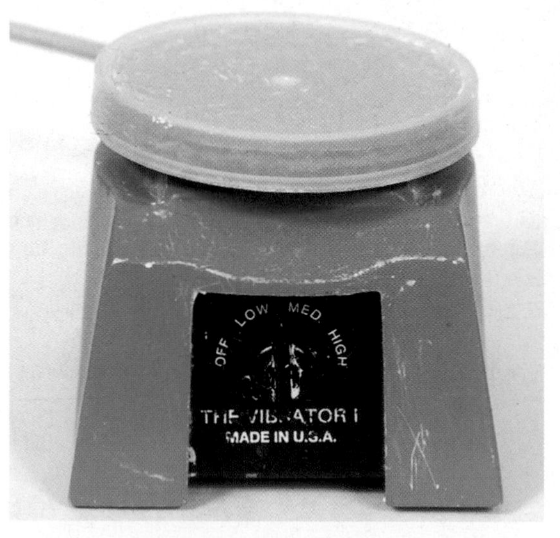
OFF
LOW
MED.
HIGH
MADE IN U.S.A.

INSTRUMENT

Vibrator for Laboratory

FUNCTION To vibrate material in mixing bowl to remove air bubbles from mixing plaster, stone, or die stone

CHARACTERISTICS Use vibrator after mixing the plaster or stone.
Use vibrator while adding plaster or stone to impression to eliminate air bubbles in impression.

PRACTICE NOTES Place plastic cover on vibrator work surface to keep vibrator free from material.

Ⓢ Disinfect Vibrator, if contaminated, according to the manufacturer's recommendation.

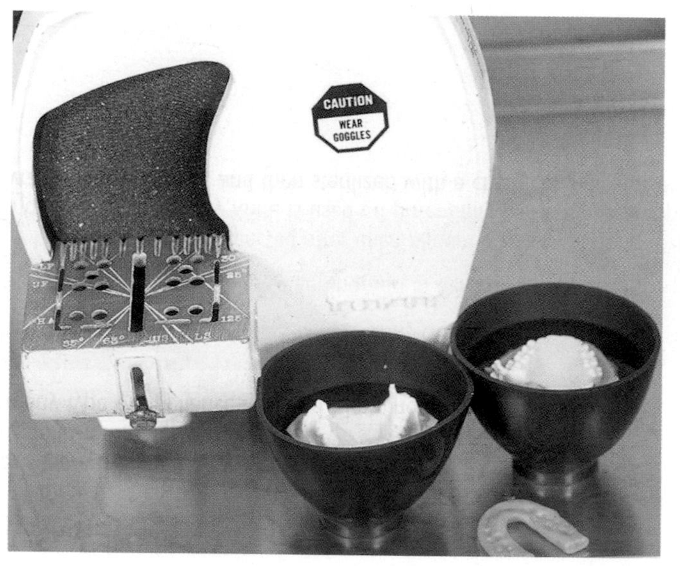
CAUTION
WEAR
GOGGLES

INSTRUMENT

Model Trimmer

FUNCTION To trim plaster, stone, or die stone models

CHARACTERISTICS Trimmer has an abrasive grinding wheel to grind excess plaster, stone, and die stone from the models.
Water runs next to the grinding wheel to reduce heat, to reduce the dust created by the grinding, and to keep the wheel clean.

PRACTICE NOTES Diagnostic models, orthodontic models, and crown and bridge models are all trimmed differently.
Glasses and mask should be worn while trimming models.

S Disinfect Model Trimmer according to the manufacturer's recommendation.

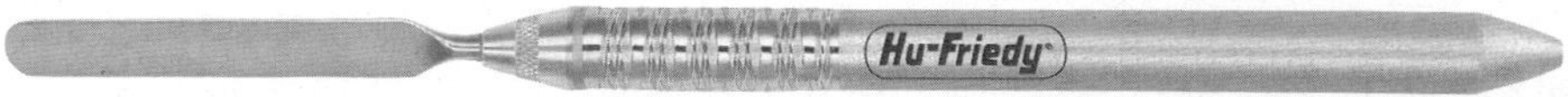

INSTRUMENT

Flexible Mixing Spatula

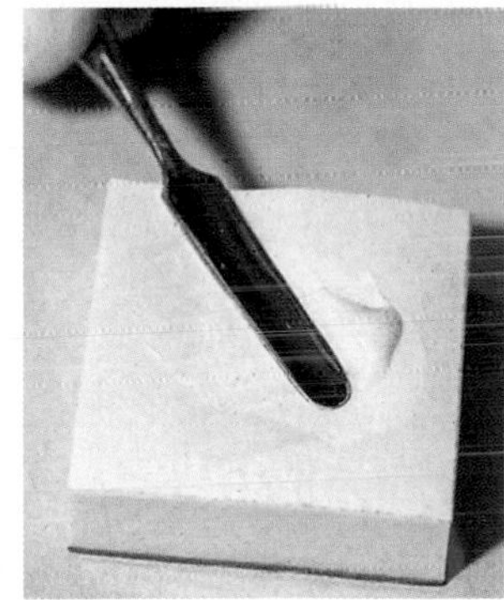

FUNCTION To mix dental materials

CHARACTERISTICS Flexible metal to allow proper manipulation
Range of sizes

PRACTICE NOTE Flexible Mixing Spatula is used on most restorative, endodontic, orthodontic, and periodontic tray setups.

Ⓢ Flexible Mixing Spatula must be cleaned, bagged individually or bagged/wrapped in a tray setup, and then sterilized. A chemical/steam indicator device should be included in the wrapping.

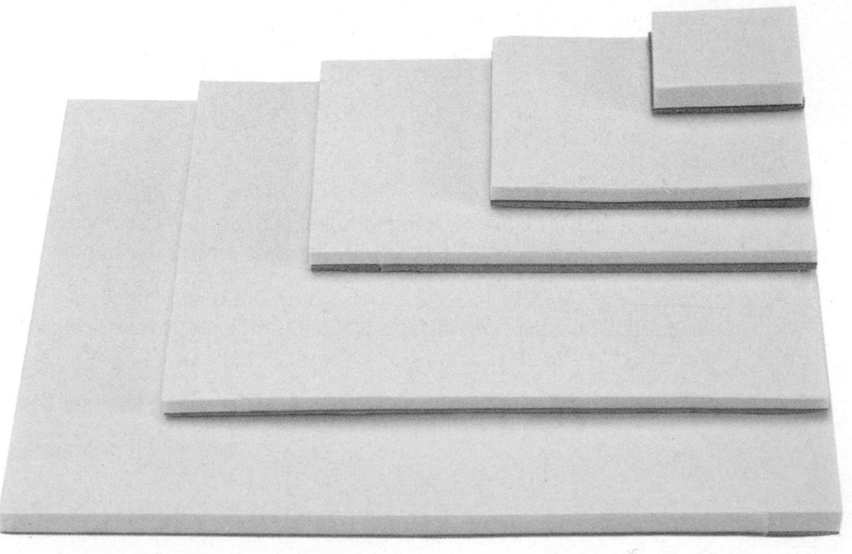

INSTRUMENT

Paper Mixing Pads

FUNCTION To mix all types of dental materials

CHARACTERISTICS Each paper on the pad is coated so material will not seep through the paper.
Many types and sizes available

PRACTICE NOTE Many materials have special paper pads that must be used when mixing certain materials.

(S) Remove one paper to mix each material and not contaminate the pad.
Entire pad should not be used to mix unless overgloves are used.

CHAPTER 20

Dental Radiography Equipment

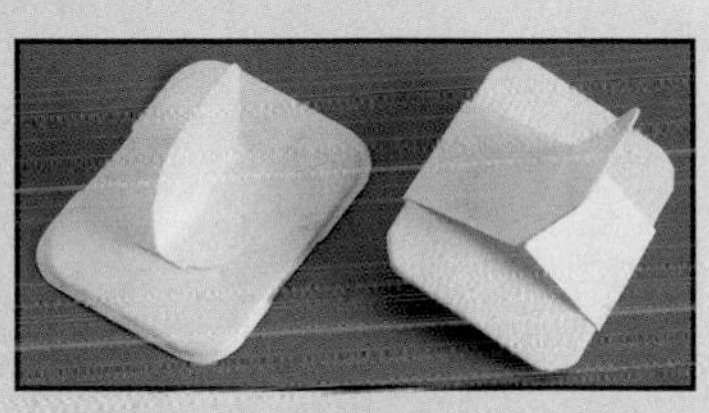

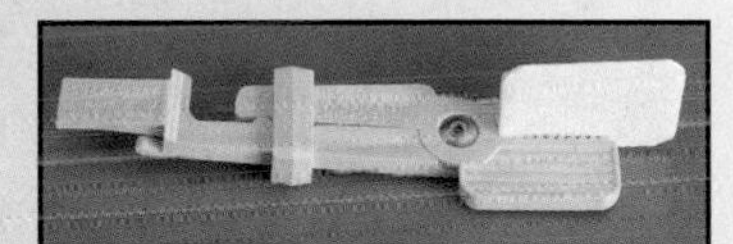

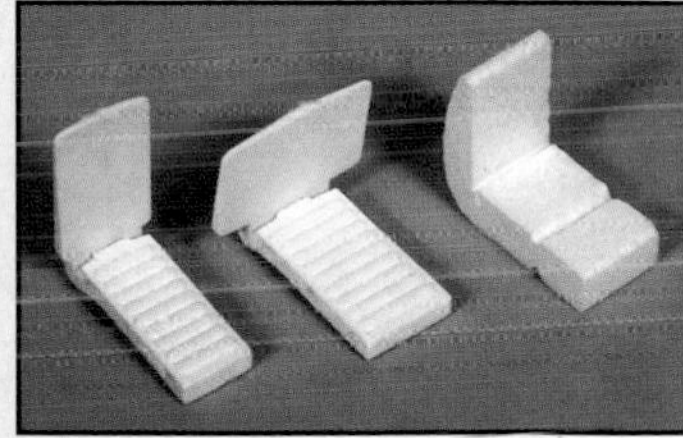

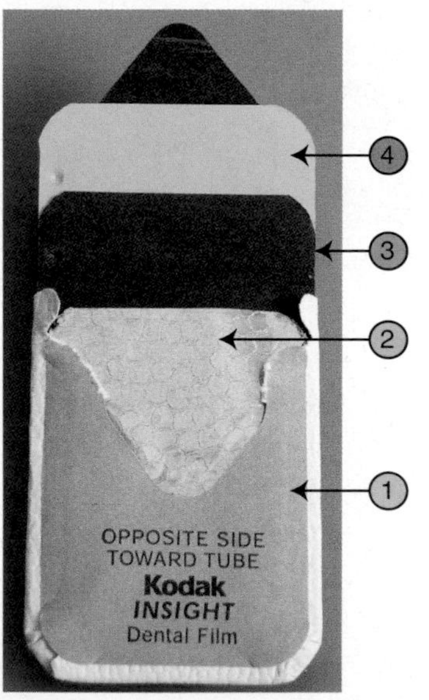
4
3
2
1
OPPOSITE SIDE
TOWARD TUBE
Kodak
INSIGHT
Dental Film

INSTRUMENT

Intraoral X-Ray Film

FUNCTION To use to project the patient's teeth through x-ray onto the film

CHARACTERISTICS

① Outside covering of film—Soft plastic or paper (both waterproof)
② Sheet of lead foil to stop the radiation from extending beyond the film
③ Black paper to protect the film from light penetration x-ray film
④ Film—Single or double film

Film speed indicated on each packet—Set by American National Standards Institute (ANSI)
Film speed A through F—D, E, F used intraorally
Faster speed of the film reduces the amount of radiation exposure; F speed is faster than D speed
Film speed determines amount of radiation needed to produce a quality radiograph—Settings are on x-ray unit

PRACTICE NOTE Intraoral x-ray film is used in all phases of dentistry.

S Follow standard precautions and cross-contamination protocol when exposing and processing film for developing. Outer packet and black paper may be disposed of in the garbage. Correct disposal of lead foil must be checked within your state. In some states lead foil is considered a hazardous waste and must be collected and disposed of properly. Refer to Department of Environmental Health in the state in which you practice for proper recycling program.

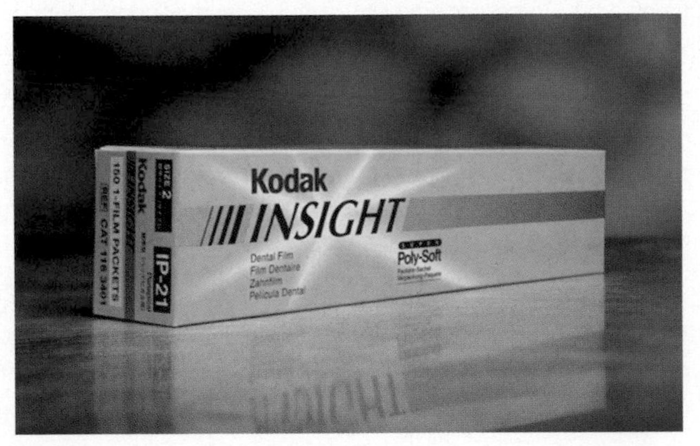
Kodak
INSIGHT
Dental Film
Film Dentaire
Zahnfilm
Película Dental
Poly-Soft
IP-21
SIZE 2
Kodak
150 1-FILM PACKETS
CAT 116 3401

INSTRUMENT

Package of X-Ray Film

FUNCTION To use to project the patient's teeth through x-ray onto the film

CHARACTERISTICS Box labeled:

- Type of film
- Film speed (picture shows F speed film)
- Number of film in each individual film packet
- Number of film packets in the box
- Expiration date of film

Film packets—Single or double film

PRACTICE NOTES Each film has an identification dot. It is a raised bump—concave on one side and convex on the other—important in taking and mounting film. Convex/bump goes toward the teeth when placing the x-ray.

Film storage is important to the integrity of the film. Refer to package instructions for storage recommendations.

S Follow standard precautions and cross-contamination protocol when processing film for developing. Outer packet and black paper may be disposed of in the garbage. Correct disposal of lead foil must be checked within your state. In some states lead foil is considered a hazardous waste and must be collected and disposed of properly. Refer to Department of Environmental Health in the state in which you practice for proper recycling program.

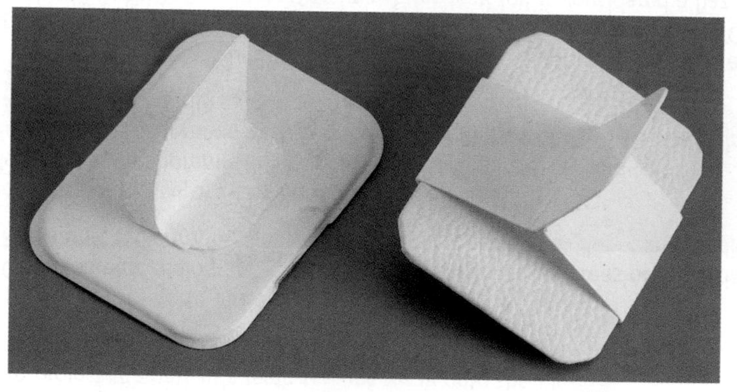

INSTRUMENT

Bite-Wing X-Ray Tabs

FUNCTION To use to take a bite-wing x-ray projection

CHARACTERISTICS Stick on or slip on tab

Tab or wing is placed on the occlusal and patient bites on the tab to secure the x-ray.

PRACTICE NOTES Slip on tabs are available in different sizes to accommodate different size film.

Size 2 film is used for adult bite-wing x-ray.

Bite-wing x-rays are mainly used for diagnosing caries on proximal surfaces (mesial and distal) of the posterior teeth.

Four bite-wings are usually taken on adult dentition—One premolar and one molar projection on each side of the mouth.

Ⓢ Follow standard precautions and cross-contamination protocol when exposing and processing film. Outer packet, black paper, and bite-wing tabs may be disposed of in the garbage. Correct disposal of lead foil must be checked within your state. In some states lead foil is considered a hazardous waste and must be collected and disposed of properly. Refer to Department of Environmental Health in the state in which you practice for proper recycling program.

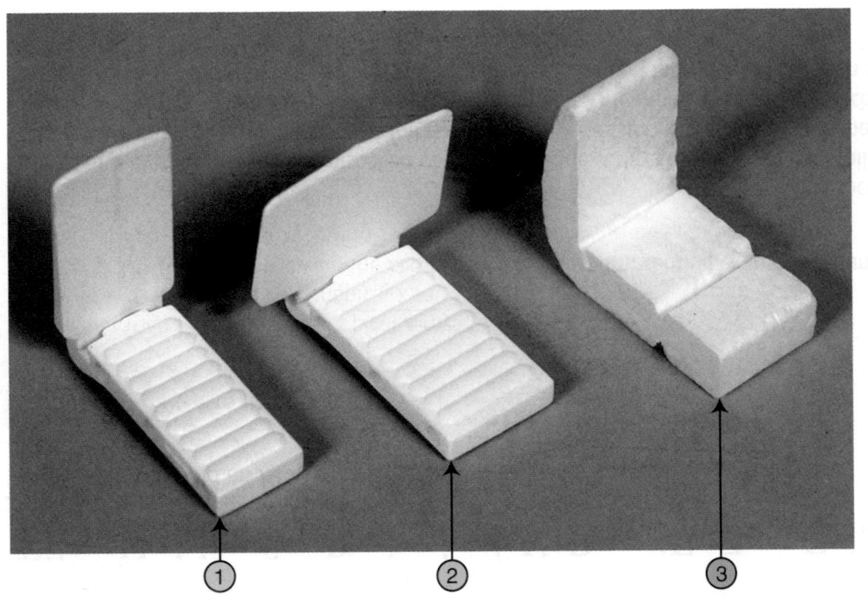
1
2
3

INSTRUMENT

Film Holders—Periapical X-Ray evolve

FUNCTION

To position and hold an x-ray in patient's mouth for periapical x-ray

To allow patient to bite on holder to keep x-ray in place while positioning the position indicating device (PID) and exposing the film

CHARACTERISTICS

① Holds film for anterior teeth projection—Plastic that can be sterilized

② Holds film for posterior teeth projection—Plastic that can be sterilized

③ Holds film for anterior and posterior projection—Disposable Styrofoam

Slot holds film in place

PRACTICE NOTE

Periapical x-rays are used for viewing the coronal part of the tooth, root, apex, and surrounding bone and tissue.

S Follow standard precautions and cross-contamination protocol when exposing and processing film. Outer packet and black paper may be disposed of in the garbage. Correct disposal of lead foil must be checked within your state. In some states lead foil is considered a hazardous waste and must be collected and disposed of properly. Refer to Department of Environmental Health in the state in which you practice for proper recycling program. Film Holders must be cleaned, bagged individually, and then sterilized. A chemical/steam indicator device should be included in the wrapping. Disposable Styrofoam holder may be disposed of in garbage.

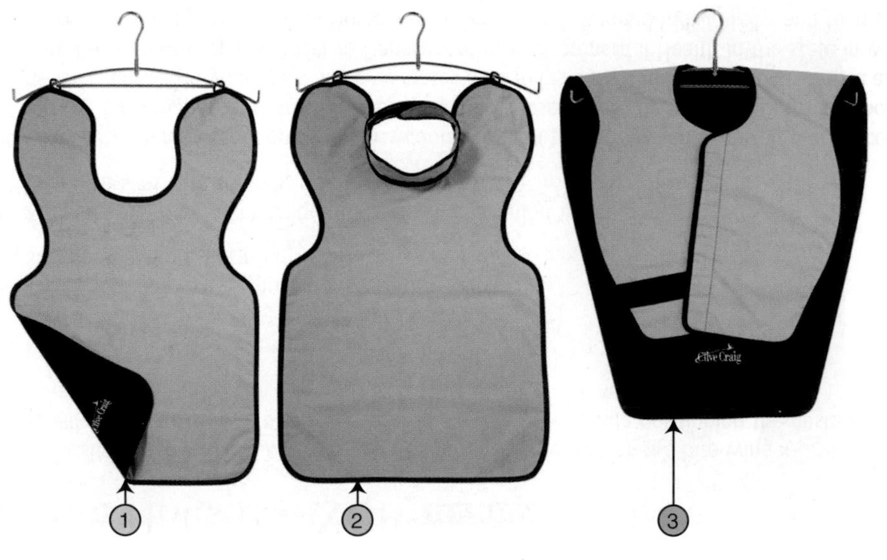
1
2
3

INSTRUMENT

Lead Aprons

evolve

FUNCTION To place on patient for protection against scattered x-rays during exposure of x-ray film

CHARACTERISTICS

① Lead apron
② Lead apron with collar to protect thyroid area
③ Lead apron poncho for front and back protection

PRACTICE NOTE Lead apron must be used when exposing patient to dental x-rays.

Ⓢ Disinfect lead apron according to the manufacturer's recommendation.

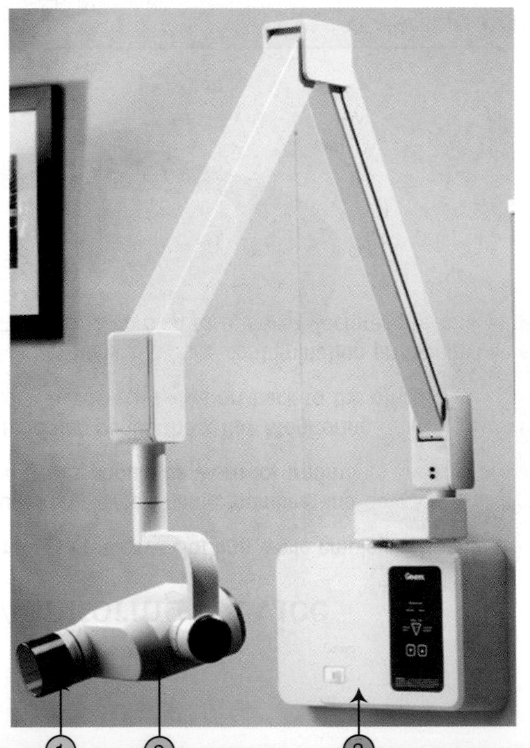

INSTRUMENT

Dental X-Ray Unit

FUNCTION To expose film with radiation that is generated in the x-ray unit

CHARACTERISTICS

① Position Indicating Device (PID)
② Tube Head
③ X-Ray Unit

Round (shown) or Rectangular PIDs available

PRACTICE NOTE Control Panel for the x-ray unit and button to expose the film are outside patient's treatment room. On some machines, you may adjust the exposure time that the x-ray is exposed. Other machines adjust the exposure time, Kilovoltage Peak (kVp), and Milliamperage mA.

Ⓢ Follow standard precautions and cross-contamination protocol when exposing and processing film. Barriers should be used on x-ray head, PID, and panel where x-ray button is pushed. Also follow manufacturer's recommendation for disinfection.

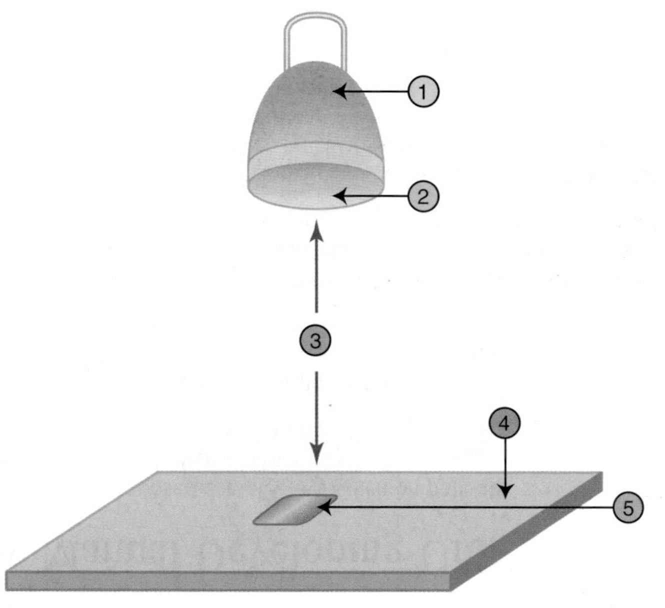
1
2
3
4
5

INSTRUMENT

X-Ray Safelight

FUNCTION To develop x-rays in a dark room with only a safelight

CHARACTERISTICS

① Safelight
② Safelight filter
③ Minimum distance (at least 4 feet) from safelight to undeveloped x-ray
④ Working area
⑤ Undeveloped and unwrapped x-ray film

PRACTICE NOTE Unwrapped film left too close to the safelight or exposed for more than 2 to 3 minutes will appear fogged.

Ⓢ Follow standard precautions and cross-contamination protocol when processing film. Outer packet and black paper may be disposed of in the garbage. Correct disposal of lead foil must be checked within your state. In some states lead foil is considered a hazardous waste and must be collected and disposed of properly. Refer to Department of Environmental Health in the state in which you practice for proper recycling program.

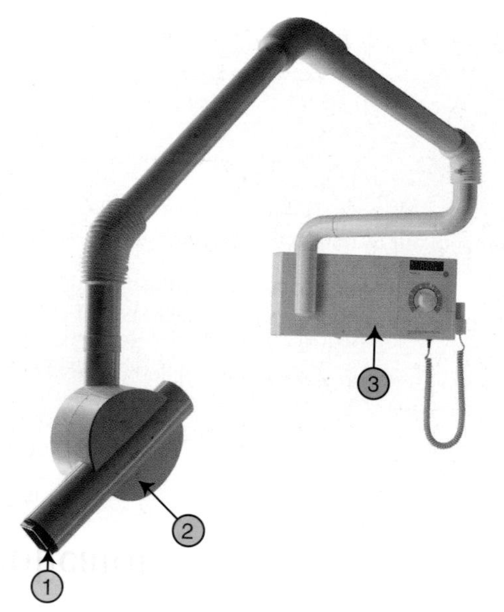
1
2
3

INSTRUMENT

Digital Intraoral Radiography X-Ray Unit

FUNCTIONS

To take digital intraoral x-rays without film or without processing the film

To project the image of the teeth by digitally projecting radiation onto an electronic sensor and then to computerized imaging system

CHARACTERISTICS

① Position Indicating Device (PID) ② Tube Head ③ X-Ray Unit with Digital Panel

Round or Rectangular (*pictured*) PIDs available

Digital radiographs use less radiation than conventional x-rays

Networks to computers in all areas of the dental office

Immediate imaging available

PRACTICE NOTES

Dental offices store digital x-rays on the computer along with patient records. Many offices have paperless charts and radiographs.

Digital Intraoral imaging is used in all phases of dentistry, especially endodontics, orthodontics, oral surgery, and implantology.

Ⓢ Follow standard precautions and cross-contamination protocol when exposing digital film. Barriers must be placed on the sensors. Barriers should be used, and the manufacturer's recommendation for disinfection followed.

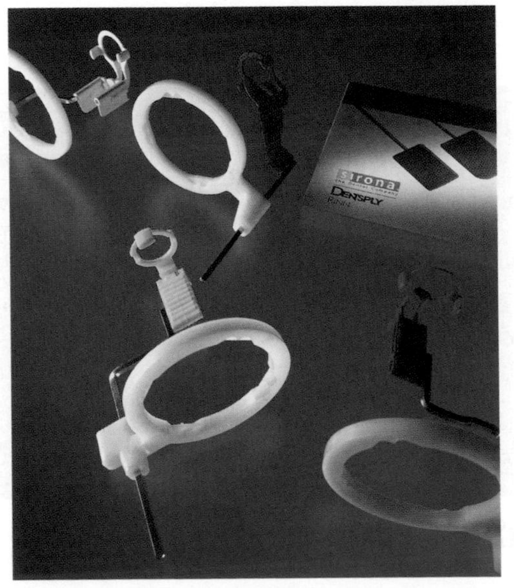
sirona
DENTSPLY

INSTRUMENT

Rinn XCP Holders for Digital Radiography

FUNCTIONS

To position and hold digital sensor in patient's mouth for periapical and bite-wing x-rays using parallel technique

To allow patient to bite on holder to keep x-ray in place while positioning the PID and exposing the electronic sensor

CHARACTERISTICS

Red—Holds film for bite-wing projection
Blue—Holds film for anterior teeth projection
Yellow—Holds film for posterior teeth projection
Slots hold electronic sensor in place

PRACTICE NOTE

Several different styles of electronic sensor holders are available.

S Follow standard precautions and cross-contamination protocol when exposing digital film. Barriers must be placed on the sensors. Barriers should be used on the x-ray unit, and the manufacturer's recommendation for disinfection should be followed. Digital Radiography XCP Holders must be cleaned, bagged individually, and then sterilized. A chemical/steam indicator device should be included in the wrapping.

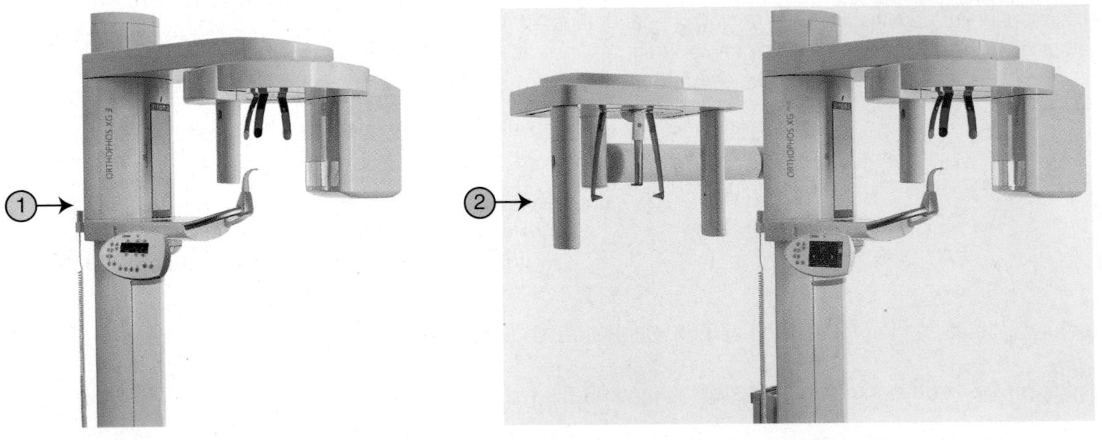
1
ORTHOPHOS XG 3
2
ORTHOPHOS XG

INSTRUMENT

Digital Panoramic Imaging Unit and Digital Cephalometric Imaging Unit

FUNCTION

To take digital panograph x-rays without film or without processing the film

To project the image of maxillary and mandibular teeth by digitally projecting radiation onto an electronic sensor and then to computerized imaging system

CHARACTERISTICS

① Digital Panoramic Imaging Unit ② Digital Cephalometric Imaging Unit

Digital radiographs use less radiation than conventional x-rays

Networks to computers in all areas of the dental office

Immediate imaging available

PRACTICE NOTE

Dental offices store digital panoramic imaging on the computer along with patient records. Many offices have paperless charts and radiographs.

Digital Panoramic and Cephalometric imaging is used in all phases of dentistry, especially orthodontics, oral surgery, and implantology.

Ⓢ Follow standard precautions and cross-contamination protocol. Barriers should be used, and the manufacturer's recommendation for disinfection followed.

Index

Entries followed by f *indicate figures.*

E

I

J

K

S

T